Essential Reviews in Geriatric Psychiatry

Rajesh R. Tampi • Deena J. Tampi
Juan J. Young • Meera Balasubramaniam
Pallavi Joshi
Editors

Essential Reviews in Geriatric Psychiatry

Springer

Editors
Rajesh R. Tampi
Creighton University School of Medicine
Omaha, NE, USA

Deena J. Tampi
Behavioral Health Advisory Group
Princeton, NJ, USA

Juan J. Young
Yale School of Medicine
New Haven, CT, USA

Meera Balasubramaniam
Department of Psychiatry
New York University Grossman School of Medicine
New York, NY, USA

Pallavi Joshi
University of Arizona College of Medicine
Phoenix, AZ, USA

ISBN 978-3-030-94959-4 ISBN 978-3-030-94960-0 (eBook)
https://doi.org/10.1007/978-3-030-94960-0

This Springer imprint is published by the registered company Springer Nature Switzerland AG
The registered company address is: Gewerbestrasse 11, 6330 Cham, Switzerland

Rajesh and Deena Tampi wish to dedicate this book to their children Alexa, Vaishnav, Julia, Olivia, Poki, Smoki, and Oreo Cookie and their parents late Dr. Rajagopalan Tampi, Sreedevi Tampi, Mr. Sam Ranani, and Marney Ranani. – Rajesh Tampi and Deena Tampi

Dr. Meera Balasubramaniam wishes to dedicate this book to her loving grandparents Mr. Ganesan and Mrs. Parvathi Ganesan. – Meera Balasubramaniam.

I dedicate this book to my wife, Jen, who has been nothing but amazing and supportive of all of my endeavors. – Juan Young

I am grateful to Dr. Tampi for his mentorship and guidance in editing this book. It is dedicated to my parents, Suhas and Vandana Joshi, my husband Robert, my brother Aditya, and Serena. – Pallavi Joshi

Foreword

In 1996, David L. Sackett and colleagues defined evidence-based medicine as the "conscientious, explicit, and judicious use of current best evidence in making decisions about the care of individual patients." Evidence-based medicine includes not only gathering the best available research to answer clinically important questions but also involves critically appraising the research—synthesizing it, understanding its strengths and limitations, gathering "take home points"—and learning how to integrate it with a particular patient's characteristics, preferences, and goals to provide the best possible care. Learning the process of evidence-based medicine is one of the most important core competencies in geriatric psychiatry education and is an indispensable practice of the best geriatric mental health professionals.

As former chair of the AAGP Scholars Program—the biggest recruitment program into geriatric psychiatry in North America—and core faculty of the UCLA geriatric psychiatry fellowship, I have often been asked by my trainees for a catalog or inventory of the most important research papers in geriatric psychiatry, as they search for tools to enhance their practice of evidence-based medicine. As a practicing geriatric psychiatrist and life-long learner, I have pored over online databases and resource tools to try to locate the exact research studies I need to solve a pressing clinical problem using an evidence-based approach. While systematic reviews and online resources provide research syntheses on specific topics in geriatric psychiatry, I have never been able to locate the perfect resource that includes all the major research in geriatric psychiatry all in one place. Furthermore, outside of journal clubs and the occasional lecture on statistics, traditional medical education and other resources rarely provide us all the necessary skills to make critical appraisals that lead to the best applications of the research literature. This book fills those gaps.

For trainees or practicing clinicians looking for the definitive collection of research in geriatric psychiatry, this book is a treasure. Rajesh "Raj" Tampi and his co-editors have compiled *the* 75 papers over the last 25 years that shaped the way we practice geriatric psychiatry. Ranging from the CATIE-AD Study Group's *New England Journal of Medicine* paper on the effectiveness of atypical antipsychotic drugs in patients with Alzheimer's disease to a systematic review from *JAMA Internal Medicine* on non-pharmacologic interventions for chronic pain in older adults, this book is a compendium of the leading research on every psychiatric disorder and every key topic—suicides, medication adverse effects, and even electroconvulsive therapy—that a geriatric mental health professional or trainee should know. The fact that Raj and his colleagues have simply compiled summaries of these important research papers is a gift to the field. However, each article summary also includes the strengths and limitations of the research, as well as key "take home points" and the article's potential applications to clinical practice—essential information to make critical appraisals and apply the findings of the article to our patients to fully achieve the practice of evidence-based medicine.

Raj and his colleagues are ideally suited to be editors of this book—among the leaders in evidence-based medicine within geriatric psychiatry. I have known Raj for nearly a decade as a valued colleague and dear friend. I therefore know that Raj has devoted much of his career to synthesizing the geriatric psychiatry research literature for trainees and colleagues such as myself. Indeed, Raj has published dozens of reviews on geriatric psychiatry topics ranging from suvorexant for insomnia in older adults to ethical and legal issues in geriatric psychiatry. Scholars in every way, the editors of this book are experts I trust to provide all the essential articles and ensure that all the "take home points" and practical applications are well-vetted and useful to readers.

The applications of this book toward furthering evidence-based medicine in geriatric mental healthcare seem endless. I will carry this book to clinic when supervising my trainees to aid our practice of evidence-based medicine. Indeed, clinician-educators everywhere can use this as a valuable resource for teaching and training in the clinics and on the wards. Psychiatry residents and fellows can look here first for a geriatric psychiatry article to present in journal club. Geriatric mental healthcare professionals who wish to apply the best evidence to their practice will find the article they need for any clinical situation in this book, regardless of whether their practice is in a community clinic, inpatient ward, nursing home, consult-liaison service, or another setting. Clinicians who are *not* geriatric mental healthcare professionals but want to practice evidence-based care of their older patients can find research on all the major topics in geriatric psychiatry here.

Essential Reviews in Geriatric Psychiatry is truly essential for practicing evidence-based medicine in geriatric mental healthcare toward our goal of better care for our older patients.

Brandon C. Yarns
Deputy Section Chief, Geriatric Mental Health
VA Greater Los Angeles Healthcare System
and Health Science Assistant Clinical Professor
Department of Psychiatry and Biobehavioral Sciences
University of California, Los Angeles
Los Angeles, CA, USA

Preface

The World Health Organization reports that between 2015 and 2050, the proportion of the world's older adults (≥60 years) will double from about 12% to almost 22% of the total population. This means that the population of older adults will increase from 900 million to approximately 2 billion. Data indicates that there will be a similar growth of the population of individuals 65 years and older in the USA from 46.2 million or 14.5% of the total population to roughly 21.7% of the US population by 2040. It is estimated that over 20% of older adults have a diagnosable psychiatric disorder. Men had higher rates of substance use disorders and any personality disorder whereas women experienced higher rates of mood and anxiety disorders. Available data indicates that approximately 20% of the community dwelling older adults have been prescribed psychotropic medications. Additionally, data indicates that treatment with psychotropic medications can result in significant functional decline, cognitive changes, cerebrovascular adverse events, and also death among older adults. In this new book we have critically appraised 75 papers published within the past 25 years that we think provides the highest knowledge-yield/impact for practicing clinicians and educators in the field of geriatric mental health. We think that these papers have shaped the way geriatric psychiatry is currently practiced. These papers have been critically appraised by experts in geriatric psychiatry using a standardized format. A summary of these papers and their practical application have also been provided by the experts. All the major psychiatric disorders in later life have been covered in this book including anxiety disorders, bipolar disorders, depressive disorders, neurocognitive disorders, psychotic disorders, sleep disorders, and substance use disorders. This book also reviews important studies on suicides in late life and on interventional procedures in geriatric psychiatry like the ECT. In addition, the adverse effects of psychotropic medications on older adults with psychiatric disorders have been reviewed. This book aspires to assist anyone who is interested learning about the care of psychiatric disorders among older adults.

Omaha, NE, USA — Rajesh R. Tampi
Princeton, NJ, USA — Deena J. Tampi
New Haven, CT, USA — Juan J. Young
Phoenix, AZ, USA — Pallavi Joshi
New York, NY, USA — Meera Balasubramaniam

Acknowledgment

Rajesh and Deena Tampi wish acknowledge the hard work and dedication of their co-editors, colleagues, and trainees in making this book possible.

Contents

Contributors

Esther Akinyemi Henry Ford Health System, Detroit, MI, USA

Sara J. Anderson University of Missouri Kansas City and The Missouri Department of Mental Health – Center for Behavioral Medicine, Kansas City, MO, USA

Gagandeep K. Bhatia Yale University School of Medicine, New Haven, CT, USA

Mary "Molly" Camp UT Southwestern Medical Center at Dallas, Dallas, TX, USA

Avee Champaneria Department of Psychiatry and Behavioral Sciences, Duke University Health System, Durham, NC, USA

Fellow in Geriatric Psychiatry, Duke University School of Medicine, Durham, NC, USA

Seetha Chandrasekhara Lewis Katz School of Medicine at Temple University, Philadelphia, PA, USA

Chloe Cheng Department of Psychiatry and Behavioral Sciences, University of California San Francisco, San Francisco, CA, USA

Miles Christensen Department of Psychiatry, Duke University School of Medicine, Durham, NC, USA

Michelle L. Conroy Yale University School of Medicine, New Haven, CT, USA

VA Connecticut Healthcare System, West Haven, CT, USA

Jennie B. Davidow Mass General Brigham Geriatric Psychiatry Fellowship, Harvard Medical School Clinical Fellow, Boston, MA, USA

Izabella Dutra de Abreu UT Southwestern Medical Center at Dallas, Dallas, TX, USA

Christa DeFries Department of Psychiatry, Baylor Scott & White Health, Temple, TX, USA

Audrey Eichenberger UT Southwestern Medical Center at Dallas, Dallas, TX, USA

Matthew Erisman University of Arizona Department of Psychiatry, Tucson, AZ, USA

Jason Gandelman Department of Psychiatry and Behavioral Sciences, University of California San Francisco, San Francisco, CA, USA

Erica C. Garcia-Pittman The University of Texas at Austin Dell Medical School, Department of Psychiatry and Behavioral Sciences, Austin, TX, USA

Clay Gueits Psychiatry Resident, Einstein Medical Center, Philadelphia, PA, USA

Aarti Gupta Yale University School of Medicine, New Haven, CT, USA

Hudaisa Hafeez Duke University, Department of Psychiatry & Behavioral Sciences, Durham, NC, USA

Tracey Holsinger Duke University, Department of Psychiatry & Behavioral Sciences, Durham, NC, USA

Durham VA Medical Center, Durham, NC, USA

Ankit Jain Hershey Medical Center, Penn State College of Medicine, Hershey, PA, USA

Pallavi Joshi University of Arizona College of Medicine, Phoenix, AZ, USA

Adan Aslam Khan Henry Ford Health System, Detroit, MI, USA

Sarah Kim Duke University, Department of Psychiatry and Behavioral Sciences, Durham, NC, USA

Marianne Klugheit Banner University of Arizona College of Medicine Department of Psychiatry, Phoenix, AZ, USA

Southern AZ VA Health Care System, Tucson, AZ, USA

Chadrick E. Lane Peter O'Donnell Jr. Brain Institute, Department of Psychiatry, UT Southwestern Medical Center, Dallas, TX, USA

Alba E. Lara The University of Texas at Austin Dell Medical School, Department of Psychiatry and Behavioral Sciences, Austin, TX, USA

Susan W. Lehmann Johns Hopkins University School of Medicine, Baltimore, MD, USA

Katherine Levine Medical College of Wisconsin, Milwaukee, WI, USA

Michael G. Li The University of Texas at Austin Dell Medical School, Department of Psychiatry and Behavioral Sciences, Austin, TX, USA

Padmapriya Marpuri Attending Geriatric Psychiatrist, Frontier Psychiatry, Billings, MT, USA

Kristin McArthur Psychiatry, Durham VA Medical Center, Durham, NC, USA

Paroma Mitra NYU School of Medicine, Bellevue Hospital Center, New York, NY, USA

Christopher Morrow Division of Geriatric Psychiatry and Neuropsychiatry, Department of Psychiatry and Behavioral Sciences, Johns Hopkins School of Medicine, Baltimore, MD, USA

Jenny Nguyen Lewis Katz School of Medicine at Temple University, Philadelphia, PA, USA

Hanadi Ajam Oughli Department of Psychiatry and Biobehavioral Sciences, University of California Los Angeles, Los Angeles, CA, USA

Paul A. Parcon Molecular Imaging Branch, National Institute of Mental Health, Bethesda, MA, USA

Vahid Pasovic Henry Ford Health System, Detroit, MI, USA

Emily B. Phelps Mount Sinai Hospital, New York, NY, USA

Elizabeth Qin Department of Psychiatry and Behavioral Sciences, University of California San Francisco, San Francisco, CA, USA

Paul A. Riordan Durham Veterans Affairs Medical Center, Department of Psychiatry and Behavioral Sciences, Duke University School of Medicine, Durham, NC, USA

Gregg A. Robbins-Welty Durham Veterans Affairs Medical Center, Department of Psychiatry, Durham, NC, USA

Charlotte M. Schwarz University of North Carolina at Chapel Hill Department of Psychiatry, Chapel Hill, NC, USA

Jasmine Singh Banner Health Tucson, Tucson, AZ, USA

Colin M. Smith Medicine and Psychiatry Combined Program, Duke University School of Medicine, Durham, NC, USA

William B. Smith Department of Psychiatry and Behavioral Sciences, University of California San Francisco, San Francisco, CA, USA

Mohamed A. Soliman University of Michigan Department of Psychiatry, Ann Arbor, MI, USA

Jasmine C. Stephens Department of Psychiatry, The University of Texas Southwestern Medical Center, Dallas, TX, USA

Sandra Swantek Rush Medical College, Chicago, IL, USA

Rajesh R. Tampi Creighton University School of Medicine, Omaha, NE, USA

Andrew Tuck Department of Psychiatry, Duke University School of Medicine, Durham, NC, USA

Jennifer Tu Duke University School of Medicine, Durham, NC, USA

Megan Tusken UT Southwestern Medical Center at Dallas, Dallas, TX, USA

Peter Ureste Department of Psychiatry and Behavioral Sciences, University of California San Francisco, San Francisco, CA, USA

Juan Carlos Urizar Department of Psychiatry Brigham and Women's Hospital, Mass General Brigham Geriatric Psychiatry Fellowship and Harvard Medical School Instructor, Boston, MA, USA

Kalya Vardi UC San Diego School of Medicine, San Diego, CA, USA

Daniela Vela UT Southwestern Medical Center at Dallas, Dallas, TX, USA

Sophia Wang Indiana University School of Medicine, Department of Psychiatry, Indianapolis, IN, USA

Indiana Alzheimer's Disease Research Center, Indianapolis, IN, USA

Maureen Waweru Hospital at University of Pennsylvania, Philadelphia, PA, USA

Martin Witkin PGY-4 Psychiatry Resident, Einstein Medical Center, Philadelphia, PA, USA

Andrew Wong Henry Ford Health System, Detroit, MI, USA

Part I
Adverse Effects of Medications

Chapter 1
Do Atypical Antipsychotics Cause Stroke?

Jasmine C. Stephens and Erica C. Garcia-Pittman

Authors of the Original Article Nathan Herrmann, Krista L Lanctôt

Name(s) of the Appraiser of the Article Jasmine C. Stephens, MD, and Erica C. Garcia-Pittman, MD

Journal Publisher *CNS Drugs*

Year of Publication 2005

Type of Study Meta-analysis review, post hoc analyses

Funding Sources No funding sources. However, they have previously received research support and speakers honoraria from Janssen Ortho Inc., Eli Lilly, Novartis, Pfizer, and AstraZeneca, all manufacturers of atypical antipsychotics.

Objectives The objective of the article was to review the data from randomized controlled trials that prompted warnings from multiple health regulatory agencies regarding the association of atypical antipsychotics and risks of cerebrovascular accidents in the geriatric population. Furthermore, the authors wanted to determine the level of evidence and how strong of a risk is associated between these factors to develop guidance on the risk-benefit analysis for the possible severity of these outcomes [1].

J. C. Stephens
Department of Psychiatry | The University of Texas Southwestern Medical Center, Dallas, TX, USA
e-mail: Jasmine.Stephens@utsouthwestern.edu

E. C. Garcia-Pittman (✉)
The University of Texas at Austin Dell Medical School, Department of Psychiatry and Behavioral Sciences, Austin, TX, USA
e-mail: ecgarcia-pittman@ascension.org

R. R. Tampi et al. (eds.), *Essential Reviews in Geriatric Psychiatry*,
https://doi.org/10.1007/978-3-030-94960-0_1

Methods The authors completed a MEDLINE search using the above indicated keywords as well as reference lists of identified papers. The authors had direct contact with Janssen and Eli Lilly for the data and materials of unpublished trials. Eleven articles were identified and an overall relative risk for cerebrovascular events in individuals was calculated based on the above results.

Results When reviewing the role of dementia and CVAEs, cognitive impairment is a strong predictor of ischemic stroke independent of vascular risk factors. Patients with Alzheimer's disease were more likely to die from cerebrovascular disease than elderly individuals without Alzheimer's disease. The rate of death from CVAEs was higher than all other causes of death in patients with vascular dementia compared to other groups of dementia. In a sample elderly of dementia patients who had a stroke and were treated with an antipsychotic for 8–12 weeks, CVAEs and death were possible outcomes. The authors postulated that if patients with Alzheimer's disease and vascular dementia are at an increased risk of CVAEs, then treatment with an antipsychotic would also be associated with CVAEs and death. Throughout the reviewed articles, CVAEs included stroke, transient ischemic attacks (TIAs), cerebrovascular accidents (CVA), cerebral ischemia, cerebral infarct, cerebrovascular disturbance, and cerebrovascular disorder.

The review of risperidone included six studies; three of which were published. The published data documented information that was included on patients with Alzheimer's disease, vascular dementia, and mixed dementia, whereas the unpublished data includes information on patients with vascular and mixed dementia. 33% of included patients had vascular and mixed dementia. Individuals with vascular dementia and mixed dementia are independently more at risk of CVAEs; in the published data, more of that at-risk population was included.

The rate of serious CVAEs in those with risperidone exposure (15 of 1009, 1.5%) was not shown to be statistically significantly different from placebo (4 of 712, 0.6%) [$p = 0.27$]. The rate of all-cause mortality was similar for risperidone and placebo exposed individuals, though the stroke rate was slightly higher with risperidone exposure. Most of these participants who experienced serious CVAEs had significant risk factors including hypertension, atrial fibrillation, and history of stroke. It was found that the stroke risk factors were poorly controlled hypertension, poorly controlled diabetes mellitus, and atrial fibrillation without anticoagulant treatment. Plus, there was a concern for miscoding of events by investigators. For example, a TIA was labeled as an accidental overdose on risperidone when documented as 5 mg instead of a 0.5 mg dose. Overall, it was found that the rates of CVAEs were low in those exposed to risperidone, though subjects were not randomized or stratified based on stroke risk factors. It was also reported that events of CVAE frequency differ for nonserious events for the risperidone versus placebo treated subjects, possibly due to low power or miscoding events.

The review of olanzapine included five studies. Two of these studies were unpublished, included individuals with Alzheimer's disease, and excluded other DSM-IV disorders. One study included approximately 500 participants with vascular dementia and mixed dementia. In another study, there was no information on the number of patients with vascular dementia or details of their characteristics. There was a statistically significant difference in mortality for CVAEs in the olanzapine (42 of 1184, 3.5%) compared to the placebo (7 of 478, 1.5%) exposed individuals, ($p = 0.015$). However, there was no statistically significant difference found when accounting for serious versus nonserious CVAEs versus all-cause mortality.

There was no statistically significant difference in CVAEs or all-cause mortality rates for olanzapine (5 of 204, 2.5%) exposed individuals compared to risperidone (4 of 196, 2.0%) exposed individuals. There was no statistically significant difference in CVAEs or all-cause mortality for olanzapine exposed individuals (5 of 149, 3.4%) compared to first-generation antipsychotic exposed individuals (6 of 141, 4.3%). These values are reported without p values. It was noted that the sample sizes of the studies were small. Randomized controlled trials did indicate a significant increased risk of CVAEs with olanzapine compared to placebo. However, there was a small sample size and it is unclear if these were serious versus nonserious events.

Of the published risperidone articles, none reviewed differences in blood pressure and orthostatic blood pressure for individuals receiving risperidone compared to placebo. There were no statistically significant differences in vital signs and "clinically meaningful" orthostatic hypotension for individuals receiving olanzapine compared to individuals receiving placebo. Specifically, one article noted ≥ 30 mm HG decreases in systolic blood pressure were similar for olanzapine (7.2%) and placebo (7.0%) [Fisher's exact test, $p > 0.99$].

Discussion The authors acknowledged that no formal studies have determined casualty in this patient population. Potential mechanisms that contribute to the occurrence of CVAEs were discussed which included interactions between a patient's physiology, past medical history, and risk factors that were not better accounted for by the presence of an atypical antipsychotic:

1. Typical and atypical antipsychotics increased risk for venous thromboembolism. Possible mechanisms discussed included enhanced aggregation of platelets and presence of anticardiolipin antibodies. Yet, risperidone has not been shown to influence fibrinolysis, plasma coagulation, arachidonic acid metabolism, or platelet function reactions.
2. Cardiac effects causing CVAEs may be due to antipsychotics. Risperidone is a potent α1-adrenoreceptor blocker and olanzapine is a potent muscarinic M1 receptor antagonist. Despite these potential mechanisms, data has not shown within group differences in heart rate changes, vital signs, and EKG parameters in risperidone and olanzapine exposed groups compared to placebo groups.
3. Orthostatic hypotension from α1-adrenoreceptor blockade may cause cerebral perfusion impairment and thus CVAEs.
4. Excessive sedation and stiffness due to extrapyramidal symptoms (EPS), especially parkinsonism and dystonia, could lead to venous stasis, dehydration, and

hemoconcentration. This could put individuals at risk for CVAEs, which is another potential for miscoded events. Some individuals with EPS have been reported to experience more frequent CVAEs with atypical antipsychotics in comparison to placebo, which was a dose-dependent trend in the risperidone exposed group.

The authors revealed that the risperidone trials were longer (12 weeks) than olanzapine trials (6 weeks), and this time frame may account for CVAEs in risperidone trials. Lilly Pharmaceuticals suggested that the incidence of CVAEs with olanzapine exposure is no greater than with risperidone or typical antipsychotics.

The authors noted many studies did not have a priori hypotheses which prevented them from stratifying or randomizing patients to treatment or placebo groups. This made it difficult for these studies to delineate a cause and effect relationship. As a result, most CVAEs were detected post hoc.

Lastly, data from observational studies offered more information on the impact of multiple risk factors with longer periods of patient review. From this perspective, the odds ratio was not statistically significant for the following: hospitalization for stroke and TIAs due to risperidone exposure; all class atypical antipsychotics; and all class typical antipsychotics after adjusting for confounders. There was no difference in rates of CVAE occurrence in risperidone groups compared to olanzapine or quetiapine groups. There were an increased risk for CVAE-related admissions in the haloperidol group compared to the risperidone group and an increased risk for CVAE-related admissions in the benzodiazepine group compared to risperidone group. However, this is based on data from unpublished articles. Published data from one article found no increased risk for CVAEs with atypical antipsychotics compared to typical antipsychotics. Another published article suggested no increased risk for CVAEs associated with atypical antipsychotics compared to no antipsychotic treatment at all.

Conclusions Studies of risperidone report an increased risk for CVAEs when it is prescribed. These studies have also indicated that these CVAEs were mostly nonserious events and were more likely to occur in individuals with multiple risk factors for CVAEs. There does not seem to be an increased risk of CVAEs with atypical antipsychotics when compared to typical antipsychotics, benzodiazepines, and no exposure to antipsychotics. The association of these adverse outcomes with atypical antipsychotics is possible due to other factors like sedation, lethargy, and hypotensive episodes.

Strengths of the Study This was a well-designed meta-analysis study that appropriately elucidated concern for power, reviewed how cerebrovascular adverse events were classified, and took into consideration the multiple static and/or preexisting risk factors for cerebrovascular events. This is important in helping to counsel patients on the risks of these classes of medications and for clinicians to better understand the synergistic impact of these medications upon a patient's health.

Limitations of the Study This study used data and articles that were unpublished. Those articles did not go through the strenuous critique, feedback, validation, and fine tuning of peer-reviewed articles. Additionally, some information used in the analysis were obtained directly from pharmaceutical companies which could have provided biased information.

Take-Home Points Clinicians should continue to be mindful of the effects of polypharmacy, continue to take thorough medical and psychiatric histories from patients, and understand that use of atypical antipsychotics in the geriatric population likely has an additive role of contributing to various CVAEs rather than being the sole agent responsible for these episodes.

Practical Applications of the Take-Home Points There is some risk of CVAEs with antipsychotic use. However, this occurs mostly in individuals with preexisting risk factors and is not found to be consistently statistically significant when reviewing the data. Thus, one should weigh the risks and benefits of antipsychotics when treating geriatric patients with a neurocognitive disorder.

Reference

1. Herrmann N, Lanctôt KL. Do atypical antipsychotics cause stroke? CNS Drugs. 2005;19(2):91–103.

Chapter 2
Risk of Death with Atypical Antipsychotic Drug Treatment for Dementia: Meta-analysis of Randomized Placebo-Controlled Trials

Sara J. Anderson and Peter Ureste

Authors of the Original Article Lon S Schneider, Karen S Dagerman, Philip Insel

Name(s) of the Appraiser of the Article Sara J. Anderson, MD-MPH, and Peter Ureste, MD

Journal Publisher *The Journal of the American Medical Association*

Year of Publication 2005

Type of Study Meta-analysis of randomized placebo-controlled trial

Funding Sources Alzheimer's Disease Centers of California (grant 03-75274) and University of Southern California Alzheimer's Disease Research Center (NIH AG 05142)

Objectives To evaluate the data of increased mortality from atypical antipsychotic drug treatment for older adults with dementia [1].

Methods The authors' search included randomized placebo-controlled clinical trials (RCTs) utilizing MEDLINE (1966 to April 2005) and Cochrane Controlled Trials Register (2005, Issue 1) and non-peer-reviewed documents such as conference

S. J. Anderson
University of Missouri Kansas City and The Missouri Department of Mental Health – Center for Behavioral Medicine, Kansas City, MO, USA

P. Ureste (✉)
Department of Psychiatry and Behavioral Sciences, University of California San Francisco, San Francisco, CA, USA
e-mail: Peter.Ureste@ucsf.edu

R. R. Tampi et al. (eds.), *Essential Reviews in Geriatric Psychiatry*,
https://doi.org/10.1007/978-3-030-94960-0_2

programs, conference proceedings, abstracts of books, publication abstracts, poster presentations, slides from geriatric medicine, and psychiatric, neurological, and geriatric psychiatric professional society meetings since 1999. Pharmaceutical companies manufacturing atypical antipsychotics were contacted, and information was requested as needed. Search terms used included aripiprazole, clozapine, olanzapine, quetiapine, risperidone, ziprasidone, dementia, Alzheimer disease, and clinical trial.

RCTs were eligible for inclusion if they met the following criteria: parallel, double-blind, and placebo-controlled group with random assignment to an orally administered antipsychotic or placebo; the patients were diagnosed with Alzheimer disease, vascular dementia, mixed dementia, or a primary dementia; the numbers were randomized (with obtainable randomization methodology, dropout, and death figures).

The primary outcome assessed was mortality, with a secondary review of dropout rates. The authors included comparisons of several atypical antipsychotic drugs (aripiprazole, olanzapine, quetiapine, and risperidone) given orally and oral placebo. Exclusions were based on not meeting the above criteria and redundant publication. The assessment method formed part of the process by which papers were selected for the review, but the authors did not state who performed the validity assessment.

Additional selection criteria and review processes are not discussed, excepting the delineation between data extraction and confirmation as separate functions performed by distinct reviewers. Data were extracted on all-cause dropouts and deaths occurring within the trial period or 30 days of its conclusion. Dosage groups were aggregated within trials. Odds ratios (ORs) and absolute risk differences were calculated for dropouts and deaths.

Authors combined studies using DerSimonian and Laird random effects model for dropout outcomes and the Mantel-Haenszel fixed-effects model for deaths. A funnel plot analysis assessed potential retrieval bias in comparing published trials with the nonpublished trials (analysis results not included). Outcomes were based on standard assessment methods (with random or fixed-effects models) that calculated ORs, and risk differences included randomized and relative risks for total exposure in patient treatment.

Chi-squared tests and the I-squared statistic examined statistical heterogeneity between studies. Subgroups for sensitivity analyses included patients with diagnosis of psychosis of dementia; outpatients versus nursing home patients; whether mean baseline cognitive severity measured on the Mini-Mental State Examination (MMSE) was less than or equal to 10 or greater than 10; or by drug used.

Results Fifteen trials (9 unpublished), involving a total of 5387 patients, were included in the review. These trials were approximately 10–12 weeks in duration and included 16 comparisons between placebo and the following antipsychotic drugs: aripiprazole ($n = 3$), olanzapine ($n = 5$), quetiapine ($n = 3$), and risperidone ($n = 5$). There were a greater number of deaths in the atypical antipsychotic drug groups compared to the placebo groups (118 versus 40 deaths). The combined OR for all 15 trials by meta-analysis for death in patients treated with antipsychotic drugs compared with placebo was 1.54 (95% confidence interval (CI), 1.06, 2.23; $P = 0.02$) in favor of placebo, with no significant heterogeneity among the studies. A funnel plot graphing log ORs against sample size did not demonstrate any evidence of selection bias.

The risk differences for death were favorable for placebo than atypical antipsychotic drugs in all trials except three RCTs. Table 2.1 shows risk differences between drugs compared to placebo.

The authors found 1079 all-cause dropouts (32.2%) among the drug-treated groups and 551 (31.4%) among the placebo groups. Table 2.2 shows the risk differences for dropouts in patients treated with atypical antipsychotic drugs compared to placebo. Overall, there were no significant differences in dropouts between the drug and placebo groups, although there was significant heterogeneity among the trials and between drugs ($X^2 = 30.89$, $P = .009$; $I^2 = 51.4\%$). When the risk of death was compared to the risk of dropouts, no association was identified.

Subgroup analyses did not reveal heterogeneity in any of the trials comparing cognitive severity, trials that selected patients with psychosis of Alzheimer disease versus without, or inpatients compared with outpatients or among the four drugs.

In their ad hoc analysis, the authors found that the relative risk of mortality by length of exposure favored placebo when looking at available data on total exposure to drug or placebo in patient-years. An overall relative risk of 1.65 (95% CI, 1.19–2.29; $P = .003$) was calculated for atypical antipsychotics as a group, but weaker trends in risk of mortality were found when analyzing individual drugs.

Conclusions Atypical antipsychotic drugs may be associated with a small increased risk for death compared with placebo. One should compare the risks and benefits when determining whether to start an antipsychotic medication in the setting of dementia.

Table 2.1 Risk differences for death in patients treated with atypical antipsychotics compared to placebo

Drug	Risk difference	Confidence interval (CI)
Aripiprazole	0.01	95% CI, −0.01–0.03; $P = .20$
Olanzapine	0.01	95% CI, −0.00–0.03; $P = .07$
Quetiapine	0.02	95% CI, −0.01–0.05; $P = .22$
Risperidone	0.01	95% CI, −0.01–0.02; $P = .33$

Table 2.2 Risk differences for dropouts in patients treated with atypical antipsychotics compared to placebo

Drug	Risk difference	Confidence interval (CI)
Aripiprazole	−0.07	95% CI, −0.15–0.01; $P = .10$
Olanzapine	0.06	95% CI, −0.02–0.15; $P = .12$
Quetiapine	0.02	95% CI, −0.08–0.11; $P = .73$
Risperidone	0.03	95% CI, −0.03–0.08; $P = .31$

Strengths of the Study

1. The review question and the inclusion criteria were clear.
2. The search was adequate and included unpublished material.
3. The statistical analysis, including meta-analysis, was appropriate, thorough, and well-conducted.
4. A funnel plot graphing log ORs against sample size did not show evidence of selection bias.
5. The inclusion and exclusion material were clear.
6. Authors utilized meta-analysis to study variation of effect across RCTs, overcome the limits of small sample sizes, and examine differences from conflicting data thoroughly.
7. The unpublished RCTs, manuscripts, technical trial reports, posters, letters, and slide-formatted information could be standardized into the meta-analysis.
8. The study sample included only older adults (≥60 years of age).

Limitations of the Study

1. The authors did not elaborate in detail how the papers were selected for the review, or how many reviewers performed the selection.
2. The authors also did not report using methods to minimize bias and error when selecting studies for their review, and the validity assessment inherent in this process, although such methods were employed in the data extraction.
3. Utilization of posters and presentations with partial data which had to be reconstructed may have contributed to bias.
4. They provide little supporting data on which to base extrapolation using short-term data to longer periods from a 1% number of excess deaths at 8–12 weeks to a 4–5% risk difference over 1 year indicating it is probable that this initial risk is primarily expressed during the initial 12-week drug exposure.
5. The mortality events were negligible and the RCTs were not powered to detect a significant dose response.
6. There was insufficient information available on individual cases, causes or circumstances, baseline clinical characteristics, medical conditions, and concurrent medications.
7. They did not look at individual drugs in response to side effects but looked at overall category.
8. Few observational studies have reported that the mortality risk associated with antipsychotic use in the geriatric patients and older adults with dementia may have a dose-dependent effect.
9. Summarizing large amounts of varying information using a single number is a controversial aspect of meta-analysis as it ignores the fact that treatment effects may vary from study to study.
10. Some data presented with incomplete information and required additional information through other data presentations or from sponsors.

Take-Home Points Overall, the use of atypical antipsychotic drugs for relatively brief periods of less than 8–12 weeks was associated with a small increased risk for death compared with placebo. The number needed to harm, using an inverse of the absolute risk difference, proposes that there may be 1 death due to atypical drug use for every 100 patients treated over 10–12 weeks. The increased risk only could be identified when the atypical drugs were combined in a meta-analysis. The meta-analyses of each drug were not statistically significant, although the point estimates of the ORs ranged between 1.3 and 1.9. The upper bounds of the CIs, however, ranged from 2.2 to 4.6 and are compatible with the possibility of moderately increased risks.

Practical Applications of the Take-Home Points Older adult patients are more likely to experience adverse reactions as the result of age-related pharmacodynamic changes, and it is likely that any given medication may have the potential to both benefit and harm the patient. Although atypical antipsychotic drugs may be associated with a small increased risk for death compared with placebo, this risk should be reflected within the setting of medical need for the drugs, evidence of efficacy, medical comorbidity, and the efficacy and safety of alternatives.

It has been shown that antipsychotic drugs have been dispensed frequently to patients with dementia and used for long periods [2]. The findings within this meta-analysis emphasize the need to consider changes in clinical practices with an understanding that the established risks for cerebrovascular adverse events together with the present observations suggest that antipsychotic drugs should be used with care in these patients.

Many of these studies demonstrated increased mortality and cerebrovascular adverse events within 10–12 weeks after initiating atypical antipsychotic medication. It was also noted that within the individual clinical trials, there was substantial improvement for both drug and placebo groups within 1–4 weeks, indicating that when antipsychotic medication is prescribed, it is necessary to modify the dose with the understanding that clinical improvement emerges within this time frame. It is also essential to discontinue the medication if there is no improvement within this time frame to decrease the risk of ongoing adverse effects and increased risk of mortality.

Practicing physicians should understand that improvement in an older adult patient may not only be due to medication additions and/or changes but may also be the result of increased nursing support and care within the nursing facility, environmental changes, or changes in medical status. Naturally, starting and stopping an atypical antipsychotic medication might expose patients to greater risk. As the risks of serious adverse events are often related to initiation of medication than to continuation of medication, providers should assess the patient more frequently in this time period.

References

1. Schneider LS, Dagerman KS, Insel P. Risk of death with atypical antipsychotic drug treatment for dementia: meta-analysis of randomized placebo-controlled trials. JAMA. 2005;294(15):1934–43.
2. Gustafsson M, Karlsson S, Lövheim H. Inappropriate long-term use of antipsychotic drugs is common among people with dementia living in specialized care units. BMC Pharmacol Toxicol. 2013;14:10.

Chapter 3
Meta-analysis of the Impact of Nine Medication Classes on Falls in Elderly Persons

Jason Gandelman and Peter Ureste

Authors of the Original Article John C Woolcott, Kathryn J Richardson, Matthew O Wiens, Bhavini Patel, Judith Marin, Karim M Khan, Carlo A Marra

Journal Publisher *Archives of Internal Medicine*

Year of Publication 2009

Type of Study Meta-analysis

Funding Sources Supported in part by the Canadian Institutes of Health Research, the Michael Smith Foundation for Health Services Research, and the Government of Canada Research Chair in Pharmaceutical Outcomes.

Objectives To update a previously completed meta-analysis by Leipzig et al. [1, 2] with new studies and statistical methods in order to evaluate the association between medication use among older adults (age >60) and the risk for falls [3].

Methods This meta-analysis looked at a total of nine different drug classes. Four of the nine drug classes were primarily psychiatric drugs: (1) sedatives and hypnotics, (2) neuroleptics and antipsychotics, (3) antidepressants, and (4) benzodiazepines. The other five drug classes were cardiac and analgesic-related: (5) antihypertensive agents, (6) diuretics, (7) β-blockers, (8) narcotics, and (9) nonsteroidal anti-inflammatory drugs (NSAIDs). This meta-analysis looked purely for

J. Gandelman · P. Ureste (✉)
Department of Psychiatry and Behavioral Sciences, University of California San Francisco, San Francisco, CA, USA
e-mail: Jason.Gandelman@ucsf.edu; Peter.Ureste@ucsf.edu

R. R. Tampi et al. (eds.), *Essential Reviews in Geriatric Psychiatry*,
https://doi.org/10.1007/978-3-030-94960-0_3

statistical association via estimated odds ratio (OR) and did not attempt to discuss causation or other biological mechanisms that may contribute to falls.

New relevant studies were identified through a systematic search of English-language articles published from 1996 to 2007 in EBM, CINAHL, Embase, and MEDLINE databases.

Search criteria included MeSH terms: therapeutic uses, accident, falling, accidental fall, and home accident. These were combined with MeSH terms for the nine drug classes. Additionally, the MeSH terms epidemiology and pharmacoepidemiology were combined with "accidental fall" or "home accident" to identify studies in which exposure to drugs was not the primary objective, but may have been a secondary objective.

Eligibility criteria for studies included in the meta-analysis were as follows: original data from randomized controlled trial, case-control, cohort, or cross-sectional studies and that the study only included persons with age older than 60 years old. Exclusion criteria were as follows: studies were ultimately excluded if the authors could not obtain the data required from original study authors.

Studies were assessed independently by at least two authors and disagreements were resolved by a third author. A total of 22 new studies were identified by the search strategy.

This meta-analysis combined the 22 newly identified studies with 69 studies that were analyzed in the previously completed meta-analysis by Leipzig et al. in order to calculate an updated Bayesian pooled odds ratios (OR) and 95% credible intervals (95% CrIs). This Bayesian methodology was used as it allows for adjustment of greater uncertainty and other information known about the prior ORs (ORs calculated in the previous Leipzig et al. meta-analysis).

To provide a contrast to the Bayesian pooled OR and a more direct comparison to the Leipzig et al. previous findings, the authors also estimated a random-effects pooled OR (using frequentist ORs) and 95% confidence intervals (95% CIs), which was done by weighting each study by the inverse of its variance.

A secondary subgroup analysis was also completed that analyzed subgroups of the 22 studies by residential type (long-term care, community, or others), falling frequency (>35% or <35%), mean age of participants (>75 years old or <75 years old), study design, and method of ascertainment of falls. This subgroup analysis was meant to determine whether the above factors changed the estimated OR of falls in the nine drug classes.

Results A total of 22 new studies met the inclusion criteria for this meta-analysis. The investigators added these new studies to the previously identified 69 studies in the meta-analysis by Leipzig et al. The 22 studies included a total of 10 prospective cohort studies, 5 case-control studies, 7 cross-sectional studies, and 0 randomized controlled trials. Only six studies were considered to have "good" medication and falls ascertainment (not reliant on retrospective report bias). The meta-analysis ultimately included a total of 79,081 participants.

Meta-analyses were completed on the nine unique drug classes, with the primary outcome of Bayesian pooled OR estimates and 95% CrIs listed below. Due to Bayesian methodology, when the entire 95% CrI >1, it is considered a statistically significant increased likelihood for falling.

For the four primarily psychiatric drug classes:

1. Sedatives and hypnotics had a Bayesian pooled OR of 1.47 (95% CrI: 1.35–1.62)
2. Neuroleptics and antipsychotics had a Bayesian pooled OR of 1.59 (95% CrI: 1.37–1.83)
3. Antidepressants had a Bayesian pooled OR of 1.68 (95% CrI: 1.47–1.91)
4. Benzodiazepines had a Bayesian pooled OR of 1.57 (95% CrI: 1.43–1.72)

For the other five drug classes:

5. Antihypertensives had a Bayesian pooled OR of 1.24 (95% CrI: 1.01–1.50)
6. Diuretics had a Bayesian pooled OR of 1.07 (95% CrI: 1.01–1.14)
7. Beta-blockers had a Bayesian pooled OR of 1.01 (95% CrI: 0.86–1.17)
8. Narcotics had a Bayesian pooled OR of 0.96 (95% CrI: 0.78–1.18)
9. NSAIDs had a Bayesian pooled OR of 1.21 (95% CrI: 1.01–1.44)

All four of the psychiatric drug classes had statistically significant association with increased falls. Antidepressants had the strongest association with falls with a Bayesian pooled OR of 1.68. Narcotics had the least association with falls and were not statistically significant at Bayesian pooled OR of 0.96. All of the above associations remained significant even when decreasing the weight of the Leipzig prior meta-analyses. Some original studies reported adjusted ORs and the authors were thus able to calculate adjusted Bayesian pooled ORs. This did not change significance of association with falls with drug classes, except for neuroleptics and antipsychotics, where the association became not statistically significant with an adjusted Bayesian pooled OR of 1.39 (95% CrI: 0.94–2.00).

Subgroup analysis also in general did not change the statistical significance of the above results. Subgroup analysis by residential type, falling frequency, mean age of participants, or study design did not significantly affect the above Bayesian pooled OR estimates. In fact, even when only incorporating the six studies with "good" medication and falls ascertainment, all four psychiatric drug classes still had significantly significant association with increased falls.

Conclusion The use of sedatives and hypnotics, neuroleptics and antipsychotics, antidepressants, and benzodiazepines demonstrated a significant association with falls in older adults.

Strengths of the Study

1. While meta-analyses of systematically searched randomized controlled trials (RCTs) are often ranked as the highest available category of evidence (i.e., Category Ia), this is a meta-analysis of studies with case-control, cohort, or cross-sectional designs (no RCTs met criteria) [4].

2. Systematic reviews with meta-analyses are theoretically less susceptible to bias. Given the pooling of multiple studies and subjects, it can enhance the precision of estimated ORs (tighter confidence intervals) and thus may reduce the probability of false negative results.
3. The study sample included only older adults (≥60 years).
4. The study attempted to control for confounding by using a subgroup meta-analysis that is stratified by residential type, falling frequency, mean age of participants, study design, and method of ascertainment of falls and medications.
5. The quality of meta-analyses is discussed by Higgins et al. [5] using a qualitative list of 43 questions that are grouped into 4 categories (see table below for our evaluation of this meta-analysis).

Questions **1. Yes** **2. Probably yes** **3. Unclear** **4. Probably no** **5. No** **6. Not applicable**	**(A) Data sources:** Were the review methods adequate such that biases in location and assessment of studies were minimized or able to be identified?	**(B) Analysis of individual studies by the meta-analyst:** Were the individual studies analyzed appropriately and without avoidable bias?	**(C) General meta-analysis:** Were the basic meta-analysis methods appropriate?	**(D) Reporting and interpretation:** Are the conclusions justified and the interpretations sound?
Score	Yes	Yes	Unclear	Probably yes

Limitations of the Study

1. This study does not include the most recent studies and drugs, as it only includes studies prior to 2007.
2. Meta-analysis included multiple study designs; however none were RCTs. Additionally, studies were from multiple settings and used multiple methods of ascertaining a fall. Some studies used recall from participants, which the authors admit is a "poor" method of ascertaining falls and medication compliance.
3. This meta-analysis combines data from earlier meta-analyses by Leipzig et al. [1, 2] with the study data from 22 new studies between 1996 and 2007 to create a Bayesian pooled (posterior-adjusted) OR. As this is not generally used in meta-analyses, it is unclear if this method could provide biased results.
4. While the meta-analysis does attempt to control for confounding by using a subgroup meta-analysis, it is unclear whether this is an appropriate way to analyze for confounding and whether their conclusion that the confounders of residential type, falling frequency, mean age of participants, study design, and method of ascertainment of falls and medications actually did not significantly bias the results.
5. This meta-analysis does not control for "confounding by indication," i.e., those who take antidepressants are more likely to have depressive, anxiety, or trauma-related disorders and it is conceivable that the effect on falls is due to the psychiatric condition and that antidepressants are only a marker of disease and not causative of falls.

6. It is unclear which medications are included in which classes and many of the nine "unique" drug classes could conceivably overlap. For example, the article does not specify or attempt to specify whether trazodone is considered an antidepressant or a sedative and hypnotic. Thus, certain medications within a "unique" drug class may drive the statistical association with falls for that class.

Take-Home Points Despite some limitations, this high-quality meta-analysis showed that all psychiatric drug classes that were analyzed such as (1) sedatives and hypnotics, (2) neuroleptics and antipsychotics, (3) antidepressants, and (4) benzodiazepines were associated with an increased risk of falls among older adults. Notably, antidepressants had the strongest association with risk for falls.

Practical Applications of the Take-Home Points Be cautious when prescribing medications to older adults, and always consider reducing polypharmacy whenever possible to make it safer for the patient. While most clinicians consider antidepressants to confer lower relative risk for falls, this study may indicate that this group of medications appear to have a similar or stronger risk for falls among older adults when compared to benzodiazepines, antipsychotics, and narcotics.

References

1. Leipzig RM, Cumming RG, Tinetti ME. Drugs and falls in older people: a systematic review and meta-analysis: I. Pychotropic drugs. J Am Geriatr Soc. 1999;47(1):30–9.
2. Leipzig RM, Cumming RG, Tinetti ME. Drugs and falls in older people: a systematic review and meta-analysis: II. Cardiac and analgesic drugs. J Am Geriatr Soc. 1999;47(1):40–50.
3. Woolcott JC, Richardson KJ, Wiens MO, Patel B, Marin J, Khan KM, Marra CA. Meta-analysis of the impact of 9 medication classes on falls in elderly persons. Arch Intern Med. 2009;169(21):1952–60.
4. Shekelle PG, Woolf SH, Eccles M, Grimshaw J. Clinical guidelines: developing guidelines. BMJ. 1999;318(7183):593–6.
5. Higgins JP, Lane PW, Anagnostelis B, Anzures-Cabrera J, Baker NF, Cappelleri JC, Haughie S, Hollis S, Lewis SC, Moneuse P, Whitehead A. A tool to assess the quality of a meta-analysis. Res Synth Methods. 2013;4(4):351–66.

Chapter 4
The Efficacy and Safety of Atypical Antipsychotics for the Treatment of Dementia: A Meta-analysis of Randomized Placebo-Controlled Trials

Peter Ureste and Chloe Cheng

Authors of the Original Article Hui Ma, Yinglin Huang, Zhengtu Cong, Yuan Wang, Wenhai Jiang, Shuhe Gao, Gang Zhu

Journal Publisher *Journal of Alzheimer's Disease*

Year of Publication 2014

Type of Study Meta-analysis of randomized placebo-controlled trials

Funding Sources The National Natural Science Foundation

Objectives To evaluate the efficacy, safety, and tolerability of second-generation antipsychotic (SGA) medications from a meta-analysis of randomized placebo-controlled trials (RCTs) for the treatment of psychological and behavioral symptoms of dementia [1].

Methods The authors conducted a literature search using the primary search terms ("dementia"; "psychological, psychiatric, or behavioral symptoms"; "double-blind"; "placebo"; "random") which were used together with one of the following: "atypical antipsychotic," "quetiapine," "aripiprazole," "risperidone," "olanzapine," "amisulpride," or "ziprasidone." Combinations of terms were searched in the following databases: MEDLINE, PsycINFO, and the Cochrane Central Register of Controlled Trials. Articles were excluded if they were not written in English, trials were presented at meetings but not published, drugs were administered by

P. Ureste (✉) · C. Cheng
Department of Psychiatry and Behavioral Sciences, University of California San Francisco, San Francisco, CA, USA
e-mail: Peter.Ureste@ucsf.edu; Chloe.Cheng@ucsf.edu

R. R. Tampi et al. (eds.), *Essential Reviews in Geriatric Psychiatry*,
https://doi.org/10.1007/978-3-030-94960-0_4

intramuscular injection, and effect evaluations were immediate. Only papers of double-blind, placebo-controlled, randomized controlled trials comparing SGAs with placebo that used any of the following scales as outcome measures were included: Neuropsychiatric Inventory (NPI), Brief Psychiatric Rating Scale (BPRS), Cohen-Mansfield Agitation Inventory (CMAI), Clinical Global Impression of Change (CGI-C), and Clinical Global Impression of Severity (CGI-S). The quality of the randomized controlled trials (RCTs) was assessed using various assessment scales.

The authors reported obtaining the following data from individual studies: study design, key inclusion criteria, subject nationality, mean age, gender ratio, study group size, drug dose(s), trial duration, baseline rating scores, endpoint outcomes, dropouts, mortality, and adverse events (AEs). Trials that utilized a study design involving subgroups with different fixed doses were represented in the meta-analysis by the sum of observed events in all subgroups (e.g., the total number of AEs from all subgroups was calculated and used to represent an individual trial's data in the meta-analysis) or by the total change in means and standard deviations (SDs) of rating scale scores calculated from data derived from all subgroups. Notably, the authors indicated that they primarily utilized the data from the subgroup with the most effective dose for neuropsychiatric symptoms of dementia to represent an individual trial, although they would also compare each subgroup's data with a control group during their analysis. Categorical variables like attrition and death were analyzed by calculating odds ratios (ORs), while standardized mean differences (SMDs) or weighted mean differences (WMDs) were calculated for analysis of continuous data measurements obtained from rating scales like the NPI, CGI-S, BPRS, CMAI, and CGI-C. The main endpoints evaluated from each trial included overall antipsychotic treatment efficacy as measured by the BPRS, total NPI, CGI-C, CGI-S, and CMAI, as well as safety and tolerability measures for SGA administration compared to placebo. In addition to investigating the overall efficacy, safety, and tolerability of SGAs as a class, individual SGAs (aripiprazole, olanzapine, quetiapine, and risperidone) were examined separately as subgroups.

Results The search yielded a total of 22 studies, of which 3 were excluded due to use of intramuscular injections and 3 were excluded for not using the pre-selected scales. The remaining 16 trials included 19 comparisons of SGAs versus placebo. Of these, three studied aripiprazole, two olanzapine, five quetiapine, four risperidone, one olanzapine and risperidone, and one olanzapine, quetiapine, and risperidone. Taken together, the authors were able to conduct a meta-analysis of data from a total of 3343 drug-treated and 1707 placebo-treated dementia patients. All trials were reported to be randomized, double-blind, and placebo controlled. However, the methods of randomization were reported in only five studies, while methods regarding blinding patients or investigators were described in only two studies. Most of these 16 trials were conducted in multicenter sites. The quality of trials included in the meta-analysis was high based on mean scores of the Brown, Jadad, and van Tulder scales being above the cutoff [2–4].

Patients receiving various SGAs had significantly improved NPI, BPRS, CMAI, CGI-C, and CGI-S total scores when compared to placebo. Subgroup analyses showed aripiprazole and quetiapine significantly improved NPI and BPRS; aripiprazole and risperidone significantly improved CMAI; aripiprazole, olanzapine, quetiapine, and risperidone significantly improved differences in CGI-C; and risperidone significantly improved CGI-S. Table 4.1 provides the efficacy of antipsychotics on various outcome scales and heterogeneity of studies with second-generation antipsychotics for dementia.

In terms of attrition, 35.6% of patients (1190 of 3343) in the drug groups dropped out prematurely when compared to the placebo groups (41.5% [865 of 2085] before removal of duplicates in placebo groups; 35.4% [604 of 1707] after removal of duplicates). No statistically significant difference in dropout rates between drug and placebo groups was found (pooled OR = 0.99; 95% CI, 0.82–1.20; $P = 0.92$). In their subgroup meta-analysis, differences among the individual SGAs were observed. Specifically, the odds of dropping out in patients treated with aripiprazole were less when compared to placebo (OR = 0.71; 95% CI, 0.52–0.96; $P = 0.03$). However, groups treated with olanzapine, quetiapine, and risperidone did not exhibit a statistically significant increase in odds of dropout compared to placebo. The authors reported that reasons for dropout included all of the following death, AEs, withdrawn consent, failure to follow up, noncompliance, lack of efficacy or response, intolerability, protocol deviation, physician decision, and investigator discretion.

About 15% of drug-treated patients experienced extrapyramidal side effects (EPS) when compared to 8.4% in the placebo group. Patients receiving SGAs appeared to have a significantly higher risk of experiencing EPS compared to placebo (OR = 1.74; 95% CI, 1.41–2.14; $P < 0.00001$). Individually, odds of EPS was higher for olanzapine ($P = 0.01$) and risperidone ($P < 0.00001$) subgroups. In terms of somnolence, this was found in 17% of patients in the pooled drug group compared to 7.3% (7.2% after duplicates were removed) in the placebo group. Groups prescribed SGAs exhibited higher odds of experiencing somnolence compared to those receiving placebo (OR = 2.95; 95% CI, 2.33–3.75; $P < 0.00001$). Individually, all SGAs reported increased the odds of somnolence.

Cerebrovascular events (CVAEs) occurred in 2.1% of patients in the pooled drug group compared to 0.8% (0.9% after duplicate correction) in the pooled controlled group. Higher odds of CVAEs were reported in the pooled antipsychotic group (OR = 2.50; 95% CI, 1.36–4.60; $P = 0.003$) and in the risperidone subgroup. In terms of agitation, this was experienced in 10.6% of subjects in the drug groups when compared to 12.7% (13.3% after correction) in the pooled placebo group. Patients receiving SGAs exhibited lower odds of agitation compared to those receiving placebo (OR = 0.80; 95% CI, 0.65–0.98; $P = 0.03$), with a specific decrease in odds of agitation in the aripiprazole subgroup. In terms of self-injury or accidental injury, this was experienced by 22.2% of patients in the pooled drug group when compared to 22.5% (23.5% after correction) in the pooled placebo group. Patients treated with SGAs demonstrated no significant higher odds of injury risk when compared to placebo.

Table 4.1 Efficacy of antipsychotics on various outcome scales and heterogeneity of studies with second-generation antipsychotics for dementia

	Outcome scale				
SGA	NPI	BPRS	CMAI	CGI-C	CGI-S
Aripiprazole	WMD = −3.81 95% CI: −6.36 to −1.26 $P = 0.003$	WMD = −2.41 95% CI: −4.24 to −0.58 $P = 0.01$	WMD = −4.09 95% CI: −7.52 to −0.66 $P = 0.02$	WMD = −0.30 95% CI: −0.59 to −0.01 $P = 0.04$	WMD = −0.12 95% CI: −0.25 to 0.02 $P = 0.08$
Olanzapine	WMD = −2.12 95% CI: −4.89 to 0.65 $P = 0.13$	WMD = −1.24 95% CI: −2.69 to 0.22 $P = 0.10$	WMD = −0.40 95% CI: −1.33 to 0.53 $P = 0.40$	WMD = −0.32 95% CI: −0.56 to −0.07 $P = 0.01$	Not evaluated
Quetiapine	WMD = −3.45 95% CI: −6.78 to −0.11 $P = 0.04$	WMD = −2.70 95% CI: −5.24 to −0.16 $P = 0.04$	WMD = −0.34 95% CI: −4.87 to 4.20 $P = 0.88$	WMD = −0.29 95% CI: −0.53 to −0.04 $P = 0.02$	WMD = −0.13 95% CI: −0.42 to 0.16 $P = 0.37$
Risperidone	WMD = −0.53 95% CI: −4.93 to 3.86 $P = 0.81$	WMD = −0.37 95% CI: −2.55 to 1.81 $P = 0.74$	WMD = −2.37 95% CI: −4.18 to −0.57 $P = 0.01$	WMD = −0.35 95% CI: −0.56 to −0.14 $P = 0.001$	WMD = −0.41 95% CI: −0.61 to −0.20 $P < 0.0001$
Overall heterogeneity	$\chi^2 = 11.93$ $P = 0.53$ $I^2 = 0\%$	$\chi^2 = 10.83$ $P = 0.29$ $I^2 = 17\%$	$\chi^2 = 17.07$ $P = 0.02$ $I^2 = 59\%$	$\chi^2 = 17.41$ $P = 0.07$ $I^2 = 43\%$	$\chi^2 = 6.28$ $P = 0.18$ $I^2 = 36\%$

WMD weighted mean difference

A total of 6.9% of patients in the pooled drug groups experienced gait abnormalities when compared to 1.9% (1.7% after duplicated data removed) in the pooled placebo groups. Higher odds of gait abnormality were reported in the pooled antipsychotic group (OR = 3.35; 95% CI, 2.06–5.46; $P < 0.00001$). Patients treated with olanzapine and risperidone had higher odds of gait abnormalities. Subjects in the pooled and placebo drug groups experienced edema (9.3% versus 4.8% [5.2% after correction]), urinary tract infections (14.9% versus 10.9%), falls (15.2% versus 17.2%) [18.8% after correction]), insomnia (5.7% versus 5.4% [5.4% after correction]), and vomiting (8.5% versus 4.9%). Patients receiving SGAs had higher odds of experiencing edema (OR = 1.80; 95% CI, 1.29–2.49; $P = 0.0005$) and urinary tract infections (OR = 1.35; 95% CI, 1.07–1.71; $P = 0.01$), but did not exhibit higher odds for other conditions.

For mortality, 3.6% of drug-treated patients died during the studies or within 30 days of discontinuation when compared to 2.2% (2.3% after correction) in the pooled placebo group. Of the few studies that reported cause of death, the most frequent were pneumonia, stroke, and cardiac arrests. Groups receiving any SGA exhibited higher odds of death when compared to those receiving placebo (OR = 1.52; 95% CI, 1.06–2.18; $P = 0.02$); however, subgroup analysis for aripiprazole, olanzapine, quetiapine, or risperidone revealed no individual SGA was associated with higher odds of death.

Conclusions Evidence from this meta-analysis of 16 published double-blind placebo-controlled randomized trials indicates that individual SGAs showed some efficacy for improving neuropsychiatric symptoms of dementia as measured by BPRS, CMAI, NPI, CGI-C, or CGI-S. In terms of individual drugs, risperidone was associated with elevated risks of somnolence, edema, EPS, gait abnormalities, and CVAEs; olanzapine with somnolence, EPS, and gait abnormalities; quetiapine with somnolence and vomiting; and aripiprazole only with somnolence. Dementia patients on any SGA did not show higher rates of discontinuation.

Strengths of the Study

1. The study was a meta-analysis of randomized, double-blind, placebo-controlled trials.
2. There was minimal evidence of selection bias, as indicated by symmetry around the mean overall effect in the funnel plots of most primary endpoints investigated by the trials.
3. The quality of all RCTs included in the meta-analysis was evaluated using the Brown, Jadad, and van Tulder scales. The means scores of all the scales for all the included studies were above the cut point, suggesting they were high-quality studies.
4. The study assessed on the basis of Jadad score [3] indicates that this meta-analysis was a high-quality study with a score of 4 out of 5.

Questions Yes (1) No (0)	Was the study described as random?	Was the randomization scheme described and appropriate?	Was the study described as double-blind?	Was the method of double blinding appropriate? (Were both the patient and the assessor appropriately blinded?)	Was there a description of dropouts and withdrawals?	Total score Range of score quality 0–2, low 3–5, high
Score	1	0	1	1	1	4

Limitations of the Study

1. Conclusion is limited by significant methodological differences between individual trials.
2. There is a possible publication bias regarding data about agitation (CMAI) and dropouts, as indicated by asymmetry around the mean in their respective funnel plots.
3. The effectiveness and benefits of SGAs might have been overestimated or miscalculated because studies with negative results or other languages were not published and included in this meta-analysis.
4. Some valuable information was missing, such as the CGI-S results but without standard deviations.

Take-Home Points

Despite some limitations, this high-quality meta-analysis of randomized, double-blind, and placebo-controlled trials indicates that SGAs are significantly efficacious on the treatment of psychological and behavioral symptoms of dementia. These drugs showed no difference in risk for discontinuation when compared to placebo. However, those on SGAs had higher risk for AEs (except agitation) and mortality, which might offset their benefits.

Practical Applications of the Take-Home Points

The efficacy, safety, and tolerability of SGAs should be weighed carefully against clinical needs.

References

1. Ma H, Huang Y, Cong Z, Wang Y, Jiang W, Gao S, Zhu G. The efficacy and safety of atypical antipsychotics for the treatment of dementia: a meta-analysis of randomized placebo-controlled trials. J Alzheimers Dis. 2014;42(3):915–37.
2. Brown SA. Measurement of quality of primary studies for meta-analysis. Nurs Res. 1991;40(6):352–5.

3. Jadad AR, Moore RA, Carroll D, Jenkinson C, Reynolds DJ, Gavaghan DJ, McQuay HJ. Assessing the quality of reports of randomized clinical trials: is blinding necessary? Control Clin Trials. 1996;17(1):1–12.
4. van Tulder M, Furlan A, Bombardier C, Bouter L, Editorial Board of the Cochrane Collaboration Back Review Group. Updated method guidelines for systematic reviews in the Cochrane collaboration back review group. Spine (Phila Pa 1976). 2003;28(12):1290–9.

Chapter 5
Do Antipsychotics Lead to Cognitive Impairment in Dementia? A Meta-analysis of Randomized Placebo-Controlled Trials

Sarah Kim and Tracey Holsinger

Authors of the Original Article Alexander Wolf, Stefan Leucht, Frank-Gerald Pajonk

Journal Publisher *European Archives of Psychiatry and Clinical Neuroscience*

Year of Publication 2017

Type of Study Meta-analysis

Funding Sources None

Objective To determine the association between the use of antipsychotics for the treatment of BPSD and the side effect of further decline in cognitive function from a meta-analysis of ten randomized, double-blind, placebo-controlled trials [1].

Methods The investigators of the study searched for all published and unpublished randomized controlled trials that assessed the efficacy of antipsychotics in the treatment of BPSD in the following databases: MEDLINE, Scopus, CENTRAL (last search 2014), and ClinicalStudyResults (open database for trials, last search 2008). The investigators were only looking for randomized, double-blind, placebo-controlled trials with a minimum duration of 1 week. The keywords used in the

S. Kim
Duke University, Department of Psychiatry and Behavioral Sciences, Durham, NC, USA
e-mail: kyung.kim@duke.edu

T. Holsinger (✉)
Duke University, Department of Psychiatry and Behavioral Sciences, Durham, NC, USA

Durham VA Medical Center, Durham, NC, USA
e-mail: Tracey.holsinger@duke.edu

R. R. Tampi et al. (eds.), *Essential Reviews in Geriatric Psychiatry*,
https://doi.org/10.1007/978-3-030-94960-0_5

search included antipsychotic, antipsychotics, neuroleptic, neuroleptics, aripiprazole, chlorpromazine, clozapine, flupenthixol, haloperidol, melperone, olanzapine, pimozide, pipamperone, quetiapine, risperidone, sulpiride, thioridazine, ziprasidone, and zuclopenthixol, in conjunction with the keyword searches dementia, Alzheimer, Alzheimer's, AD, vascular dementia, VD, BPSD, behavioural and psychological, behavioral and psychological, Pick, and Pick's disease. Keywords used in the search of ClinicalStudyResults included dementia or Alzheimer dementia in conjunction with antipsychotic, neuroleptic, aripiprazole, clozapine, olanzapine, quetiapine, risperidone, or ziprasidone.

The exclusion criteria for this study were studies without a placebo arm and those studies that evaluated individuals with Lewy body dementia.

The primary outcome measure of the cognitive change in all included studies was the Mini-Mental State Examination (MMSE). However, two studies provided additional data on the Alzheimer's Disease Assessment Scale-Cognitive Subscale (ADAS-Cog). A sensitivity analysis was performed using ADAS-Cog instead of MMSE where provided. A meta-regression was performed to test a correlation between baseline MMSE scores and study duration. All pooled antipsychotics were analyzed individually.

The outcome data of the studies were summarized in a meta-analysis using the random effects model to take heterogeneity among studies into account. The investigators calculated both mean differences (weighted mean difference, WMD) in MMSE raw values and standardized mean differences (SMD) as the effect size. To assess study heterogeneity, the investigators used chi-square test ($P < 0.1$ set a priori to assume presence of heterogeneity) and I-square statistic (values $\geq 50\%$ as considerable heterogeneity). The possibility of publication bias was examined using the funnel plot method.

Results The investigators screened 27,602 records from Scopus, MEDLINE, CENTRAL, and ClinicalStudyResults, of which 27,484 records were excluded from initial screening. A total of 118 records were assessed for eligibility. Of these, 103 records were excluded for reasons as follows: combined post hoc or subgroup analysis, inappropriate diagnosis or participants, inappropriate intervention or control, no allocation concealment, length less than 1 week, and no relevant outcome.

A total of 15 records referring to 10 studies with 13 arms and 1586 participants were included in this meta-analysis. Eleven studies investigated placebo versus a second-generation antipsychotic (aripiprazole, olanzapine, quetiapine, risperidone), and two investigated placebo versus a first-generation antipsychotic haloperidol. Included study participants were more often female (mean 69%; range 55–80%), with mean age of 80 (range 75–84) years and a mean baseline MMSE score of 12.7 (range 5.2–21.5).

Antipsychotic use was associated with decline in cognitive function in the pooled analysis when compared to placebo (SMD = −0.065, WMD = −0.211). However, only two studies showed significant effects, and when those two were excluded, the SMD turned zero ($P = 0.95$). As mentioned above, each antipsychotic outcome data was pooled individually.

Aripiprazole
Two included studies showed cognitive worsening with aripiprazole, being significant in one trial and not significant in the other.

Olanzapine
Three out of four included studies showed no or minimal differences between olanzapine and placebo. Of note, one trial which included participants with a particularly high MMSE (21.5 points) reported significant decline in cognitive function with olanzapine as compared to placebo.

Quetiapine
Three included studies showed no significant difference between quetiapine and placebo.

Risperidone
Two included studies showed no significant difference between risperidone and placebo.

Haloperidol
Two included studies showed no significant difference between haloperidol and placebo.

Test of heterogeneity was significant for the trials with aripiprazole, olanzapine, and risperidone, and not significant for quetiapine and haloperidol. Two included olanzapine studies also provided ADAS-Cog scores. When using the mean change in ADAS-Cog scores instead of MMSE scores, there was an enhanced effect of cognitive worsening. Furthermore, meta-regression found a significant and strong linear correlation between study length and SMD in MMSE change: the longer the study duration, the greater the cognitive decline with antipsychotic treatment when compared to placebo. There was also a high correlation between baseline MMSE and SMD: the higher the baseline MMSE, the higher the cognitive worsening with antipsychotic treatment when compared to placebo. However, in a sensitivity analysis where the two studies with the largest impact were removed, neither a correlation between study length and cognitive worsening nor a correlation between baseline MMSE score and cognitive worsening was found.

Conclusions In this meta-analysis that evaluated data from ten randomized, double-blind, placebo-controlled trials, the random effect model did not show a significant decline in cognitive function with antipsychotic use, when compared to placebo in treatment of BPSD. The meta-regression showed a significant correlation between cognitive impairment and treatment duration, and between cognitive impairment and baseline MMSE score.

Strengths of the Study

1. Meta-analysis used random effects model for the purpose of taking heterogeneity among various studies into account.
2. Included studies were randomized, double-blind, and placebo-controlled trials.
3. There was inclusion of both first-generation and second-generation antipsychotics.
4. There was comparison of each antipsychotic agent individually with placebo.

Limitations of the Study

1. Though a funnel plot was used, there might be a publication bias, as negative results are less likely to be published.
2. MMSE is a widely used cognitive assessment tool for initial detection of cognitive impairment, but MMSE is not a very sensitive tool to detect changes in cognitive functioning, especially when short study duration is not taken into account.
3. Only two studies investigated cognitive changes for more than 12 weeks, and only one more than 20 weeks.
4. Dosage and the number of antipsychotics used (if more than one medication was used) for each participant are not identified.
5. Confounding factors for cognitive function, such as general health, active medical illness, use of cognitive enhancers, variable progression, and prognosis in Alzheimer's disease vs vascular dementia vs Pick's disease, were not accounted for in this study.

Take-Home Points Despite some limitations, this meta-analysis indicates no significant difference in the potential side effect of cognitive impairment in antipsychotic treatment for BPSD when compared to placebo. There was also no significant difference found among different generations of antipsychotic and the different agents used. This is in line with the results from the CATIE-AD study [2]: antipsychotics do not seem to cause significant cognitive changes as compared to placebo, and show improvement in symptoms such as anger, agitation, and paranoia which may help with BPSD. Of note, one out of the four olanzapine studies showed a significant decline in cognitive function as compared to placebo, which suggests similarity to one of the findings from the CATIE-AD study showing worsening of functional skills with olanzapine use as compared to placebo.

Practical Applications of the Take-Home Points BPSD such as delusions, hallucinations, agitations, and aggression are common in dementia and pose a significant barrier in the care of patients with dementia. However, there are only limited options for pharmacological treatment, with limited data on efficacy of these agents. Moreover, most of the agents used carry a side effect profile that is not favorable to the elderly population. Antipsychotics should be used after careful evaluation of risks vs benefits for each individual patient, targeting the minimum effective dose being used, for as brief a time as possible, and the use of these agents should be monitored closely.

References

1. Wolf A, Leucht S, Pajonk FG. Do antipsychotics lead to cognitive impairment in dementia? A meta-analysis of randomised placebo-controlled trials. Eur Arch Psychiatry Clin Neurosci. 2017;267(3):187–98.
2. Sultzer DL, Davis SM, Tariot PN, Dagerman KS, Lebowitz BD, Lyketsos CG, Rosenheck RA, Hsiao JK, Lieberman JA, Schneider LS, CATIE-AD Study Group. Clinical symptom responses to atypical antipsychotic medications in Alzheimer's disease: phase 1 outcomes from the CATIE-AD effectiveness trial. Am J Psychiatry. 2008;165(7):844–54.

Chapter 6
A Systematic Review and Meta-analysis of the Risk of Dementia Associated with Benzodiazepine Use, After Controlling for Protopathic Bias

Paroma Mitra

Authors of the Original Article Ross Penninkilampi, Guy D Eslick

Journal Publisher *CNS Drugs*

Year of Publication 2018

Type of Study Systematic review and meta-analysis

Funding Sources None. A Summer Research Scholarship provided by the University of Sydney funded the costs of retrieving the medical records for the study.

Objectives The aim of the study was to investigate the risk of dementia associated with the use of benzodiazepines in older adults, after controlling for protopathic bias [1].

Methods The authors performed a systematic review and meta-analysis according to the Preferred Reporting Items for Systematic Reviews and Meta-Analyses (PRISMA) guidelines. Electronic searches of databases MEDLINE, PubMed, Embase, Cochrane Trials, Cumulative Index to Nursing and Allied Health Literature (CINAHL), and Literatura Latino-Americana e do Caribe em Ciências da Saúde (LILACS) were conducted. Search terms included "Alzheimer disease" *or* "dementia" *and* "benzodiazepines" *or* "hypnotics" *or* "sedatives". Screening was performed in two steps. Firstly, titles and abstracts were screened for broad inclusion into the review. Following that, manuscripts were reviewed with predetermined inclusion and exclusion criteria for final inclusion in the review and meta-analysis.

P. Mitra (✉)
NYU School of Medicine, Bellevue Hospital Center, New York, NY, USA

R. R. Tampi et al. (eds.), *Essential Reviews in Geriatric Psychiatry*, https://doi.org/10.1007/978-3-030-94960-0_6

For inclusion in the review, observational studies were required to meet the following criteria: (1) adequate case ascertainment by way of physician diagnosis or identification from a registry or database, (2) optimal assessment for benzodiazepine use in the form of patient report or a prescription database, (3) an appropriate control group, (4) documentation that benzodiazepines were used prior to the diagnosis of dementia, (5) results that either described or yielded odds ratio and 95% confidence intervals, (6) at least 50 cases studied, and (7) mean age of participants of at least 65 years.

Relevant data was extracted in a structured manner. The authors calculated pooled odds ratios and 95% confidence intervals for the risk of dementia associated with benzodiazepine use using a random effects model. The quality of included studies was assessed using Newcastle–Ottawa Quality Assessment Scale (NOS) [2]. Studies which scored at least 6 out of a possible score of 9 were considered as high-quality studies.

Results The search resulted in a total of 3730 studies. After screening of titles and abstracts, 24 studies were selected for full text review, which then culminated in 15 studies. These comprised 5 cohort studies and 10 case-control studies, cumulatively consisting of 159,090 cases. The studies varied widely in the number of cases and follow-up periods. Some studies accounted for lag time, while others did not.

The authors demonstrated that any use of benzodiazepines was associated with increased risk of dementia (OR 1.39, 95% CI 1.21–1.59; $p < 0.001$).

The authors examined the comparative impact of short-acting vs long-acting benzodiazepines. Short-acting benzodiazepines were associated with significantly increased risk of dementia (OR 1.13, 95% CI 1.02–1.26; $p = 0.01$). The association lacked statistical significance for long-acting benzodiazepines, although the estimate of the effect was greater than that of short-acting benzodiazepines (OR 1.21, 95% CI 0.99–1.49; $p = 0.06$).

The authors also explored dosing strength and duration of use. The meta-analysis of studies that examined the total use of benzodiazepines (highest cumulative dose) versus "no use" found non-significant risk of dementia (OR 1.29, 95% CI 1.00–1.66; $p = 0.052$). Longer duration of use had greater association with dementia (OR 1.47, 95% CI 1.20–1.81; $p < 0.001$), although only two studies included in the review had examined duration. When risk factors such as anxiety, depression, and insomnia were adjusted for, and a lag time was included, there was a significant risk of dementia associated with any use of benzodiazepines (OR 1.31, 95% CI 1.11–1.54; $p = 0.001$).

Studies without lag time had high strength of association (OR 1.48, 95% CI 1.17–1.89; $p = 0.001$). Studies with any lag time demonstrated positive association between benzodiazepine use and dementia (OR 1.12, 95% CI 1.03–1.323; $p = 0.012$). Interestingly, studies that consisted of a long lag time of 5 years or more, one in which protopathic bias can be considered mitigated, also showed a significant association with dementia (OR 1.30, 95% CI 1.14–1.48; $p < 0.001$).

Table 6.1 describes the strength of association of dementia with risk factors with the statistically significant factors being highlighted.

Table 6.1 The strength of association of dementia with risk factors

Timing of use	OR (odds ratio)	(95% CI)	*P* value
Any use	**1.39**	**1.21–1.59**	***P* < 0.001**
Type of benzodiazepine			
Short-acting	**1.13**	**1.02–1.26**	***P* = 0.01**
Long-acting	1.21	0.99–1.49	*P* = 0.06
Cumulative dose			
Highest dose duration vs control	1.29	1.00–1.66	*P* = 0.052
Highest duration dose	**1.47**	**1.20–1.81**	***P* < 0.001**
Adjustment for risk factors			
Adjustment for depression, anxiety, insomnia, and inclusion of lag time	**1.31**	**1.11–1.54**	***P* = 0.001**
Lag time			
No lag	**1.48**	**1.17–1.89**	***P* = 0.001**
Any lag	1.12	1.03–1.23	*P* = 0.012
>5 years' lag	**1.30**	**1.14–1.48**	***P* < 0.001**

Quality Assessment: All included studies had a quality score of 6 or more and were deemed as high-quality studies. The case-control studies had points deducted if they derived records from databases instead of physician diagnosis, used prescription databases instead of structured interview, or lacked adjustment for educational status, depression, or anxiety. The cohort studies were overall of higher quality.

Conclusion The authors conclude that benzodiazepines are associated with increased risk of Alzheimer's disease and other neurocognitive disorders while controlling for protopathic bias. They recommend reduction of inappropriate benzodiazepine use as a means to mitigate risk of dementia. Given the smaller effect size for the use of short-acting benzodiazepines when compared to long-acting benzodiazepines (although the latter lacked statistical significance), the authors advocate for prescribing short-acting benzodiazepines for limited periods, when clinically indicated.

Strengths of the Study

1. In this meta-analysis, the authors looked at almost 160,000 cases over a duration of several years.
2. The inclusion criteria were rigorous and carefully applied.
3. The authors examined a multitude of prescribing patterns, namely, the impact of short-acting and long-acting benzodiazepines, dosing strength, and duration of use.
4. The authors examined if the pattern of prescribing benzodiazepines for depression and anxiety, in those who are predisposed to cognitive decline, creates an artefactual excess of cases of dementia, thereby controlling for protopathic bias.
5. Included studies were assessed for quality.
6. Most of the studies have several years of follow-up data.

Limitations of the Study

1. Although the analysis included a large number of cases, the heterogenous nature of the included studies limits the strength of the overall findings.
2. The duration of benzodiazepine use, follow-up periods, and psychiatric comorbidities varied across studies.
3. It was unclear in some of the studies whether there was actual benzodiazepine use by patients, given that prescription registries were used instead of actual patient interviews.

Take-Home Points Benzodiazepine use is associated with an increased risk of dementia. Careful use of benzodiazepines is advised in the older population.

Practical Applications of the Take-Home Points Benzodiazepines increase the risk of developing neurocognitive disorders in older adults. If benzodiazepines are indicated, short-acting benzodiazepines should be considered for a limited duration of time.

References

1. Penninkilampi R, Eslick GD. A systematic review and meta-analysis of the risk of dementia associated with benzodiazepine use, after controlling for protopathic bias. CNS Drugs. 2018;32(6):485–97.
2. Wells G, Shea B, O'Connell D, Peterson J, Welch V, Losos M, Tugwell P. The Newcastle-Ottawa Scale (NOS) for assessing the quality of nonrandomised studies in meta-analyses. 2013. http://www.ohri.ca/programs/clinical_epidemiology/oxford.asp. Accessed 8 June 2021.

Part II
Anxiety Disorders

Chapter 7
Treatment of Panic Disorder in Older Adults: A Pilot Study Comparison of Alprazolam, Imipramine, and Placebo

Colin M. Smith and Paul A. Riordan

Authors of the Original Article Javaid I. Sheikh JI and Pamela I. Swales

Journal Publisher *The International Journal of Psychiatry in Medicine*

Year of Publication 1999

Type of Study Parallel group, double-blind, placebo-controlled, flexible-dose pilot study

Funding Sources Supported by the Veterans Affairs Palo Alto Health Care System, National Institutes of Health, US Department of Health and Human Services, and the Upjohn Company

Objectives To gather pilot data in older patients with panic disorder (DSM-III-R) to begin to determine the efficacy of imipramine and alprazolam [1].

Methods This study recruited 25 community-dwelling adults ≥55 years of age to participate in an 8-week parallel group, double-blind, placebo-controlled, flexible-dose pilot study of alprazolam, or imipramine for panic disorder. Subjects completed a pre-screen questionnaire, and those who were likely to fulfill study criteria

C. M. Smith
Medicine and Psychiatry Combined Program, Duke University School of Medicine, Durham, NC, USA
e-mail: colin.smith@duke.edu

P. A. Riordan (✉)
Durham Veterans Affairs Medical Center, Department of Psychiatry and Behavioral Sciences, Duke University School of Medicine, Durham, NC, USA
e-mail: paul.riordan@duke.edu

R. R. Tampi et al. (eds.), *Essential Reviews in Geriatric Psychiatry*,
https://doi.org/10.1007/978-3-030-94960-0_7

were clinically interviewed using the structured clinical interview for DSM-III-R-Patient Version and Mini-Mental State Exam (MMSE). Inclusion criteria included age ≥55 years who met DSM-III-R criteria for panic disorder with or without agoraphobia (n = 25; 23 females, 2 males).

Exclusion criteria included bipolar disorder, schizophrenia or other psychosis, borderline personality disorder, obsessive-compulsive disorder, or cognitive impairment (MMSE ≤23). Subjects with alcohol or other substance abuse/dependence within prior 6 months or concurrent treatment with anxiolytics or concurrent treatment for anxiety with another clinician were also excluded. Finally, patients with active unstable medical, metabolic, or cardiopulmonary conditions were also excluded.

In this 8-week study, participants completed a 2-week washout period and were then randomized to receive, in a double-blind fashion, alprazolam, imipramine, or placebo. Subjects were assessed on an outpatient basis by a psychiatrist or psychiatry fellow for clinical response and need for medication adjustment weekly for the first 4 weeks, biweekly for weeks 6–8 (week 8 = endpoint), and at withdrawal of drug (week 10).

Subjects could receive medication up to four times daily to mimic clinical prescribing of alprazolam, starting with one nightly capsule (alprazolam 1 mg, imipramine 25 mg, or placebo) and increasing to one capsule twice daily after 3 days if tolerated. Dose increases occurred at weekly visits with a target dose of ten capsules, or the maximum beneficial dose not limited by side effects, by week 4. To mimic real-world practice of flexibility in dosing, the dose per capsule was reduced to 0.5 mg in alprazolam and 10 mg in imipramine after the first 14 subjects completed the study. Mean doses for subjects were 2.87 mg/day (SD = 1.66, range 1–6) for alprazolam and 77.5 mg/day (SD = 59.4, range 10–200) for imipramine.

The primary outcome measures in this study were global change ratings using Hamilton Anxiety Rating Scale (HAM-A), Hamilton Depression Rating Scale (HAM-D), Physicians' Global Impression (PGI) ratings, and average number of panic attacks per week from self-reported daily panic diaries.

The small sample size prevented statistical analyses between the groups, so only descriptive data were reported.

Results Twenty-five participants were randomized in the study, eight to the alprazolam group, ten to the imipramine group, and seven to the placebo group. The baseline mean age and mean age of panic onset were 62.75 years and 34.88 years for subjects in the alprazolam group, 61.30 years and 38.11 years for those in the imipramine group, and 59.29 years and 38.00 years for participants in the placebo group. The mean number of panic attacks per week in the month before treatment was similar among groups (alprazolam 2.38, imipramine 3.60, and placebo 3.2). Comorbid diagnoses and dependent measures of depressed mood (HAM-D) and anxiety (HAM-A) were grossly comparable across groups as well.

Of the 25 patients randomized to the 3 treatment groups, 4 dropped out during week 1, 1 dropped out during week 2, and 1 dropped out during week 3. Six of the seven dropouts were from the placebo group and one from the imipramine group. With the dropout rate approaching 25%, the investigators terminated the study early.

As shown in Table 7.1, the number of panic attacks per week, measured by self-reported panic diaries, decreased from baseline to posttreatment in the alprazolam,

Table 7.1 Panic disorders outcomes after treatment with alprazolam, imipramine, and placebo

		Alprazolam		Imipramine		Placebo	
		Baseline	Posttreatment	Baseline	Posttreatment	Baseline	Posttreatment
N		8	8	10	9	7	1
Outcome	*Measure*						
Mean panic attacks per week (SD)	Panic diary	2.38 (2.39)	0.00 (0.00)	3.60 (4.22)	0.13 (0.35)	3.29 (3.09)	0.00[a]
Physician's mean global ratings (SD)	PGI question #1	3.00 (0.89)	1.75 (1.04)	3.40 (1.27)	1.70 (0.95)	3.50 (0.71)	3.33 (2.08)[b]
Physician's mean global clinical impression (SD)	PGI question #2	–	1.50 (0.76)	–	2.30 (1.36)	–	4.00 (2.16)[c]
Mean therapeutic effects of medication (SD)	PGI question #3	–	4.50 (0.76)	–	3.70 (1.10)	–	2.50 (1.73)[c]
Physician's mean rating of minimal severity of side effects (SD)	PGI question #4	–	0.88 (0.99)	–	0.80 (0.63)	–	0.67 (1.16)[b]
Physician's mean anxiety rating score (SD)	HAM-A	17.86 (11.74)	3.87 (5.62)	13.40 (6.24)	5.30 (3.65)	20.00 (10.00)	15.00 (10.55)[c]
Physician's mean depression rating score (SD)	HAM-D	14.00 (7.79)	3.88 (6.11)	11.40 (6.77)	3.20 (2.39)	12.71 (5.38)	9.00 (7.44)[c]

SD standard deviation

[a]Using one subject, last available data point

[b]Using three subjects, last available data point

[c]Using four subjects, last available data point

imipramine, and placebo groups, although there was only a single placebo participant at the completion of the study. Physician's mean global rating (PGI question #1), a measure of symptoms severity, for alprazolam, imipramine, and placebo groups were higher at week 1 when compared to the posttreatment period. The physician's mean anxiety rating score, as measured by the HAM-A, and mean depression rating score, as measured by the HAM-D, were also lower in the posttreatment period for all groups when compared to baseline.

Conclusions Findings suggest comparable efficacy for alprazolam and imipramine in the short-term treatment of panic disorder in adults ≥55 years old. The results also suggested that the effective dose for alprazolam and imipramine for older female adults might be about half of the usual effective dose for younger adults.

Strengths of the Study

1. The study was randomized, double-blind, and placebo controlled.
2. Medication dosing design was flexible.
3. All participants were older adults ≥55 years old.
4. The authors do not overstate their results, recognizing that the conclusions that can be drawn are limited due to the very small sample size.

Limitations of the Study

1. A very small sample size of 25 participants divided over 3 groups meant that only descriptive statistics could be provided with no statistical analyses between groups or intent-to-treat analyses performed.
2. A short treatment period of 8 weeks leaves the question of whether alprazolam leads to tolerance in the elderly unanswered.
3. The recruitment process was through self-referral.
4. The study assessed on the basis of Jadad score indicates that this was low-quality study with a score of 2 out of 5 [2].

Questions Yes (1) No (0)	**Was the study described as random?**	**Was the randomization scheme described and appropriate?**	**Was the study described as double-blind?**	**Was the method of double blinding appropriate? (Were both the patient and the assessor appropriately blinded?)**	**Was there a description of dropouts and withdrawals?**	**Total score Range of score quality 0–2, low 3–5, high**
Score	1	0	1	0	0	2

5. While described as a double-blinded study, no reference was made regarding how blinding was maintained. Also, no CONSORT statement flowchart was provided to adequately assess dropouts and withdrawals at time of recruitment as well as after study enrollment. The number of dropouts per group was provided, but no patient reported reasons.
6. Twenty-three of 25 persons in the study are women, and 24 of 25 persons in the study are white, both limiting generalizability of the study.
7. Details of random sequence generation and allocation concealment were not provided.
8. There was a 25% dropout rate and 6 of 7 patients in the placebo group withdrew early.
9. The study medications were provided by Upjohn Company, the maker of alprazolam, and conflicts of interest are unstated.
10. The short study duration of 8 weeks limits ability to assess for multiple known adverse effects of benzodiazepine use in elderly, such as dizziness, sedation, cognitive impairment, and hip fractures [3–5].

Take-Home Points Although relatively low doses of alprazolam and imipramine were tolerable and reduced self-reported and physician rated anxiety in older adults with panic disorder, generalizability of this study is severely limited by its small size and short duration.

Practical Applications of the Take-Home Point Among older adults with panic disorder, alprazolam and imipramine appear to be efficacious in the short term.

References

1. Sheikh JI, Swales PJ. Treatment of panic disorder in older adults: a pilot study comparison of alprazolam, imipramine, and placebo. Int J Psychiatry Med. 1999;29(1):107–17.
2. Jadad AR, Moore RA, Carroll D, Jenkinson C, Reynolds DJ, Gavaghan DJ, McQuay HJ. Assessing the quality of reports of randomized clinical trials: is blinding necessary? Control Clin Trials. 1996;17(1):1–12.
3. Offidani E, Guidi J, Tomba E, Fava GA. Efficacy and tolerability of benzodiazepines versus antidepressants in anxiety disorders: a systematic review and meta-analysis. Psychother Psychosom. 2013;82(6):355–62.
4. Poly TN, Islam MM, Yang HC, Li YJ. Association between benzodiazepines use and risk of hip fracture in the elderly people: a meta-analysis of observational studies. Joint Bone Spine. 2020;87(3):241–9.
5. Sithamparanathan K, Sadera A, Leung L. Adverse effects of benzodiazepine use in elderly people: a meta-analysis. Asian J Gerontol Geriatr. 2012;2:107–11.

Chapter 8
Efficacy and Tolerability of Citalopram in the Treatment of Late-Life Anxiety Disorders: Results from an 8-Week Randomized, Placebo-Controlled Trial

Pallavi Joshi and Rajesh R. Tampi

Authors of the Original Article Eric J Lenze, Benoit H Mulsant, M Katherine Shear, Mary Amanda Dew, Mark D Miller, Bruce G Pollock, Patricia Houck, Barbara Tracey, Charles F Reynolds 3rd

Journal Publisher *American Journal of Psychiatry*

Year of Publication 2005

Type of Study Randomized placebo-controlled trial

Funding Sources Forest Pharmaceuticals and National Institute of Mental Health (NIMH)

Objectives To determine the efficacy and safety of citalopram for the treatment of anxiety disorders among older adults from a double-blind, randomized, placebo-controlled trial [1].

Methods This study recruited a total of 34 adults, ≥60 years in age from the community to participate in an 8-week randomized, double-blind, and placebo-controlled trail of citalopram for anxiety disorders. Participants who screened positive for anxiety symptoms underwent assessments using the Structured Clinical Interview for DSM-IV. To be eligible, participants were required to meet the criteria

P. Joshi
University of Arizona College of Medicine, Phoenix, AZ, USA

R. R. Tampi (✉)
Creighton University School of Medicine, Omaha, NE, USA
e-mail: rajesh.tampi@yale.edu

R. R. Tampi et al. (eds.), *Essential Reviews in Geriatric Psychiatry*,
https://doi.org/10.1007/978-3-030-94960-0_8

for a DSM-IV anxiety disorder. Majority of the participants were given a principal diagnosis of generalized anxiety disorder ($n = 30$) followed by panic disorder ($n = 3$) and posttraumatic stress disorder (PTSD) ($n = 1$). In this study all the participants scored ≥17 on the structured Hamilton Anxiety Rating Scale indicating moderate to severe symptoms.

Exclusion criteria for this study were as follows: a current diagnosis of major depressive episode, a diagnosis of dementia, history of psychosis, unstable medical illness, and active alcohol or substance use disorder. Baseline assessments included the Hamilton Depression Rating Scale, the Mini-Mental State Examination, and scales for instrumental and physical activities of daily living.

The investigators made the decision to allow participants who are taking a benzodiazepine before the start of the study to continue taking an equipotent dose of lorazepam (maximum dose of 2 mg a day), as long as the dose was kept constant in order to maximize recruitment and retention of participants in the study. This decision was based on available evidence that older adults are the leading consumers of benzodiazepines and it is difficult to taper off and discontinue these medications unless the anxiety symptoms are appropriately treated using a different medication. The participants were not allowed to take any other psychotropic medication for at least 2 weeks before the beginning of the study and during the study period.

In this 8-week study, the participants were evaluated every week for the first 4 weeks and every other week thereafter. At no time during this trail period did any of the participants receive formal psychotherapy. The participants were randomly assigned to receive citalopram or placebo on the basis of a computer program that used stratified permuted block randomization. Additionally, the medication was provided in a double-blind fashion, so that that citalopram was started at 10 mg a day and increased after 1 week to 20 mg a day. If the participant did not achieve response, the dose of citalopram was increased to 30 mg after 4 weeks.

The primary outcome measures in this study were the scores on the Hamilton anxiety scale and the Clinical Global Improvement (CGI) scale, administered by independent raters who were blind to treatment condition. A response was a 50% reduction in Hamilton anxiety score or a CGI rating of 1 or 2. The scores on the Hamilton anxiety scale were obtained at all visits, whereas the CGI improvement scores were obtained only at weeks 4 and 8. The side effects from the medications were measured using the Udvalg for Kliniske Undersøgelser (UKU) Side Effect Rating Scale.

The investigators used data from the last available visit to determine response (intent-to-treat principle) for participants who dropped out of the study. The two-tailed chi-square tests and linear modeling were used to compare the rates of response and side effects between the citalopram and placebo groups. A Cochran-Mantel-Haenszel test was performed to test the group differences stratified by gender, as a greater proportion of men were randomly assigned to the placebo group.

Results

From a total of 47 individuals who signed the consent forms to participate in the study, a total of 34 individuals enrolled in the study. Ten participants refused randomization, and three were excluded for the following reason: one had spontaneous improvement of anxiety before randomization, one did not meet the diagnostic criteria for any anxiety disorder other than specific phobia, and one had a major depressive episode.

Of the 34 participants, 17 participants were randomly assigned, stratified by diagnosis to the citalopram and placebo groups respectively. Among individuals with a primary diagnosis of generalized anxiety disorder ($n = 30$), 17 individuals had at least 1 current or past comorbid psychiatric disorder, especially an anxiety disorder or depressive disorder. The demographic characteristics and baseline clinical measures were similar between the two groups, except more men were randomly assigned to the placebo group when compared to the citalopram group (11 vs 2). The mean age of the participants was 70.7 years in the citalopram group and 68.1 years in the placebo group. Eighty-eight percent of participants in the citalopram group and 100% participants in the placebo group were white.

Eighty-five percent (29 out of 34) participants completed the 8-week study. Only five individuals dropped out before week 8, of these three individuals were in the citalopram group and two were in the placebo group. Only one individual (citalopram group) dropped out because of intolerable sedation after one dose.

Eleven of the 17 participants in the citalopram group responded to treatment [65%; 95% confidence interval (CI), 42–87%] when compared to 4 of 17 individuals in the placebo group [24%; 95% CI, 3–44%]. The relative risk of response was 2.57 (95% CI, 1.05–6.27) for individuals in the citalopram group ($p < 0.02$) when compared to placebo group, and it remained significant when controlled for gender ($p < 0.04$).

Eight of the 17 individuals (47%) in the citalopram group had a Hamilton anxiety score of ≤ 10 when compared to 3 of the 17 participants (18%) in the placebo group ($p = 0.07$), at the end of 8 weeks. Additionally, the investigators found greater improvements in anxiety in the citalopram group when compared to the placebo group over time with a treatment-by-week interaction ($p = 0.05$) and with a moderate effect size (Cohen's d of 0.79; 95% CI, 0.01–1.46). Among individuals with a diagnosis of generalized anxiety disorder, 10 of 15 individuals (67%) in the citalopram group responded when compared to 4 of 15 individuals (27%) in the placebo group ($p < 0.03$).

Twelve of the 17 participants (71%) in the citalopram group complained of at least 1 side effect when compared to 9 of the 17 individuals (53%) in the placebo group. Commonest side effects in both groups were dry mouth, nausea, and fatigue, respectively (three reports for each in the citalopram group and three, two, and two reports for each in the placebo group). A mixed-effect linear model of the total scores over time indicated a reduction in side effects in the citalopram group over time, with no change over time in the placebo group ($p < 0.09$). The investigators found that 35 percent (12 of 34) individuals in the study received fixed doses of co-prescribed lorazepam with no difference noted in response attributable to this medication.

Conclusions Evidence from this 8-week randomized, double-blind, and placebo-controlled trial indicates that citalopram is more effective than placebo in reducing symptoms of anxiety disorders, especially generalized anxiety disorder among adults ≥60 years in age, and is well tolerated.

Strengths of the Study

1. The trial design was randomized, double-blind, and placebo-controlled.
2. The study assessed on the basis of Jadad score indicates that this was high-quality study with a score of 5 out of 5 [2].

Questions Yes (1) No (0)	Was the study described as random?	Was the randomization scheme described and appropriate	Was the study described as double-blind?	Was the method of double blinding appropriate? (Were both the patient and the assessor appropriately blinded?)	Was there a description of dropouts and withdrawals?	Total score Range of score quality 0–2, low 3–5, high
Score	1	1	1	1	1	5

3. The study sample included only older adults (≥60 years).
4. All participants had moderate to severe anxiety symptoms based on the Hamilton anxiety scale score.
5. There was an 85% completion rate for the study.

Limitations of the Study

1. The study had a small sample size of 34 participants.
2. It had a short duration of study period of 8 weeks.
3. The recruitment was completed through advertisements and referrals.
4. A restrictive sample excluded participants with a current diagnosis of major depressive episode, a diagnosis of dementia, history of psychosis, unstable medical illness, and active alcohol or substance use disorder.
5. There were 5.5 times more men (11 vs 2) in the placebo group when compared to citalopram group, although the authors statistically controlled for this issue.
6. Thirty-two of the 34 participants (94%) were white.
7. Thirty of the 34 participants (88%) had a diagnosis of generalized anxiety disorder.

Take-Home Points Despite some limitations, this high-quality randomized, double-blind, and placebo-controlled trial indicates that citalopram was more efficacious than placebo for the treatment of anxiety disorders among older adults over 8 weeks. Citalopram was generally well tolerated when compared to placebo with the most commonly reported side effects being dry mouth, nausea, and fatigue among both groups.

Practical Applications of the Take-Home Points Among older adults who present with a diagnosable anxiety disorder with moderate to severe symptoms, citalopram is an efficacious and well-tolerated treatment option.

References

1. Lenze EJ, Mulsant BH, Shear MK, Dew MA, Miller MD, Pollock BG, Houck P, Tracey B, Reynolds CF 3rd. Efficacy and tolerability of citalopram in the treatment of late-life anxiety disorders: results from an 8-week randomized, placebo-controlled trial. Am J Psychiatry. 2005;162(1):146–50.
2. Jadad AR, Moore RA, Carroll D, Jenkinson C, Reynolds DJ, Gavaghan DJ, McQuay HJ. Assessing the quality of reports of randomized clinical trials: is blinding necessary? Control Clin Trials. 1996;17:1–12.

Chapter 9
Efficacy and Tolerability of Duloxetine in Elderly Patients with Generalized Anxiety Disorder: A Pooled Analysis of Four Randomized, Double-Blind, Placebo-Controlled Studies

Pallavi Joshi and Rajesh R. Tampi

Authors of the Original Article Jonathan Davidson, Christer Allgulander, Mark H Pollack, James Hartford, Janelle S Erickson, James M Russell, David Perahia, Madalaine M Wohlreich, Janice Carlson, Joel Raskin

Journal Publisher *Human Psychopharmacology: Clinical and Experimental*

Year of Publication 2008

Type of Study Pooled analysis of randomized placebo-controlled trials

Funding Sources Eli Lilly and Company and Boehringer Ingelheim

Objectives To determine the efficacy and safety of duloxetine for the treatment of generalized anxiety disorder among older adults from a pooled analysis of four randomized placebo-controlled trials [1].

Methods This study combined the results of four separate multicenter, randomized, double-blind, placebo-controlled, parallel-group studies of outpatients with a diagnosis of generalized anxiety disorder (GAD) in mixed age populations and reported results from their post hoc analyses of elderly individuals.

P. Joshi
University of Arizona College of Medicine, Phoenix, AZ, USA

R. R. Tampi (✉)
Creighton University School of Medicine, Omaha, NE, USA
e-mail: rajesh.tampi@yale.edu

R. R. Tampi et al. (eds.), *Essential Reviews in Geriatric Psychiatry*,
https://doi.org/10.1007/978-3-030-94960-0_9

For this analysis, 73 individuals ≥65 years in age with a DSM-IV-TR diagnosis of GAD were included. Participants were required to have moderate–severe illness, reflected by Hospital Anxiety and Depression Scale (HADS) anxiety subscale score of ≥10, a Covi anxiety scale (CAS) score of ≥9, and clinical global impressions–severity of illness (CGI-S) score of ≥4.

Study 1 had a 9-week acute therapy phase in which participants were randomized to receive duloxetine 60 mg, duloxetine 120 mg, or placebo. Participants in both duloxetine treatment groups were started at 60 mg/day, which could initially and temporarily be lowered to 30 mg/day if a higher dose was not tolerated. Study 2 consisted of a 10-week acute therapy phase, followed by a 2-week discontinuation phase. Participants were randomized to duloxetine or placebo. Participants in the duloxetine treatment group were started at 60 mg/day, which could initially and temporarily be lowered to 30 mg/day if tolerability concerns arose. After titration to 60 mg/day, flexible dosing was allowed in weekly increments of 30 mg/day up to a maximum dose of 120 mg/day. Study 3 consisted of a 10-week acute therapy phase. Participants were randomized to receive duloxetine 60–120 mg/day, venlafaxine 75–225 mg/day, or placebo in a 1:1:1 ratio. Duloxetine treatment was initiated at 30 mg/day for 1 week, followed by an increase to 60 mg/day, after which flexible dosing was allowed in weekly increments of 30 mg/day up to a maximum dose of 120 mg/day. Study 4 consisted of a 10-week acute therapy phase, followed by a 2-week tapering phase. Participants were randomized in a 2:1:2:2 ratio to duloxetine (60–120 mg/day), duloxetine (20 mg/day), venlafaxine (75–225 mg/day), or placebo. Duloxetine treatment was initiated at 30 mg/day for 1 week and increased to 60 mg/day. After titration to 60 mg/day, flexible dosing was allowed in weekly increments of 30 mg/day up to a maximum dose of 120 mg/day. Data from the venlafaxine arms and duloxetine 20 mg/day arm were not included in the pooled analysis.

The primary outcome measure was the mean baseline-to-endpoint change in Hamilton anxiety scale (HAM-A). Secondary measures included the HADS, the CGI-I and Patient Global Impressions of Improvement scales, and the Sheehan disability scale (SDS) impairment scores. Response was defined as ≥50% reduction from baseline in HAMA total score, or a CGI-I score of ≤2 at endpoint. Sustained improvement was defined as a ≥30% reduction from baseline in HAMA total score at any visit before endpoint, sustained until the last visit; and remission was defined as a HAMA total score of ≤7 at endpoint. Two-tailed chi-square tests and linear modeling was used to compare the rates of response and side effects between the duloxetine and placebo groups.

Results Of the 1491 participants who were randomly assigned to treatments in the 4 studies, 73 (4.9%; duloxetine = 45; placebo = 28) were included in this pooled analysis. There were no significant differences between the treatment groups on the demographic variables or the severity of illness at baseline. Thirty participants in the duloxetine group (66.7%) and 20 participants in the placebo group (71.4%) completed treatment ($P = 0.610$). Significantly more participants randomized to duloxetine discontinued treatment due to an adverse event [10 (22.2%) vs. 0 (0.0%),

$P = 0.011$]. The treatment groups did not differ significantly with respect to other reasons for discontinuation. The mean age of the participants was 70.1 years in the duloxetine group and 70.9 years in the placebo group. A total of 95.6% of participants in the duloxetine group and 96.4% of participants in the placebo group were white.

The treatment groups did not significantly differ in the incidence of HAMA response (20/42 (48%) vs. 8/28 (29%), $P = 0.149$), remission (10/42 (24%) vs. 2/28 (7%), $P = 0.053$), or sustained improvement (26/42 (62%) vs. 10/28 (36%), $P = 0.05$). Compared with placebo, participants treated with duloxetine experienced significantly greater improvements on the HAMA total ($P = 0.029$), the HAMA psychic anxiety factor ($P = 0.034$), HADS anxiety ($P = 0.049$) and depression scales ($P = 0.026$), but not the HAM-A somatic anxiety factor ($P = 0.074$). The treatment groups did not significantly differ in CGI-I ($P = 0.143$) or PGI-I scores at endpoint ($P = 0.064$).

A total of 35 participants (70%) in the duloxetine group complained of at least 1 side effect when compared to 15 individuals (53.6%) in the placebo group. The most common side effects in the duloxetine group were nausea, dizziness, and hyperhidrosis (15, 7, and 6, respectively), and those in the placebo group were dizziness, constipation, and hyperhidrosis (5, 4, and 3, respectively). Participants treated with duloxetine reported significantly more nausea (30.0% vs. 7.1%, $P = 0.023$) and weight loss ($P = 0.018$). More participants treated with duloxetine discontinued treatment due to an adverse event (22.2% vs. 0%; $P = 0.011$).

Conclusions Evidence from this pooled analysis of four randomized placebo-controlled trials of duloxetine for the treatment of GAD in adults ≥65 years indicates that duloxetine is more effective than placebo in reducing overall symptoms of anxiety, but the side effects may be difficult to tolerate for some older adults.

Strengths of the Study

1. This was a pooled analysis of randomized, double-blind, and placebo-controlled trials.
2. The study assessed on the basis of Jadad score indicates that this was a high-quality study with a score of 5 out of 5 [2].

Questions Yes (1) No (0)	Was the study described as random?	Was the randomization scheme described and appropriate?	Was the study described as double-blind?	Was the method of double blinding appropriate? (Were both the patient and the assessor appropriately blinded?)	Was there a description of dropouts and withdrawals?	Total score Range of score quality 0–2, low 3–5, high
Score	1	1	1	1	1	5

3. The study sample included only older adults (≥65 years).
4. All participants had moderate to severe anxiety symptoms based on the included anxiety scale scores.
5. There was a 68% completion rate for the study.

Limitations of the Study

1. The study had a small sample size of 73 participants.
2. It had a short duration of study period of 10 weeks in the longest trial.
3. A total of 95.6% of participants in the duloxetine group and 96.4% of participants in the placebo group were white.
4. There was no significant difference in the rates of response, remission, or sustained improvement in the two groups.
5. Participants treated with duloxetine had more nausea (30.0% vs. 7.1%, $p = 0.023$) and weight loss ($P = 0.018$).
6. More participants treated with duloxetine discontinued treatment due to an adverse event (22.2% vs. 0%; $P = 0.011$).

Take-Home Points

Evidence from this pooled analysis of four randomized placebo-controlled trials of duloxetine for the treatment of GAD in adults ≥65 years indicates that duloxetine is more effective than placebo in reducing overall symptoms of anxiety, psychic anxiety, and depression. Its tolerability in older adults needs to be explored further.

Practical Applications of the Take-Home Points Among older adults who present with a diagnosable anxiety disorder with moderate to severe symptoms, duloxetine is an efficacious treatment option.

References

1. Davidson J, Allgulander C, Pollack MH, Hartford J, Erickson JS, Russell JM, Perahia D, Wohlreich MM, Carlson J, Raskin J. Efficacy and tolerability of duloxetine in elderly patients with generalized anxiety disorder: a pooled analysis of four randomized, double-blind, placebo-controlled studies. Hum Psychopharmacol. 2008;23(6):519–26.
2. Jadad AR, Moore RA, Carroll D, Jenkinson C, Reynolds DJ, Gavaghan DJ, McQuay HJ. Assessing the quality of reports of randomized clinical trials: is blinding necessary? Control Clin Trials. 1996;17:1–12.

Chapter 10
Escitalopram for Older Adults with Generalized Anxiety Disorder: A Randomized Controlled Trial

Pallavi Joshi and Rajesh R. Tampi

Authors of the Original Article Eric J Lenze, Bruce L Rollman, M Katherine Shear, Mary Amanda Dew, Bruce G Pollock, Caroline Ciliberti, Michelle Costantino, Sara Snyder, Peichang Shi, Edward Spitznagel, Carmen Andreescu, Meryl A Butters, Charles F Reynolds 3rd

Journal Publisher *Journal of the American Medical Association*

Year of Publication 2009

Type of Study Randomized placebo-controlled trial

Funding Sources The National Institute of Mental Health (NIMH), Center for Mental Health Services Research, Advanced Center for Interventions and Services Research in Late Life Mood Disorders, John A. Hartford Center of Excellence in Geriatric Psychiatry, University of Pittsburgh Medical Center, and Forest Laboratories Inc.

Objectives To determine the efficacy and safety of escitalopram for the treatment of generalized anxiety disorder among older adults from a double-blind, randomized, placebo-controlled trial [1].

P. Joshi
University of Arizona College of Medicine, Phoenix, AZ, USA

R. R. Tampi (✉)
Creighton University School of Medicine, Omaha, NE, USA
e-mail: rajesh.tampi@yale.edu

R. R. Tampi et al. (eds.), *Essential Reviews in Geriatric Psychiatry*,
https://doi.org/10.1007/978-3-030-94960-0_10

Methods This study recruited a total of 177 adults, ≥60 years in age from primary care practices and related subspecialty clinics to participate in a 12-week randomized, double-blind, and placebo-controlled trail of escitalopram for GAD. Participants who screened positive for anxiety symptoms underwent assessments using the Structured Clinical Interview for DSM-IV. To be eligible, participants were required to meet DSM-IV criteria for GAD. In this study all the participants scored ≥17 on the structured Hamilton Anxiety Rating Scale indicating moderate to severe symptoms.

Exclusion criteria for this study were as follows: lifetime psychosis or bipolar disorder, a diagnosis of dementia, current suicidal ideation, medical instability, ongoing psychotherapy, and current antidepressant or anxiolytic use with the exception of benzodiazepine equivalent to lorazepam 2 mg a day. The investigators made the decision to allow participants who are taking a benzodiazepine before the start of the study to continue taking an equipotent dose of lorazepam (maximum dose 2 mg a day), as long as the dose was kept constant in order to maximize recruitment and retention of participants in the study. This decision was based on available evidence that older adults are the leading consumers of benzodiazepines and it is difficult to taper off and discontinue these medications unless the anxiety symptoms are appropriately treated using a different medication.

Baseline assessments included the Hamilton Anxiety and Depression Rating Scales and the Mini-Mental State Examination (MMSE).

In this 12-week study, the participants were evaluated every week for the first 4 weeks and every other week thereafter. At no time during this trail period did any of the participants receive formal psychotherapy. The participants were randomly assigned to receive escitalopram or placebo on the basis of a computer program that used stratified permuted block randomization. Additionally, the medication was provided in a double-blind fashion, so that that escitalopram was started at 10 mg a day. If the participant did not achieve response, the dose of escitalopram was increased to 20 mg after 4 weeks.

The primary outcome measures in this study were the scores on the Hamilton Anxiety Rating Scale and the Clinical Global Improvement (CGI) scale, administered by independent raters who were blind to treatment condition. A response was a 50% reduction in Hamilton anxiety score or a CGI rating of 1 or 2. The self-report Penn State Worry Questionnaire was done at weeks 4, 8, and 12, and the Late Life Function and Disability Instrument and Medical Outcome Survey 36-item Short Form were done at baseline and week 12. The scores on the Hamilton Anxiety Rating Scale were obtained at all visits, whereas the CGI improvement scores were obtained only at weeks 4 and 8.

The investigators used data from the last available visit to determine response (intent-to-treat principle) for participants who dropped out of the study. The two-tailed chi-square tests and linear modeling was used to compare the rates of response and side effects between the escitalopram and placebo groups.

Results From a total of 257 individuals who signed the consent forms to participate in the study, a total of 179 individuals enrolled in the study. A total of 43 participants refused randomization and 35 were ineligible for the study. Of the 179 participants, two participants withdrew consent before receiving study medication and were excluded from all analyses. Seven participants withdrew consent after receiving study medication but without providing any follow-up data and were included in the ITT analysis but excluded from the modified ITT analysis.

Of the 177 participants, 85 were randomized to escitalopram and 92 to placebo. The demographic characteristics and baseline clinical measures were similar between the two groups. The mean age of the participants was 71.7 years in the escitalopram group and 72.2 years in the placebo group. A total of 80% of participants in the escitalopram group and 84.8% participants in the placebo group were white. A total of 80% (69 out of 86) of participants in the escitalopram group and 80% (75 out of 93) in the placebo group completed the 12-week study. Only three participants in the escitalopram group and four in the placebo group dropped out because of adverse effects.

A total of 69% of participants in the escitalopram group responded to treatment [95% confidence interval (CI), 58–80%] when compared to 51% in the placebo group [95% CI, 40–62%]. In the ITT analysis, the response was not different (57%; 95% CI, 46–67% for escitalopram; vs 45%; 95% CI, 35–55% for placebo; $P = 0.11$). However, in a modified ITT analysis, response was higher in the escitalopram group than in the placebo group (60%; 95% CI, 50–71%; vs 45%; 95% CI, 36–56%; $P = 0.048$). Time to response (6 weeks median in the escitalopram group vs 10 weeks in placebo) did not significantly differ ($P = 0.19$).

The investigators found the largest effect sizes with Clinical Global Impressions Improvement scale (0.93; 95% CI, 0.50–1.36; $P < 0.001$) and role emotional impairment subscale (0.96; 95% CI, 0.03–1.90; $P = 0.04$). Small to moderate effect sizes were seen in Penn State Worry Questionnaire (0.30; 95% CI, 0.23–0.48; $P = 0.01$) and activity limitations subscale (0.32; 95% CI, 0.01–0.63; $P = 0.04$). Mean score difference in Hamilton Anxiety Rating Scale was −0.43 (SD = 0.04) for the escitalopram group and −0.32 (SD = 0.04) for the placebo group ($P = 0.06$).

A total 65 of the 85 participants (76.5%) in the escitalopram group complained of at least one side effect when compared to 59 out of 64 individuals (64%) in the placebo group. The most common side effects in both groups were fatigue, gastrointestinal upset, and headache, respectively (35, 22, and 13 reports for each in the escitalopram group and 10, 26, and 7 reports for each in the placebo group). The escitalopram group reported fatigue significantly more than the placebo group ($P < 0.001$). The only single time point in which a significantly higher proportion of participants receiving escitalopram had adverse effects ($P = 0.007$) was at week 6, which was after most participants had a dosage increase from 10 to 20 mg/day.

Conclusions Evidence from this 12-week randomized, double-blind, and placebo-controlled trial indicates that escitalopram is more effective than placebo in reducing symptoms of anxiety and improving self-reported role functioning among adults ≥60 years in age with GAD and is well tolerated.

Strengths of the Study

1. The trial design was randomized, double-blind, and placebo-controlled.
2. The study assessed on the basis of Jadad score indicates that this was high-quality study with a score of 5 out of 5 [2].

Questions Yes (1) No (0)	Was the study described as random?	Was the randomization scheme described and appropriate?	Was the study described as double-blind?	Was the method of double blinding appropriate? (Were both the patient and the assessor appropriately blinded?)	Was there a description of dropouts and withdrawals?	Total score Range of score quality 0–2, low 3–5, high
Score	1	1	1	1	1	5

3. The study sample included only older adults (≥60 years).
4. All participants had moderate to severe anxiety symptoms based on the Hamilton Anxiety Rating Scale score.
5. There was an 80% completion rate for the study.

Limitations of the Study

1. The study had a small sample size of 179 participants.
2. It had a short duration of study period of 12 weeks.
3. The recruitment was completed through advertisements and referrals.
4. A restrictive sample excluded participants with a history of psychosis or bipolar disorder, a diagnosis of dementia, unstable medical illness, and active alcohol or substance use disorder.
5. 80% of participants in the escitalopram group and 84.8% participants in the placebo group were white.

Take-Home Points Despite some limitations, this high-quality randomized, double-blind, and placebo-controlled trial indicates that escitalopram was more efficacious than placebo for the treatment of GAD among older adults over 12 weeks. Escitalopram was generally well tolerated when compared to placebo with the most commonly reported side effects being fatigue, gastrointestinal upset, and headache in both groups.

Practical Applications of the Take-Home Points Among older adults who present with GAD with moderate to severe symptoms, escitalopram is an efficacious and well-tolerated treatment option.

References

1. Lenze EJ, Rollman BL, Shear MK, Dew MA, Pollock BG, Ciliberti C, Costantino M, Snyder S, Shi P, Spitznagel E, Andreescu C, Butters MA, Reynolds CF 3rd. Escitalopram for older adults with generalized anxiety disorder: a randomized controlled trial. JAMA. 2009;301(3):295–303.
2. Jadad AR, Moore RA, Carroll D, Jenkinson C, Reynolds DJ, Gavaghan DJ, McQuay HJ. Assessing the quality of reports of randomized clinical trials: is blinding necessary? Control Clin Trials. 1996;17:1–12.

Chapter 11
Meta-analysis Comparing Different Behavioral Treatments for Late-Life Anxiety

Hudaisa Hafeez and Tracey Holsinger

Authors of the Original Article Steven R Thorp, Catherine R Ayers, Roberto Nuevo, Jill A Stoddard, John T Sorrell, Julie Loebach Wetherell

Journal Publisher *Elsevier via ScienceDirect*

Year of Publication 2009

Type of Study Meta-analysis

Funding Source The National Institute of Mental Health (NIMH) Grant

Objectives To examine the efficacy of different types of behavioral treatments including cognitive behavioral therapy (CBT) alone, CBT with relaxation training (RT), and RT alone in geriatric patients with anxiety [1].

Methods Selection of studies for inclusion was done by utilizing Internet databases (i.e., MEDLINE, PsycINFO) with the use of keywords, examining reference lists, and consulting geriatric anxiety experts. For inclusion, studies must (1) be published in English before September 2007, (2) report a mean sample age of 65+ years or have a lower age limit of 55+ years, (3) provide a prospective test of psychotherapeutic interventions for anxiety disorders, (4) include at least five subjects,

H. Hafeez
Duke University, Department of Psychiatry & Behavioral Sciences, Durham, NC, USA
e-mail: hudaisa.hafeez@duke.edu

T. Holsinger (✉)
Duke University, Department of Psychiatry & Behavioral Sciences, Durham, NC, USA

Durham VA Medical Center, Durham, NC, USA
e-mail: Tracey.holsinger@duke.edu

R. R. Tampi et al. (eds.), *Essential Reviews in Geriatric Psychiatry*,
https://doi.org/10.1007/978-3-030-94960-0_11

(5) include subjects with subjective anxiety symptoms, (6) include treatments which are done for at least two sessions, and (7) have sufficient data for calculation of effect size. Approximately 300 abstracts were screened, and 83 articles were reviewed. Nineteen studies met the inclusion criteria.

Of the 19 included studies, 8 included subjects with generalized anxiety disorder (GAD), 5 included subjects with mixed anxiety disorders (predominantly GAD and panic disorder (PD)), 5 included subjects who complained of anxiety symptoms but had no diagnosis, and 1 included subjects with diagnosis of panic disorder (PD). Four of the studies had no control condition for comparison, but the remaining 15 studies had 1 or 2 active control conditions which in the included studies meant supportive psychotherapy, "nonformal" CBT or relaxation instruction, group discussion, psychoeducation, or weekly medication management.

Only anxiety and depressive measures were used for this analysis.

Thirteen of the 19 studies utilized the trait anxiety measure to measure anxiety symptoms. Ten studies included worry measures such as Penn State Worry Questionnaire. Nine studies reported clinician-rated as well as self-reported instruments. Sixteen studies included at least one depressive measure to measure depressive symptoms. Most used was Beck Depression Inventory (BDI). The Hamilton Rating Scale for Depression was used in three studies.

Overall, 24 treatment samples along with 8 active control and 8 waitlist control groups were constructed from 19 studies and were categorized into 5 sample groups:

1. Waitlist/no treatment control groups (8 samples)
2. CBT with RT (12 samples)
3. CBT without RT (5 samples)
4. RT only (7 samples)
5. Active controls (8 samples)

The above five groups were defined by the review authors and based on rater's determinations of whether relaxation training was sufficient to classify a treatment in this group or whether it was to be considered "traditional CBT strategies" only. CBT delivery was not standardized. Relaxation training included different modalities. Some treatment was given in groups and some individually. Three studies appear to have included recent widows without anxiety diagnoses only. Two other included studies required "moderate depression and trait anxiety" and "uncomfortable anxiety," respectively.

The effect sizes were calculated using the standardized mean difference statistics (Hedges's g) for anxiety and depressive measures between and within groups, and the results were then averaged among all studies. The Q statistics were calculated to test for heterogeneity among effect sizes of treatment groups. In cases where standard deviations were not available and could not be obtained, review authors substituted standard deviations from similar populations.

The effect sizes were calculated for uncontrolled conditions in which treatment modalities were not compared with active controls. Effect sizes were also calculated for controlled conditions in which treatment modalities were compared with active controls. Positive effect sizes meant a reduction in anxiety and depressive symptoms.

Results The mean uncontrolled effect sizes (defined as comparison of active treatment or active control against no treatment) for all treatment groups were RT alone (0.91), CBT with RT (0.86), and CBT alone (1.18). All were larger than active controls (0.50) and no treatment group (0.05) effect sizes on anxiety measures.

For depressive measures, the effect sizes were RT alone (0.77), CBT with RT (0.77), CBT alone (0.78), active controls (0.53), and waitlist group (0.20).

The mean controlled effect sizes (defined as comparison of active treatment against active control) for RT were 0.90, CBT with RT were 0.33, and CBT alone were 0.00. There were no apparent outcome differences among the three types of treatments on depressive symptoms and all effect sizes were small (0.23, 0.12, 0.23). For anxious subjects, the 95% confidence interval included zero for both CBT conditions. On depressive measures, the 95% confidence interval included zero for all three conditions.

The results suggest that RT may be somewhat more effective than CBT on anxiety measures. Relaxation training had no significant advantage over the other behavioral treatments on depressive measures. Two of the three studies comparing CBT without RT to an active alternative treatment found that the alternative condition led to greater gains than did CBT alone suggesting that CBT alone could be a relatively weak intervention for geriatric anxiety.

Conclusions The results suggest that anxious older adults are unlikely to spontaneously stop feeling anxious. Both relaxation training and cognitive behavioral therapy appear to be more effective than no treatment for older adults with subjective anxiety. Relaxation training (RT) provided the most benefit when provided as a stand-alone treatment. To understand the roles of RT and CBT in addressing anxiety and depression in older adults, better definition of treatment delivered and populations receiving it would be necessary.

Strengths of the Study

1. Standardized instruments were used to conduct analysis, and Q statistics were used to test heterogeneity among individual studies and treatment groups.
2. Per authors, the study represents the closest approximation to a dismantling study and thus can be used in clinical and research application of psychotherapeutic studies.

Limitations of the Study

1. Data was extracted from a limited number of studies with variable sample sizes and populations studied. Individual studies were parsed into different samples for comparison with such subsets from other studies. When standard deviations were not available, the review authors estimated them based on other samples.
2. Four out of 19 studies did not have a control arm of any kind.
3. The randomization of study samples was not noted.
4. The demographic differences between studies were not examined.
5. The scales to measure anxiety/depressive measures were not consistent among all studies.

6. The authors chose their own taxonomy to define treatment modalities which could be different from used or intended by the authors of the original studies. For example, included studies with psychosocial treatments were considered to be RT if components of RT were included. Sometimes techniques such as mindfulness training were included. The fidelity of treatments to standards was not clear. Some treatments were done in group formats and this analysis combines them with treatments delivered individually.
7. Heterogeneity in effect sizes was found within treatment group RT, suggesting that effectiveness of RT may differ in real-life situation based on how RT is administered, or the type of relaxation training used.

Take-Home Points Despite the limitations, this analysis suggests that CBT, RT, and "active control" treatments are more efficacious in late-life anxiety than no treatment. Among CBT, a variety of active control treatments and relaxation therapy, relaxation therapy appeared most beneficial in decreasing anxiety in a geriatric population. However, the method of administration of RT was not similar in all included studies. The author suggests that more research is needed in this area to identify specific RT which would be most beneficial in geriatric anxiety.

Practical Applications Relaxation training can be a less complex intervention than other forms of behavioral interventions for anxiety in geriatric population. RT alone or with CBT could be an attractive option to treat late-life anxiety.

Reference

1. Thorp SR, Ayers CR, Nuevo R, Stoddard JA, Sorrell JT, Wetherell JL. Meta-analysis comparing different behavioral treatments for late-life anxiety. Am J Geriatr Psychiatry. 2009;17(2):105–15.

Chapter 12
Cognitive Behavior Therapy for Generalized Anxiety Disorder Among Older Adults in Primary Care: A Randomized Clinical Trial

Jenny Nguyen and Seetha Chandrasekhara

Authors of the Original Article Melinda A Stanley, Nancy L Wilson, Diane M Novy, Howard M Rhoades, Paula D Wagener, Anthony J Greisinger, Jeffrey A Cully, Mark E Kunik

Journal Publisher *The Journal of the American Medical Association*

Year of Publication 2009

Type of Study Randomized controlled trial

Funding Sources The National Institute of Mental Health (NIMH) and Houston Veteran Affairs Health Services Research and Development Center of Excellence

Objectives To examine the effects of cognitive behavioral therapy (CBT) relative to enhanced usual care (EUC) in older adults with general anxiety disorder (GAD) in the primary care setting [1].

Methods For this trial, 134 older adults (age 60 years or older) were recruited from 2 primary care settings from March 2004 to August 2006. Participants who scored positive for the two anxiety screening questions from the Primary Care Evaluation of Mental Disorders were further screened using the Structured Clinical Interview for the DSM-IV and Mini-Mental State Examination (MMSE). Those with a principal or coprincipal diagnosis of GAD were included. Individuals who scored less than 24 on the MMSE and had active substance use, psychosis, or bipolar disorder were excluded from this study.

J. Nguyen · S. Chandrasekhara (✉)
Lewis Katz School of Medicine at Temple University, Philadelphia, PA, USA
e-mail: Seetha.Chandrasekhara@tuhs.temple.edu

R. R. Tampi et al. (eds.), *Essential Reviews in Geriatric Psychiatry*,
https://doi.org/10.1007/978-3-030-94960-0_12

Primary outcomes consisted of worry severity measured by the Penn State Worry Questionnaire (PSWQ) with a change of 8.5 points demonstrating "meaningful change" and GAD severity measured by the GAD Severity Scale (GADSS) with a change of 2 points being "meaningful." Secondary outcomes included evaluating coexisting anxiety and depression symptoms with the Structured Interview Guide for the Hamilton Anxiety Scale (SIGH-A) and Beck Depression Inventory II (BDI-II), and the physical component score (PCS) and mental component score (MCS) of the 12-Item Medical Outcomes Short Study Form for assessing quality of life. Antianxiety and antidepressant medication use was evaluated based on self-report for the prior 3 months, along with the number of outpatient visits (physical and mental health) to determine if the participants had discussed emotional issues with or received a mental health referral from their primary care physician (PCP).

Participants were treated for 3 months with either CBT or EUC. CBT was provided by therapists for up to ten sessions over 12 weeks, with telephone booster sessions at 4, 7, 10, and 13 months. Therapists were trained in CBT, and 20% of the sessions were independently rated to determine treatment integrity. Participants receiving EUC were telephoned biweekly during the first 3-month interval with support being provided by therapists and notification of the PCP if a participant required immediate psychiatric care. Data collection was conducted via a blinded phone interview, but participants and the therapists were not blinded. Assessments were conducted at baseline, 3 months posttreatment, and over 12 months of follow-up, with assessments at 6, 9, 12, and 15 months. Ten percent of these assessments also had independent raters to determine integrity with the GADSS and SIGH-A and had an intraclass correlation coefficient of 0.99 and 0.95, respectively. Two CBT manual authors evaluated treatment adherence (7.7, range 0–8 [SD, 0.55]) and competence (7.3, range 0–8 [SD, 0.67]). All EUC calls were recorded and twenty percent were reviewed by first author noting only three protocol deviations.

Communication with the PCP occurred through research notes in the written medical record which included diagnoses assigned and reasons for inclusion or exclusion. Participants who were excluded received potential psychiatric referrals. Those participants included in the study had PCP notes encouraging continued care and the designation of the treatment type they were receiving. Of the 134 older adults, 70 were randomized to receive CBT in primary care clinics (mean completed sessions = 7.4), and 64 participants were randomized to receive EUC (mean telephone check-ins = 4.3). At the study midpoint, the EUC group was noted to have a disproportionately large assignment of Hispanic participants, and a stratified randomization schedule was used.

Pre-treatment demographics, clinical characteristics, and medications were compared using a chi-square and t-test. Posttreatment outcomes were compared using the pre-treatment assessment as the covariant. Initial analyses used intention-to-treat (ITT) to address missing data. These were repeated with observed data using a random regression method. Secondary analyses of long-term outcomes used a repeated-measure analysis of covariance. In order to control for multiple comparisons (primary outcomes, coexisting anxiety-depression, health quality of life), the critical alpha was set as $p < 0.025$ with two-sided significance. Changes in antidepressant and antianxiety medications were analyzed using a chi-square method.

Treatment responders were determined at 3 and 15 months. Those with missing data used for ITT analyses were considered nonresponders. To determine the power needed for this study, scores from the PSWQ were used with a median standard deviation of 10.1. A moderate effect size of Cohen's d = 0.6 (minimal detectable difference 6.2), power of 80%, and alpha = 0.025 was used to determine the study goal of 150 participants to have 53 subjects in each group.

Results Of the 986 referred potential participants, 381 provided consent to participate in the study. Of the 381, 68 individuals dropped out or were excluded prior to the initial diagnostic evaluation due to negative responses on screening questions (14 individuals), lack of interest (35 individuals), or logistic issues (19 individuals). The remaining 313 were assessed for eligibility with 154 individuals excluded for not meeting inclusion criteria and 11 individuals separately grouped as nonclinical training cases not included in analyses. A total of 148 participants met inclusion criteria, and 134 participants (with principal or coprincipal GAD) were randomized after 14 dropped out before this step.

Participants who were randomized had a mean age of 66.9 years [95% confidence interval (CI), 65.9–67.9] and a mean education time of 15.9 years [95% CI, 15.4–16.4] and were likely to be women (75% [105/134], $p = 0.04$) compared to those not randomized. Also, they had a higher baseline PSWQ of 57.2 [95% CI, 55.4–59]. The active treatment phase of 0–3 months had lower dropouts for the CBT group compared to EUC (5.9% [4/70] vs 21.9% [14/64], $p = 0.006$) due to reported dissatisfaction (CBT $n = 0$ vs EUC $n = 9$) with random assignment. Long-term follow-up attrition between 3 and 15 months was comparable for CBT and EUC (CBT 12.9% [9/70]; EUC 9.4% [6/64]; $p = 0.52$), and total attrition over the 15 months was 24.6% ($n = 33$) and did not show significant difference between groups ($p = 0.09$). Participants in CBT and EUC differed with regard to baseline PSWQ scores, but this was included as a covariate during analyses.

ITT analyses showed significantly larger improvement of PSWQ in the CBT group compared to EUC (45.6 [95% CI, 43.4–47.8] vs 54.4 [95% CI, 51.4–57.3], $p < 0.001$). A mean change of 7.7 points was measured with CBT group on the PSWQ and 3.2 points in the EUC group. The GADSS did not demonstrate a significant difference between CBT (2.8 points) and EUC (1.4 points). ITT analyses also showed significant improvement on the BDI-II for those completing CBT compared to EUC (10.2 [95% CI, 8.5–11.9] vs 12.8 [95% CI, 10.5–15.1], $p = 0.02$) along with the MCS (CBT 49.6 [95% CI, 47.4–51.8], $p = 0.008$ compared to EUC). Scores on the SIGH-A and PCS were not statistically significant.

No significant increase in medications was noted during the active treatment phase (antianxiety, $p = 0.45$; antidepressant, $p = 0.25$). Similarly, the rates of dose reduction and discontinuation across the groups were not significant (antianxiety, $p = 0.41$; antidepressant, $p = 0.17$). Both groups had similar number of outpatient medical visits ($p = 0.85$) and infrequent mental health visits ($p = 0.82$). Of those included in the completed analyses, very few participants received a mental health referral (CBT 5/65, EUC 4/50) or spoke to their PCP about emotional issues (CBT 13/65, EUC 9/50).

Continued improvement in PSWQ scores over long-term follow-up was seen in both groups with no significant changes (time effect and group effect) seen with covariate posttreatment analyses indicating no differences between groups, and that treatment response after the active period was maintained. Scores on the MCS and BDI-II were significant on 12-month follow-up indicating that posttreatment effects were maintained. Additionally, rates of medication dose increase, or additions (antianxiety, $p = 0.53$; antidepressant, $p = 0.56$) along with rates of dose reductions or discontinuations (antianxiety, $p = 0.7$; antidepressant, $p = 0.37$) were not different across groups during the long-term follow-up period.

ITT analyses demonstrated a higher treatment response rate at 3 months with the PSWQ. This was not demonstrated with completed analyses at 3 and 15 months. Treatment expectancies were higher in CBT participants compared to those in the EUC group ($p = 0.007$). When added as covariates, the treatment effects were significantly maintained with PSWQ scores ($p < 0.001$). The scores on the BDI-II ($p = 0.05$) and MCS ($p = 0.04$) were close to significance.

Conclusions CBT significantly improved worry severity, depressive symptoms, and general mental health for older adults with GAD in primary care when compared to EUC. Increased GAD severity did not correlate with greater improvement with CBT.

Strengths of the Study

1. The study did careful selection and diagnosis of patients.
2. There was large breadth of outcome assessment.
3. It had excellent treatment integrity using independent rating assessments (GADSS intraclass correlation coefficient = 0.99; SIGH-A intraclass correlation coefficient = 0.95; CBT adherence = 7.7; range 0–8 [SD, 0.55]; CBT competence = 7.3; range 0–8 [SD, 0.67]; EUC calls (20%) reviewed by first author noting only three protocol deviations).
4. There was low attrition in CBT during active treatment phase (0–3 months) [4 dropouts (out of 70 participants) in CBT group compared to 14 dropouts (out of 64 participants) in EUC group; $p = 0.006$].
5. There was significant improvement in PSWQ (score = 45.6, $p < 0.001$), BDI-II (score = 10.2, $p = 0.02$), and MCS (score = 49.6, $p = 0.008$) scale scores in the CBT compared to EUC.
6. Study quality has a Jadad score of 3, which indicates a high quality [2].

Questions Yes (1) No (0)	Was the study described as random?	Was the randomization scheme described and appropriate?	Was the study described as double-blind?	Was the method of double blinding appropriate? (Were both the patient and the assessor appropriately blinded?)	Was there a description of dropouts and withdrawals?	Total score Range of score quality 0–2, low 3–5, high
Score	1	1	0	0	1	3

Limitations of the Study

1. Use of GADSS did not demonstrate treatment effects and may not include appropriate questions to measure late-life GAD.
2. There was limited generalizability due to the participant pool (given age, sex, and education of randomized group).
3. The study had limited reproducibility in a primary care setting due to access to CBT clinicians.
4. The randomized sample was not double-blinded.
5. Communication with the PCP was limited to written notes in a research section of the medical record, and no EMR was available to facilitate treatment integration with ongoing care.

Take-Home Points CBT is beneficial for older adults with GAD in primary care. It can significantly improve worry severity, depressive symptoms, and general mental health for this population.

Practical Applications of the Take-Home Points Primary care centers should consider the integration of CBT into the treatment of GAD in older adults and look into expanding collaborative models of care that incorporate both CBT and medication. Future studies should use an EMR to identify patients and communicate with providers to recruit a more diverse and robust patient population from which more generalizable results may be drawn.

References

1. Stanley MA, Wilson NL, Novy DM, Rhoades HM, Wagener PD, Greisinger AJ, Cully JA, Kunik ME. Cognitive behavior therapy for generalized anxiety disorder among older adults in primary care: a randomized clinical trial. JAMA. 2009;301(14):1460–7.
2. Jadad AR, Moore RA, Carroll D, Jenkinson C, Reynolds DJ, Gavaghan DJ, McQuay HJ. Assessing the quality of reports of randomized clinical trials: is blinding necessary? Control Clin Trials. 1996;17:1–12.

Chapter 13
Stepped-Care Prevention of Anxiety and Depression in Late Life: A Randomized Controlled Trial

Jenny Nguyen and Seetha Chandrasekhara

Authors of the Original Article Petronella J van't Veer-Tazelaar, Harm W J van Marwijk, Patricia van Oppen, Hein P J van Hout, Henriëtte E van der Horst, Pim Cuijpers, Filip Smit, Aartjan T F Beekman

Journal Publisher *Archives of General Psychiatry*

Year of Publication 2009

Type of Study Randomized controlled trial

Funding Sources Netherlands Health Research Council

Objectives To determine the effectiveness of an indicated stepped-care prevention program for anxiety and depression disorders in older adults [1].

Methods This study consisted of 170 consenting adults from 33 primary care practices in the northwestern part of the Netherlands. Participants were aged 75 or older, with subthreshold symptom levels of depression or anxiety who did not meet the full diagnostic criteria for these disorders. They were recruited between October 1, 2004, and October 1, 2005, from the study population of a large prevention project called the Preventive Intervention for Frail Elderly (PIKO). A total of 5207 older adults were sent the PIKO self-rated health inventory, including the Center for Epidemiologic Studies Depression Scale (CES-D Scale).

J. Nguyen · S. Chandrasekhara (✉)
Lewis Katz School of Medicine at Temple University, Philadelphia, PA, USA
e-mail: Seetha.Chandrasekhara@tuhs.temple.edu

R. R. Tampi et al. (eds.), *Essential Reviews in Geriatric Psychiatry*,
https://doi.org/10.1007/978-3-030-94960-0_13

Individuals aged 75 or above from the PIKO database with a CES-D score of 16 or greater were asked whether they would be interested in a stepped-care prevention project. Of 886 individuals who qualified, 325 individuals with a CES-D score of 16 or greater who did not meet the criteria for depressive or anxiety disorder according to the Mini International Neuropsychiatric Interview (MINI) during the past 12 months were approached for the trial. "Anxiety disorder" encompassed panic disorder, agoraphobia, social phobia, or generalized anxiety disorder. Ultimately, 170 individuals met the inclusion criteria and were randomized. Of these participants, 86 were assigned to receive stepped-care intervention, while 84 were assigned to receive usual care.

The stepped-care intervention consisted of four steps, each lasting 3 months. Symptoms were measured using the CES-D every 3 months for 1 year. Step 1 was watchful waiting, during which those with a minimum CES-D score of 16 were invited to complete a second CES-D questionnaire after 3 months. If the score was at or above the cutoff point, participants underwent a diagnostic MINI. If that was negative, it was concluded that those participants had subthreshold levels of depression or anxiety and were randomized to a period of watchful waiting until they passed the threshold score.

Those with continuous depressive and anxiety symptoms (CES-D $\geq$ 16) were moved to Step 2 – cognitive behavior therapy-based bibliotherapy. A phone call explaining each step of the intervention was conducted, and participants were visited by a specially trained home care nurse who provided them with a brochure explaining mild depression, anxiety, as well as anxiety and depression coping strategies. Subsequent visits offered a self-help course on coping with depression and anxiety, which improved their social skills, addressed depressogenic or anxiogenic thinking, and increased pleasant activities and relaxation. Progress at the end of 3 months was evaluated.

Step 3 consisted of brief cognitive behavioral therapy-based problem-solving therapy (PST), which focused on practical skill-building for seven sessions. All nurses were trained in the PST protocol during a 2-day workshop and attended monthly supervision appointments. Treatment integrity was monitored with audio session recordings, and nurses filled out an evaluation form at the end.

Step 4 consisted of a written referral to primary care to discuss suitable medications. Those who met the MINI diagnosis criteria for depression and anxiety at baseline or at 6 and 12 months were referred to their primary care physician. Those in the usual-care group had unrestricted access to usual care. A primary outcome of the study was the cumulative incidence of DSM-IV major depressive disorder or anxiety disorder after 12 months as measured using the MINI.

An intention-to-treat (ITT) principle was used for analyses. Predictors of outcomes and missingness were identified in order to obtain the most precise values and help correct for differential loss to follow-up bias, respectively. A worst-case scenario was applied, and missing scores were replaced with scores indicating depression or anxiety. In order to test the hypothesis (intervention would be more successful than usual care), a logistic regression analysis of the outcome on the treatment indicator to obtain an odds ratio (OR) describing reduction of risk of

MINI for depression or anxiety disorders in the intervention group relative to the control group was used. Superiority of this was determined if the OR < 1 and had a two-tailed significance $p < 0.05$. Number needed to treat (NNT) was obtained with the inverse of the risk difference (obtained from the linear probability model of the outcome on treatment regression).

Results This study showed that the stepped-care intervention halved the 12-month incidence of depressive and anxiety disorders from 23.8% (20 of 84) in the usual-care group to 11.6% (10 of 86) in the stepped-care group, giving a relative risk of 0.49 (95% confidence interval [CI], 0.24–0.98). It reduced the chances of developing a depressive or anxiety disorder by 57.9% (OR, 0.42%; 95% CI, 0.18–0.96%). The null hypothesis of no effect was rejected (SE = 0.18; $z = -2.05$; $P = 0.04$). The analysis was then repeated based on multiple imputation, yielding an OR of 0.34 (95% CI, 0.20–0.61) which was significant (SE = 0.252; $t = 4.227$; $P < 0.001$). The worst-case analysis showed an OR of 1.19 (95% CI, 0.63–2.23), which was no longer significant (SE = 0.38; $z = -0.53$; $P = 0.60$). A Poisson regression analysis showed that the risk of disease onset is more than halved by the intervention due to a person-time-based incidence rate ratio of 0.47 (95% CI, 0.22–1.00 rounded) and was significant (SE = 0.181; $z = -1.97$; $P = 0.049$). The risk difference was 0.12 in favor of the intervention (95% CI, −0.236 to −0.007; SE = 0.058; $t = -2.10$; $P = 0.04$). The NNT was also calculated, which was 8.2. The generalized estimating equation model showed the following coefficients for the group X time interactions for each of the time points on the CES-D scores: 8.2, 11.11, 12.1, and 12.2, indicating that the intervention was substantially clinically superior compared with care as usual. The interaction terms were significant for 3 months at $P = 0.008$, and $P < 0.001$ for all other time points. After 1 year, the intervention group showed four depressive disorders, three anxiety disorders, and two co-occurrences of depression and anxiety. The usual-care group had ten depressive disorders, five anxiety disorders, and five co-occurrences. There was no significance of the distribution across the two groups.

During the first year, 23 participants in the usual-care group received antidepressant or anxiolytic-sedative medications, compared to 28 in the intervention group ($P = 0.28$). Two participants in the usual-care group mentioned that they had read information about depression or anxiety.

During the first 6 months, 13 intervention participants (10 refusals) and 3 usual-care participants dropped out of the study. During the second 6 months, four and one dropped out, respectively. Dropout occurred at a significantly higher rate in the intervention group ($P = 0.009$). Some dropout was due to mortality. In the intervention group, 3 of 79 active participants died, and 2 of 80 participants died from the usual-care group. Mortality was not related to either condition ($P = 0.99$).

Conclusions For older adults, indicated stepped-care prevention is an effective means of reducing the risk of onset of depression and anxiety disorders by half. Stepped-care interventions are time- and cost-effective in the long run as they start off with low-cost interventions and outcomes are monitored to ensure proper resource allocation.

Strengths of the Study

1. The trial design was randomized controlled.
2. This study had a Jadad score of 3, indicating that it was a high-quality study [2].

Questions Yes (1) No (0)	Was the study described as random?	Was the randomization scheme described and appropriate?	Was the study described as double-blind?	Was the method of double blinding appropriate? (Were both the patient and the assessor appropriately blinded?)	Was there a description of dropouts and withdrawals?	Total score Range of score quality 0–2, low 3–5, high
Score	1	1	0	0	1	3

3. This study's screen test identified older adults with depression and anxiety disorders who may not have been identified by their primary care physicians.
4. The study was grounded in the US Preventive Services Task Force recommendation that screening improves identification of depressed patients in primary care settings, and the empirically supported Improving Mood: Promoting Access to Collaborative Treatment (IMPACT) study.
5. It was able to focus on depressive symptoms in older adults who were 75 years or older.
6. This study also addressed anxiety, which strengthens its value because there is a high comorbidity between mood disorders and anxiety disorders.
7. This is relevant to clinical practice because it encompassed a representative sample of subclinically depressed or anxious older adults through the use of random sampling and screening and they had good controls in place to minimize confounding factors.
8. The study tried to replicate real-life conditions by giving participants the opportunity to decline each step of the stepped-care program.
9. It is likely feasible to implement this in large medical practices such as HMOs because they often already include behavioral specialists on their staff and their services are reimbursable under existing Medicare codes.
10. There was standardized training and supervision for the nurses who provided participants with each step of the stepped-care program, which helped control for variability between providers.
11. This study exhibited a decent duration of follow-up which went to 12 months, and the intervals were 3-month points for their follow-up appointments, which gave the psychotherapy sessions and pharmacotherapy treatments time to start having an impact before participants were re-evaluated.
12. They used three different imputation strategies in order to help correct for the bias of the differential loss of participants to follow-up.

Limitations of the Study

1. It was impossible to assess the specific contributions of each of the various elements of the stepped-care program because the intervention had to be treated as a whole in the analysis.
2. There were different dropout rates between the groups, indicating that perhaps the intervention required a significant amount of effort from some participants.
3. A large portion of the participants were women (73.5% [125/170] of total participants) from rural locations (44.1% [75/140] of total participants), which can limit generalizability in other patient populations.

Take-Home Points Indicated stepped-care interventions are an effective way of preventing depressive and anxiety disorders in people who are 75 years or older when compared to usual care alone. Indicated stepped-care interventions halved the 1-year cumulative incidence rate of the disorders.

Practical Applications of the Take-Home Points Many cases of depression and anxiety can be avoided through the adoption of an indicated stepped-care intervention program in those who are 75 or older. Primary care settings can be a strategic target in identifying individuals with subclinical depression and anxiety. Collaborative care by trained staff can lead to earlier remission than usual care and should be more widely implemented given that large medical practices such as HMOs often already include behavioral specialists on their staff and their services are already reimbursable under existing Medicare codes. Primary care practices can be trained to recognize the different factors that would indicate whether individuals would benefit from indicated stepped-care interventions.

References

1. van't Veer-Tazelaar PJ, van Marwijk HWJ, van Oppen P, van Hout HPJ, van der Horst HE, Cuijpers P, Smit F, Beekman ATF. Stepped-care prevention of anxiety and depression in late life: a randomized controlled trial. Arch Gen Psychiatry. 2009;66(3):297–304. https://doi.org/10.1001/archgenpsychiatry.2008.555.
2. Jadad AR, Moore RA, Carroll D, Jenkinson C, Reynolds DJ, Gavaghan DJ, McQuay HJ. Assessing the quality of reports of randomized clinical trials: is blinding necessary? Control Clin Trials. 1996;17(1):1–12.

Chapter 14
A Randomized Controlled Study of Paroxetine and Cognitive Behavioral Therapy for Late-Life Panic Disorder

Charlotte M. Schwarz and Tracey Holsinger

Authors of the Original Article G.-J. Hendriks, G. P. J. Keijsers, M. Kampman, R. C. Oude Voshaar, M. J. P. M. Verbraak, T. G. Broekman, C. A. L. Hoogduin.

Journal Publisher *Acta Psychiatrica Scandinavica.*

Year of Publication 2010.

Type of Study Single-blind randomized control trial.

Funding Sources Not noted.

Objectives To examine the effectiveness of paroxetine and cognitive behavioral therapy (CBT) in patients aged 60+ with a primary diagnosis of panic disorder with or without agoraphobia [PD(A)]. These treatments were compared with each other as well as with patients randomized to a waitlist. An additional objective was to examine the feasibility of these treatments [1].

Methods Adults aged 60+ with a principal diagnosis of PD(A) were recruited from an outpatient anxiety disorder clinic. Exclusion criteria were comorbid severe psychiatric disorder, severe somatic disorder, contraindication to paroxetine, current adequate antidepressant or psychological treatment, past failure of paroxetine or

---

C. M. Schwarz
University of North Carolina at Chapel Hill Department of Psychiatry, Chapel Hill, NC, USA

T. Holsinger (✉)
Duke University Department of Psychiatry and Behavioral Sciences and Durham VA Medical Center, Durham, NC, USA
e-mail: Tracey.holsinger@duke.edu

R. R. Tampi et al. (eds.), *Essential Reviews in Geriatric Psychiatry*,
https://doi.org/10.1007/978-3-030-94960-0_14

CBT, substance use disorder, dementia, and a score of 23 or less on the Mini-Mental State Examination (MMSE). Participants using benzodiazepines were asked to adhere to a fixed daily dose.

PD(A) diagnoses were verified using the Anxiety Disorder Interview Schedule-Revised (ADIS-IV). The patients were randomly assigned to 3 study conditions: 30 patients to 14 weeks of protocolized CBT, 30 patients to paroxetine (dose titrated up to 40 mg daily by week 4 and maintained for 26 weeks), and 15 patients to a waitlist. The patients had assessments at baseline, week 8, week 14, and week 26.

The primary outcomes of anxiety cognitions and phobic avoidance were measured with the Agoraphobic Cognitions Questionnaire (ACQ) and Mobility Inventory Avoidance scale (MI-A). The MI-A is comprised of 2 subscales to gauge the severity of phobic avoidance of 27 situations, avoidance when alone (MI-AAL) and avoidance when accompanied (MI-AAC), and 1, single-item subscale to assess the frequency of panic attacks (MI-PF). Panic-free status was a secondary outcome measured. General psychopathology was another secondary outcome assessed using the Symptom Checklist-90 (SCL-90).

A mixed-model statistical analysis was conducted. A priori contrast between paroxetine and waitlist groups and CBT and waitlist groups was investigated. Post hoc contrast between paroxetine and CBT groups was also evaluated. Cohen's *d* was calculated for effect size per treatment and between groups. More than 30% improvement on one of the primary outcome scales was deemed clinically relevant improvement.

Results A total of 49 patients (out of 153 patients screened) met criteria for the study. Among these patients, 67.3% had a chronic somatic disorder, 46.9% had cardiovascular disease, 10.2% had chronic obstructive pulmonary disease, and 28.6% had another psychiatric disorder. Psychiatric comorbidities were higher in the paroxetine treatment arm; otherwise, there were no significant between-group differences.

Of patients randomized, 10.2% (five patients in total) did not complete the 14-week treatment protocol (three for paroxetine due to side effect, protocol violation, and broken hip, respectively; one in CBT due to protocol violation; one on waitlist due to severe somatic illness). Of those who did complete CBT, eight patients were terminated after completing the treatment at week 14. At week 26, 6.1% (two in paroxetine, one in CBT) refused participation in the follow-up assessment.

At 8 weeks and 14 weeks, the ACQ and MI-A scores showed significant improvement in both the paroxetine (both $P < 0.05$) and CBT groups ($P < 0.05$ and $P < 0.01$, respectively) when compared to the waitlist group. These improvements persisted at follow-up during week 26. Between-group effects compared with the waitlist group as well as effect for within-group primary outcomes were moderate to large for both treatment arms. A clinically relevant improvement was found in 7/14 (50%) of patients in the paroxetine group, 9/18 (50%) in the CBT group, and 1/10 (9%, $P = 0.057$) of the waitlist group.

A significant change was found in the paroxetine condition ($P < 0.05$) for the SCL-90 score, whereas the change in the CBT condition ($P = 0.052$) did not reach significance. The frequency of self-reported panic attacks fluctuated greatly. Therefore, the proportion of patients who had not experienced any panic attacks the week prior to the assessment was used to calculate the panic-free ratio. At week 14, the panic-free ratio in the paroxetine condition ($P < 0.05$) showed significant improvement that was sustained at week 26 ($P < 0.05$); there was also improvement in the CBT condition ($P = 0.16$ and $P = 0.06$, respectively), although it did not reach significance.

Conclusions Protocolized CBT and paroxetine were each effective for patients aged 60+ with PD(A). Patients in each of these two treatment conditions showed significant improvement in catastrophic thinking about anxiety and panic, as measured by the ACQ, and phobic avoidance, as measured by the MI-A. There was good effect size compared to patients who had been placed on a waitlist for treatment. The interventions showed good tolerability, with only four patients withdrawing from treatment due to reasons related to intolerance. In the paroxetine group, there was also a significant reduction in general symptoms of psychopathology, as measured in the secondary outcome of the SCL-90 score.

Strengths of the Study

1. This study had relatively low attrition rates, which not only suggests good tolerability of the interventions but also allows their effects to be assessed over the course of the entire experimental period of 26 weeks.
2. The mixed-model analysis helped preclude bias that would have arisen from the method of last observation carried forward.
3. The CBT used was protocolized and PD(A)-specific.
4. Benzodiazepine use, if concomitant, was held at fixed dose throughout the study so as to minimize their effect on outcome.
5. The study assessed on the basis of Jadad score indicates that this was a high-quality study with a score of 3 out of 5 [2].

Questions Yes (1) No (0)	Was the study described as random?	Was the randomization scheme described and appropriate?	Was the study described as double-blind?	Was the method of double blinding appropriate? (were both the patient and the assessor appropriately blinded?)	Was there a description of dropouts and withdrawals?	Total score Range of score quality 0–2, low 3–5, high
Score	1	1	0	0	1	3

Limitations of the Study

1. This study was limited by small sample size, namely, 49 patients in total were randomly assigned to the three experimental arms.
2. Generalizability was limited by the exclusion criterion that participants could not be on an antidepressant in an "adequate dose," which was not defined in the paper.
3. The sample included 60-year-old people and above living in the community, thus representing a relatively healthy sample of the geriatric population. More severe medical and psychiatric comorbidities were excluded.
4. After randomization, psychiatric comorbidity was higher in the paroxetine arm of the condition, such that baseline patient characteristics were not uniform in all groups.
5. This study did not distinguish between PD and PDA. Since the DSM-5, agoraphobia is considered a distinct diagnosis rather than a qualifier of panic disorder. As such, its presentation and treatment may also benefit from being considered independently.
6. The protocols and instruments used are those that have been validated in patients 18–65 years, so their validity for this study's population has not been tested. The instruments may be less suitable for assessing anxiety cognitions in the elderly.

Take-Home Points

1. Panic disorder with and without agoraphobia in patients aged 60+ showed clinically significant improvement with paroxetine and with protocolized CBT within 14 weeks, as measured by decrease in the primary outcomes of anxiety cognitions and phobic avoidance.
2. Both these treatments showed good feasibility.

Practical Applications of the Take-Home Points

Older adults with PD(A) can benefit from pharmacological intervention or protocolized CBT within a relatively short period of time. This should encourage providers to intervene early so as to mitigate the consequences of untreated anxiety in the elderly.

References

1. Hendriks GJ, Keijsers GP, Kampman M, Oude Voshaar RC, Verbraak MJ, Broekman TG, Hoogduin CA. A randomized controlled study of paroxetine and cognitive-behavioural therapy for late-life panic disorder. Acta Psychiatr Scand. 2010;122(1):11–9.
2. Jadad AR, Moore RA, Carroll D, Jenkinson C, Reynolds DJ, Gavaghan DJ, McQuay HJ. Assessing the quality of reports of randomized clinical trials: is blinding necessary? Control Clin Trials. 1996;17(1):1–12.

Chapter 15
Antidepressant Medication Augmented with Cognitive Behavioral Therapy for Generalized Anxiety Disorder in Older Adults

Megan Tusken, Izabella Dutra de Abreu, Audrey Eichenberger, Daniela Vela, and Mary "Molly" Camp

Authors of the Original Article Julie Loebach Wetherell, PhD; Andrew J. Ptekus, MA; Kamila S. White, PhD; Hoang Nguyen, MD; Sander Kornblith, PhD; Carmen Andreescu, MD; Sidney Zisook, MD; Eric J. Lenze, MD.

Journal Publisher *The American Journal of Psychiatry.*

Year of Publication 2013.

Type of Study Randomized controlled trial.

Funding Sources The National Institute of Mental Health (NIMH) and National Institute on Aging.

Objectives To examine the efficacy of a sequential approach to treating GAD among older adults using escitalopram and CBT for augmentation and relapse prevention [1].

Methods Eligible study participants included adults ≥60 years old with a DSM-IV principal diagnosis of GAD as determined by the Structured Clinical Interview for DSM-IV and Hamilton Anxiety Rating Scale (HAM-A). Participants were recruited between 2008 and 2010, via primary care practices, mental health clinics, and advertisements at sites in Pittsburgh, San Diego, and St. Louis.

M. Tusken (✉) · I. D. de Abreu · A. Eichenberger · D. Vela · M. M. Camp
UT Southwestern Medical Center at Dallas, Dallas, TX, USA
e-mail: Megan.Tusken@PHHS.org; Izabella.DeAbreu@UTSouthwestern.edu; Audrey.Eichenberger@PHHS.org; Daniela.Vela@UTSouthwestern.edu; Molly.Camp@UTSouthwestern.edu

R. R. Tampi et al. (eds.), *Essential Reviews in Geriatric Psychiatry*,
https://doi.org/10.1007/978-3-030-94960-0_15

Patients with comorbidities, such as unipolar depression, other anxiety disorders, or substance abuse/dependence, were included if GAD was the principal diagnosis and they had been in full remission from substance use for at least 6 months. Exclusions were made for anyone with a lifetime history of psychosis or bipolar disorder, cognitive impairment, current suicidal ideation, ongoing psychotherapy, or unstable medical illness.

Patients taking psychotropic medications were tapered off of these at least 2 weeks before entering the study; however, some patients taking benzodiazepines or prescription sleep medication remained on a consistent, but usually lower, daily dose throughout the study.

Outcomes were anxiety, as measured by the HAM-A, and pathological worry, as measured by the Penn State Worry Questionnaire. The HAM-A was chosen due to its status as the gold standard outcome measure in pharmacotherapy studies for GAD. The Penn State Worry Questionnaire was chosen due to its common use as an outcome measure in psychotherapy studies of GAD.

The study utilized a sequential approach to treatment, with three noted phases: acute, augmentation, and maintenance. In the acute phase, all participants were treated with 12 weeks of open-label escitalopram, starting at 10 mg/day with titration to 20 mg/day after 4 weeks if not improved. If a participant exhibited at least 20% improvement in HAM-A, then they were randomized to one of the four conditions:

1. Sixteen weeks of escitalopram augmented with 16 sessions of CBT, followed by 28 weeks of escitalopram.
2. Sixteen weeks of escitalopram without CBT, followed by 28 weeks of escitalopram.
3. Sixteen weeks of escitalopram plus CBT, followed by 28 weeks of placebo.
4. Sixteen weeks of escitalopram without CBT, followed by 28 weeks of placebo.

CBT consisted of 16 manualized sessions targeting worry and anxiety. For ongoing assessment, participants completed the HAM-A every 4 weeks during augmentation and every 2 weeks during maintenance. The Penn State Worry Questionnaire was given only at the start and conclusion of the augmentation and maintenance phases.

Intent-to-treat analysis was used for evaluation of the augmentation and maintenance phases. The augmentation effect of CBT was defined by a HAM-A score ≤10 and a decrease of ≥8.5 points on the Penn State Worry Questionnaire, based on previous research definitions of treatment response. Kaplan-Meier survival analyses were employed to compare cumulative incidence of relapse across the four conditions in analysis of the maintenance phase.

Results One hundred fifty-eight patients were screened, 86 were started on open-label escitalopram, and 73 were randomized. Sixty-three out of 73 (95%) participants completed the 13-month protocol following randomization. Patient attrition occurred in the acute phase due to side effects or lack of efficacy. Participants withdrew during the augmentation phase due to dissatisfaction with medication or loss to follow-up.

The four treatment groups did not differ demographically; however, the group assigned to the placebo arm had a statistically significant higher proportion of participants with a baseline comorbid anxiety disorder ($P = 0.03$). There were also differences across study sites in age, education level, and mean Penn State Worry Questionnaire scores. Differences were not included as covariates because the presence of comorbid anxiety and differences across sites in age, education, etc. did not predict outcomes on HAM-A or Penn State Worry Questionnaire scores in the augmentation or relapse prevention stages.

During the augmentation phase, there was no statistically significant difference in response based on HAM-A between the escitalopram-plus-CBT group (75%; 95% confidence interval (CI), 60.2–87.6) and the escitalopram-only group (67.6%; 95% CI, 52.5–81.8). However, a statistically significant improvement was found when measured by Penn State Worry Questionnaire, with participants receiving CBT approximately three times more likely to respond than those who did not receive CBT [odds ratio (OR) = 3.19; 95% CI, 1.00–10.14; $P < 0.05$). When measuring response with the Penn State Worry Questionnaire, participants in the escitalopram-plus-CBT group had greater symptomatic improvement of pathological worry.

In maintenance, there were differences across the four conditions as measured by cumulative incidence of relapse. Participants given maintenance escitalopram had significantly lower relapse rates than those receiving placebo, regardless of CBT assignment (2.7%; 95% CI, 0.3–17.7). This finding was considered so robust that the effect of CBT was only examined within the group receiving placebo. In this subset, those receiving CBT had lower rates of relapse (25.0%; 95% CI, 10.2–31.9) than those without CBT (66.4%; 95% CI, 44.0–87.1).

Conclusions Results from this sequential study of CBT augmentation of escitalopram pharmacotherapy from a RCT of older adults with GAD support the use of CBT for patients, after starting a selective serotonin reuptake inhibitor (SSRI), for augmentation and/or maintenance treatment.

Strengths of the Study

1. The study had RCT design.
2. It used sequential study approach to model real clinical practice.
3. The study sample included only older adults (≥60 years).
4. The study adds to a limited body of evidence examining CBT for augmentation of medication in anxiety disorders.
5. The study is unique among prior research in examining evidence for the relapse prevention benefits of CBT.
6. There was 95% completion rate for the study.
7. Intention-to-treat analysis was used.
8. Study findings on SSRIs for maintenance in GAD are consistent with prior research findings in younger populations.

Limitations of the Study

1. It has small sample size.
2. It has low power for HAM-A effect size.
3. It has limited generalizability (demographically, participants were mostly white).
4. There is no active control condition for CBT.

Take-Home Points Although small in size, this RCT trial provides evidence to support the use of sequenced escitalopram and CBT for augmentation and maintenance treatment of GAD in older adults. CBT augmentation was found to reduce pathological worry. Both escitalopram and CBT prevented relapse. Furthermore, efficacy and safety of CBT indicate that it is a more acceptable strategy than other strategies such as augmentation and maintenance with benzodiazepines, which have a poor risk-benefit ratio.

Practical Applications of the Take-Home Points Among older adults with GAD, referral to CBT may be beneficial for augmentation and maintenance of therapy with an SSRI.

Reference

1. Wetherell JL, Petkus AJ, White KS, Nguyen H, Kornblith S, Andreescu C, Zisook S, Lenze EJ. Antidepressant medication augmented with cognitive-behavioral therapy for generalized anxiety disorder in older adults. Am J Psychiatry. 2013;170(7):782–9.

Chapter 16
A Meta-Analysis of Cognitive Functioning in Older Adults with PTSD

Avee Champaneria and Kristin McArthur

Authors of the Original Article Sage Schuitevoerder, Jay W Rosen, Elizabeth W Twamley, Catherine R Ayers, Heather Sones, James B Lohr, Elizabeth M Goetter, Greg A Fonzo, Kathryn J Holloway, Steven R Thorp

Journal Publisher *Journal of Anxiety Disorders.*

Year of Publication 2013.

Type of Study Meta-analysis.

Funding Sources Clinical Science R&D Program of the Veterans Health Administration.

Objectives The investigators conducted a meta-analysis to examine cognitive functioning in older adults with PTSD and without PTSD, with the hypothesis that older adults with PTSD would exhibit poorer performance in the cognitive domains studied [1].

Methods The authors used established guidelines for systematic reviews of the evidence for public health issues [2]. They queried PubMed, PsycINFO, and PILOTS to find eligible articles by combining the terms "posttraumatic stress

A. Champaneria
Department of Psychiatry and Behavioral Sciences, Duke University Health System, Durham, NC, USA
e-mail: ac540@duke.edu

K. McArthur (✉)
Psychiatry, Durham VA Medical Center, Durham, NC, USA
e-mail: Kristin.mcarthur@va.gov

R. R. Tampi et al. (eds.), *Essential Reviews in Geriatric Psychiatry*,
https://doi.org/10.1007/978-3-030-94960-0_16

disorder" or "PTSD" with "neuropsychology," "neurocognitive," or "cognitive impairment." They used the following inclusion criteria: journal articles had to be peer-reviewed, had to be in the English language, and should have human subjects over the age of 65, and articles had to provide data from which an effect size could be calculated for at least one neuropsychological test. They used the following exclusion criteria: search engine results lacking an abstract (including letters to the editor), articles focused on maladaptive thinking patterns/cognitive distortions rather than cognitive deficits, and articles that did not include a discussion of the words "elderly," "aged," "older adults," or "senior," or did not make any statistical inferences about participants older than 60 years.

Investigators used a priori method to identify ten categories of cognitive domains to be studied: global cognitive functioning, premorbid intelligence, processing speed, attention and working memory, learning, memory, language, visuospatial abilities, executive functioning, and fine motor skills.

Established test interpretation guidelines and recommendations were used to identify the potential challenges in the interpretation of the cognitive status in older adults with PTSD. Potential confounds included age; premorbid cognitive functioning and education; ethnicity/culture; severity, chronicity, and onset of PTSD symptoms; psychiatric disorders other than PTSD; drug and alcohol use; sleep disorders and fatigue; pain; medical conditions; exercise; cigarette smoking; and medications. The investigators examined the statistical control of these variables in the articles.

Investigators examined three levels of trauma exposure: PTSD positive (PTSD+), trauma exposed but PTSD negative (PTSD−), and non-trauma-exposed healthy comparison (HC) samples.

Investigators calculated effect sizes for two comparisons: PTSD+ vs. PTSD− and PTSD+ vs. HC. Effect sizes were calculated using the standardized mean difference statistic (Hedges' g), and they subtracted the mean of the comparison group from the mean of the PTSD+ group; therefore, negative effect size (ES) suggests poorer cognitive performance. Investigators used a well-documented way of standardizing measures within each study and across the studies for each of the cognitive domains, in essence, making standardized composite scores based on relevant measures for each domain before calculating the mean effect size across studies, allowing for comparisons between measures that are otherwise on different scales. They used fixed-effects model to control for unobserved study-specific variation. They prevented for preferential weighing by averaging the effect sizes in studies which used data from various cognitive measures from the same group of participants.

Results Eleven articles met the criteria for the systematic review; 77 were excluded according to the exclusion criteria. Total sample sizes in the identified articles ranged from 25 to 114, and mean age range was 62–80 years. Six studies examined participants who identified as Jewish or Israeli and had experienced Holocaust-related trauma; and five studies included veterans from the United States with trauma from combat and captivity as POWs.

All studies utilized PTSD-specific structured clinical interviews and self-report measures to assess for PTSD symptoms/diagnosis and trauma exposure. Ten studies included a trauma inventory—Trauma History Questionnaire, Combat Exposure Scale, Childhood Trauma Questionnaire, and Live Events Questionnaire. One study conducted a chart review of previously administered trauma inventories to assess for traumatic events. Nine studies used the Clinician Administered PTSD Scale to assess for current and lifetime PTSD symptoms. One of these studies administered a version of the CAPS that assessed symptoms in a 1-week period, rather than the 1 month required to meet diagnosis of PTSD. Two of the studies used self-report measures of PTSD—the Mississippi Scale for Combat-Related PTSD and the Posttraumatic Stress Diagnostic Scale.

The meta-analysis included 72 tests or subtests measuring cognitive functioning utilized in the studies. The potential confound of age was controlled in all studies using age-related test norms, evaluation of age-equivalency between groups with statistical tests, or matched comparison samples using methodological control. Ten studies (91%) accounted for the severity of PTSD, major comorbid psychiatric conditions, and the impact of medical, neurological, or cerebrovascular conditions. Nine studies (82%) assessed past drug or alcohol use. Education and medications were accounted for less consistently in the studies, 64% and 55%, respectively. Only 36% of the studies established statistical equivalency of ethnicities between comparison groups or the age of index trauma. The potential confounding factors of sleep disorder, cigarette smoking, exercise, pain, or impact of the effort on testing results were not accounted for in any of the studies.

All studies used means comparisons to evaluate the impact of trauma exposure or PTSD on neurocognition. Seven studies compared three groups: PTSD+, PTSD−, and HC. Three studies compared PTSD+ and PTSD− groups. One study compared two PTSD+ samples, with and without comorbid schizophrenia to a sample of HC. Almost all the studies used a cross-sectional design.

Five of the 11 studies utilized a shared sample of participants who were survivors of the Holocaust. Two of the studies reported data from the same cohort of combat veterans. Ultimately, six unique samples were considered in the calculations of effect size.

The investigators calculated effect sizes for each cognitive domain (refer to Table 16.1) and for comparison between Holocaust survivors and combat veterans as well (refer to Table 16.2). They tested for heterogeneity when determining the effect sizes and, when appropriate, made adjustments to correct for between and within study variances.

Conclusion Investigators found that older adults with PTSD exhibited poorer performance in all cognitive domains in comparison to trauma-exposed older adults without PTSD and healthy controls. Memory showed a large effect size when comparing the PTSD+ and PTSD− samples. Effect size was larger for the cognitive domain of learning in the PTSD+ vs. HC than with PTSD+ vs. PTSD− samples. When comparing the samples of PTSD+ to PTSD− and PTSD+ to HC, the effect sizes were moderate to large in the combat veteran samples. In the samples of the

Table 16.1 Cognitive domain ES for comparison samples PTSD+ vs. PTSD and PTSD+ vs. HC

Domain	Comparison sample	Mean effect size	95% CI for mean ES
All cognitive domains	PTSD+ vs. PTSD−	− 0.58	− 1.05, − 0.10
	PTSD+ vs. HC	− 0.72	− 0.90, − 0.54
Global cognitive functioning	PTSD+ vs. PTSD−	N/A (no measures provided)	N/A
	PTSD+ vs. HC	− 1.01	N/A
Premorbid intelligence	PTSD+ vs. PTSD−	− 0.71	− 1.47, 0.04
	PTSD+ vs. HC	− 0.98	− 1.15, − 0.82
Processing speed	PTSD+ vs. PTSD−	− 1.17	N/A
	PTSD+ vs. HC	− 0.87	N/A
Attention and working memory	PTSD+ vs. PTSD−	− 0.67	− 1.66, 0.88
	PTSD+ vs. HC	− 0.28	N/A
Learning	PTSD+ vs. PTSD−	− 0.40	− 0.54, − 0.26
	PTSD+ vs. HC	− 0.72	− 1.09, − 0.35
Memory	PTSD+ vs. PTSD−	− 0.97	− 1.83, 0.48
	PTSD+ vs. HC	− 0.73	− 1.02, − 0.44
Language	PTSD+ vs. PTSD−	− 0.34	− 0.86, 0.18
	PTSD+ vs. HC	N/A (no measures provided)	N/A
Visuospatial abilities	PTSD+ vs. PTSD−	− 0.61	− 0.81, − 0.42
	PTSD+ vs. HC	− 0.61	− 0.77, − 0.44
Executive functioning	PTSD+ vs. PTSD−	− 0.80	− 1.79, 1.04
	PTSD+ vs. HC	− 1.49	N/A
Fine motor skill	PTSD+ vs. PTSD−	N/A (no measures provided)	N/A
	PTSD+ vs. HC	− 0.47	N/A

Table 16.2 ES for comparison groups PTSD+ vs. PTSD- and PTSD+ vs. HC for Holocaust survivors and combat veterans

	Comparison sample	Effect size	95% CI for mean ES
Holocaust survivors	PTSD+ vs. PTSD−	− 0.47	N/A
	PTSD+ vs. HC	− 0.66	− 0.70, − 0.62
Combat veterans	PTSD+ vs. PTSD−	− 0.74	− 1.21, − 0.03
	PTSD+ vs. HC	− 0.91	N/A

Holocaust survivors, however, the effect sizes were small to moderate. This poses a question whether combat traumas impact the cognitive abilities differently in older adults and if there are combat-specific factors at play, or whether there are some protective factors in the Holocaust survivors, warranting further research. In the cognitive domain of learning, the effect size was about half the magnitude for PTSD+ vs. PTSD− comparison group as the PTSD+ vs. HC, suggesting that trauma exposure may be a contributing factor to poorer performance in learning. The largest differences between older adults with PTSD and HC were in the areas of processing speed, learning, memory, and executive functioning; thus, cognitive training may be an appropriate intervention. Additional research is needed to examine the impact of cognitive deficits on treatment interventions in older adults with PTSD.

Strengths of the Study

- The investigators used a priori method to identify ten cognitive domains and classify the neuropsychological measures by sub-scales to facilitate systematic comparison.
- The investigators examined methodological challenges across the studies to inform future efforts in research.
- This meta-analysis highlights the scarcity of peer-reviewed empirical studies on cognitive functioning in older adults with PTSD.

Limitations of the Study

- Almost all the studies employed a cross-sectional design; therefore, the impact of course of PTSD and symptom fluctuation on cognitive status could not be assessed.
- Study samples were restricted to groups of Holocaust survivors and combat veterans, limiting its generalizability.
- The combat veteran samples comprised entirely of men, limiting generalizability.
- Cohort effects have been well established in psychological studies of intelligence and other cognitive structures [3, 4], which may also limit generalizability.
- Sample sizes were relatively small in many of the studies and may have provided insufficient statistical power.
- Many of the studies which examined memory deficits failed to account premorbid level of functioning or for the effects of attention/learning.
- The potential confounds like sleep disorder, exercise, pain, cigarette smoking, or the impact of effort on the test results were not accounted of controlled for in any of the studies.
- There was inconsistency in reporting of the neuropsychological test scores—raw, scaled, and standard formats—likely impacting indices of heterogeneity.
- There was infrequent reporting of premorbid IQ, which is an established risk factor for developing PTSD prior to trauma exposure in younger adult samples [5].

Take-Home Points

There is scarcity of peer-reviewed empirical research on cognitive function of older adults with PTSD. This meta-analysis provides evidence that older adults with PTSD perform more poorly on tests of memory in comparison with older adults without PTSD; however, the generalizability of these results is limited. Cognitive training could be an appropriate intervention to help improve processing speed, learning, memory, and executive functioning in older adults with PTSD.

Practical Applications of the Take-Home Points

Further empirical research is needed to assess for cognitive function in older adults with PTSD.

References

1. Schuitevoerder S, Rosen JW, Twamley EW, Ayers CR, Sones H, Lohr JB, Goetter EM, Fonzo GA, Holloway KJ, Thorp SR. A meta-analysis of cognitive functioning in older adults with PTSD. J Anxiety Disord. 2013;27(6):550–8.
2. Centre for Reviews and Dissemination. Systematic reviews: CRD's guidance for undertaking reviews in health care. 2009. Retrieved from: http://www.york.ac.uk/inst/crd/. Accessed January 25, 2021.
3. Gerstorf D, Ram N, Hoppmann C, Willis SL, Schaie KW. Cohort differences in cognitive aging and terminal decline in the Seattle longitudinal study. Dev Psychol. 2011;47(4):1026–41.
4. Schaie KW, Willis SL, Pennak S. An historical framework for cohort differences in intelligence. Res Hum Dev. 2005;2(1–2):43–67.
5. Weintraub D, Ruskin PE. Posttraumatic stress disorder in the elderly: a review. Harv Rev Psychiatry. 1999;7(3):144–52.

Chapter 17
Anxiety as a Predictor for Cognitive Decline and Dementia: A Systematic Review and Meta-Analysis

Aarti Gupta and Gagandeep K. Bhatia

Authors of the Original Article Bernice Gulpers, Inez Ramakers, Renske Hamel, Sebastian Köhler, Richard Oude Voshaar, Frans Verhey

Journal Publisher *The American Journal of Geriatric Psychiatry.*

Year of Publication 2016.

Type of Study Systematic review and meta-analysis.

Funding Sources NA.

Objectives

1. To determine if anxiety is predictive of cognitive decline, cognitive impairment, and/or dementia among individuals in the community.
2. To determine whether anxiety predicts the conversion of mild cognitive impairment (MCI) to dementia among individuals at specialized memory clinics [1].

Methods The investigators searched PubMed, PsycINFO, Embase, and CINAHL databases until January 2015 for relevant cohort studies that evaluated the association between anxiety and cognitive decline or conversion to dementia using various search terms.

The investigators included longitudinal cohort studies that evaluated clinically relevant anxiety that was based on either a validated scale or an anxiety disorder according to either the International Classification of Diseases or the Diagnostic and

A. Gupta (✉) · G. K. Bhatia
Yale University School of Medicine, New Haven, CT, USA
e-mail: aarti.gupta@yale.edu

R. R. Tampi et al. (eds.), *Essential Reviews in Geriatric Psychiatry*,
https://doi.org/10.1007/978-3-030-94960-0_17

Statistical Manual of Mental Disorders criteria in specialized care and International Classification of Primary Care criteria or equivalent in primary care.

The investigators excluded studies where anxiety was only assessed as a trait or personality characteristic, the participants had dementia at baseline, and a cohort of individuals restricted to specific somatic diseases at baseline like diabetes, stroke, or depression and individuals with mild cognitive disorder with established underlying neurodegenerative pathology were included. Only studies published in English, German, French, and Dutch language were included.

The two authors independently extracted the following information from the relevant studies: the number and percentage of cognitive decline or dementia, the cross table for anxiety and cognitive decline or dementia, the odds ratios, hazard ratios, relative risks or β, 95% confidence intervals, p values, the covariates, and the overall conclusion of the study. They also extracted the following information from each of the studies: the cohort, baseline diagnosis, definition of cognitive status at baseline, setting, included ages, inclusion and exclusion criteria, cognition scale, anxiety scale, number of subjects, mean age and standard deviation, number of women and men, education in years, mean score of Mini-Mental State Examination (MMSE) and standard deviation, mean score on the anxiety scale and the standard deviation, and the mean of follow-up years and the standard deviation. They used a third author to resolve any disagreements regarding the data that was obtained. The investigators also contacted the corresponding authors of relevant studies when the data was incomplete for the meta-analysis.

To access the quality of the studies, the 2 authors independently rated a total of 26 items from each of the included studies that were related to the following: sample of patients, the follow-up of patients, the loss to follow-up, the outcome, the prognostic variable, and the analysis. These items were rated being present (1), questionable (0.5), or absent (0). To obtain a global measure of the quality of the study, these scores were then summed and divided by the total number of items (range, 0–1.0). Pooled relative risks were calculated when it was possible to evaluate anxiety as a possible risk factor for cognitive decline, cognitive impairment, and dementia in community studies and for conversion of individuals with mild cognitive impairment (MCI) to dementia at specialized memory clinics.

Results The investigators included a total of 20 studies in the systematic review and meta-analysis. There was no evidence for possible publication bias across all studies.

Objective 1: Data from Community-Based Studies

A. Anxiety and Rate of Cognitive Decline.

The investigators included data from 7 studies with 23,871 participants that evaluated the relation between anxiety and decline on individual cognitive domains. The average methodological quality of these studies was 0.74. Given the heterogeneity in the cognitive domains and the cognitive tests used in these studies, a meta-analysis could not be conducted. Only one out of seven studies showed an association between anxiety and significant memory decline. Three of the five studies that evaluated executive functioning indicated that anxiety is predictive of a decline in executive functioning. The findings on all other cognitive domains were found to be nonsignificant.

B. Anxiety and Risk for Incident Cognitive Impairment.

There were 4 studies with 4155 participants that evaluated the association between anxiety and the risk for incident cognitive impairment. The average methodological quality of the studies was 0.80. The investigators did not find any heterogeneity found among studies. A significant association was noted between anxiety and incident cognitive impairment among community-dwelling individuals [pooled relative risk (RR) = 1.77, $p < 0.001$]. When only studies with adjusted relative risks ($n = 2$) were included, the association remained significant (RR = 1.92, $p < 0.001$). The Population Attributable Risk (PAR) was 6.5% of the risk for incident cognitive impairment that was attributable to anxiety indicating a causal relationship.

C. Anxiety and Risk for Incident Dementia.

There were 6 studies with 6004 participants that evaluated the association between anxiety and the risk for incident dementia. The average methodological quality score for these six studies was 0.75. There was significant heterogeneity noted among the studies. The meta-analysis showed that anxiety was a significant predictor for incident dementia with a RR = 1.57 ($P = 0.040$). The mean age of the study sample had a significant effect on the heterogeneity. The association with anxiety and risk for incident dementia was greater among individuals aged ≥80 years when compared to individuals ≤80 years in age (RR = 2.51 vs 1.23). The two studies with a mean of participants ≥80 years that used clinician-based anxiety scales showed stronger associations with anxiety and incident dementia. The PAR suggested that 7.9% of the risk for dementia was attributable to anxiety with the assumption that anxiety and dementia are causally related. In a meta-analysis of the data from a subgroup analysis of three studies that included individuals with MCI at baseline and had a mean methodological quality of 0.78, the investigators found a nonsignificant risk for anxiety and the development of incident dementia [RR = 1.35; 95% confidence interval (CI), 0.84–2.15; $P = 0.213$].

Objective 2: Data from Memory Clinics

A meta-analysis of the data from 6 studies with 2589 subjects and an average methodological quality of 0.77 found a nonsignificant risk for anxiety and the conversion rate from MCI to dementia in clinical samples [RR = 1.21; 95% CI, 0.90–1.63; $P = 0.200$]. There was significant heterogeneity across the studies, and the heterogeneity was caused by the use of a clinician-rated anxiety scale in one study. It was also noted that the studies that did not use a clinician-rated anxiety scale reported a greater effect for anxiety.

A meta-analysis of the data from 4 studies and 2364 participants that only used adjusted measurements showed a nonsignificant risk for anxiety and the conversion rate from MCI to dementia in clinical samples [RR = 1.16; 95% CI, 0.75–1.81; $P = 0.512$]. There was significant heterogeneity across studies, and the heterogeneity was caused by the use of a clinician-rated anxiety scales and the mean differences of the Mini-Mental State Examination (MMSE). The effect of anxiety was greater in studies with a lower MMSE at baseline when compared to higher MMSE at baseline (RR, 1.47 versus 0.98).

Conclusions The data from this systematic review and meta-analysis indicates that anxiety is associated with a greater risk for incident cognitive impairment and possibly for incident dementia among individuals living in the community. The overall risk for incident cognitive impairment and dementia among community-dwelling individuals that was attributable to anxiety was 6.5% and 7.9%, respectively. Additionally, the association between anxiety and incident dementia appears to be higher among individuals ≥80 years in age. The association between anxiety and cognitive decline among community-dwelling individuals was not identified. Among individuals with MCI, the association between anxiety and the progression to dementia could not be established among individuals evaluated in specialized memory clinics. It remains uncertain whether the association between anxiety and cognition is a result of reverse causality as there was no consistent association between anxiety and cognitive aging.

Strengths of the Study

1. This study provides a comprehensive review of the available literature by including studies that evaluated individuals from both the community and specialized memory clinics.
2. The risk of referral bias was minimized including individuals from the community and specialized memory clinics.
3. There is Quality of Meta-analysis [2]:

   (i) Study question clearly stated: yes.
   (ii) Comprehensive literature search: yes.
   (iii) Complete data abstraction: yes.
   (iv) Appropriate evaluation of results: yes.
   (v) Evaluation for publication bias: yes.
   (vi) Applicability of results: yes.
   (vii) Funding sources/conflicts of results noted: unclear.

Limitations of the Study

1. The number of studies available for the final review is small.
2. Meta-analysis could not be limited to studies reporting fully adjusted relative risk due to limited number of available studies.
3. Studies used different scales to measure symptoms of anxiety resulting in significant heterogeneity between studies.
4. The association between any specific subtype of anxiety and cognitive changes could not be evaluated as the number of studies was small.
5. Only 5 of the 20 articles included in the review were corrected for co-occurring depressive symptoms. Depression is an identified risk factor for the progression of MCI to dementia.

Take-Home Points

1. Anxiety is associated with a greater risk for incident cognitive impairment among individuals living in the community.
2. Anxiety is possibly associated with a greater risk for incident dementia among individuals who live in the community, especially among individuals ≥80 years in age.
3. The association between anxiety and cognitive decline could not be established among individuals living in the community.
4. The association between anxiety and the progression of MCI to dementia could not be established among individuals evaluated in memory clinics.

Practical Applications of the Take-Home Points Clinicians who evaluate older adults for psychiatric symptoms including anxiety should also assess their cognitive functioning as there may be evidence for incident cognitive impairment and dementia among these individuals. It may also be prudent to serially monitor cognition among these individuals so as to detect any progression of cognitive decline.

References

1. Gulpers B, Ramakers I, Hamel R, Köhler S, Oude Voshaar R, Verhey F. Anxiety as a predictor for cognitive decline and dementia: a systematic review and meta-analysis. Am J Geriatr Psychiatry. 2016;24(10):823–42.
2. Russo MW. How to review a meta-analysis. Gastroenterol Hepatol (N Y). 2007;3(8):637–42.

Part III
Bipolar Disorder

Chapter 18
A Pilot Study of Standardized Treatment in Geriatric Bipolar Disorder

Hanadi Ajam Oughli and Kalya Vardi

Authors of the Original Article Ariel G. Gildengers, Benoit H. Mulsant, Amy E. Begley, Mary McShea, Jacqueline A. Stack, Mark D. Miller, Andrea Fagiolini, David J. Kupfer, Robert C. Young, Charles F. Reynolds 3rd.

Journal Publisher *The American Journal of Geriatric Psychiatry.*

Year of Publication 2005.

Type of Study Prospective, open-label, pilot study.

Funding Sources Public Health Service grants, MH19986, MH52247, MH01684, MH01613, and MH067028, and the Commonwealth of Pennsylvania Department of Health grant ME-02385.

Objectives The objective of this study is to assess the feasibility of recruiting, assessing, treating, and monitoring older adults (aged ≥60 years) with a diagnosis of bipolar disorder under standardized treatment conditions [1].

Methods This study recruited subjects by approaching patients aged ≥60 years with bipolar disorder who were either inpatients at the University of Pittsburgh Medical Center (UPMC) Western Psychiatric Institute and Clinic or outpatients at

H. A. Oughli
Department of Psychiatry and Biobehavioral Sciences, University of California Los Angeles, Los Angeles, CA, USA
e-mail: hanadiajamoughli@mednet.ucla.edu

K. Vardi (✉)
UC San Diego School of Medicine, San Diego, CA, USA
e-mail: kvardi@health.ucsd.edu

R. R. Tampi et al. (eds.), *Essential Reviews in Geriatric Psychiatry*,
https://doi.org/10.1007/978-3-030-94960-0_18

the UPMC Intervention Research Center for Late-Life Mood Disorders. The diagnosis of bipolar disorder was then confirmed through the Structured Clinical Interview for the DSM-IV (SCID) which was reviewed by at least three geriatric psychiatrists.

The primary outcome measure was the number of "days well" which was defined as a score of ≤10 on the 17-item Hamilton Rating Scale for Depression (Ham-D-17) and ≤7 on the Young Mania Rating Scale (YMRS). Both measures were administered during the acute, continuation, and maintenance phases of the study. A straight line connected successive assessment points, and any day on the line that was below the cutoff was counted as a "day well." Trough levels of lithium and valproate were measured during each clinical assessment. Medication side effects were evaluated using the UKU Side Effect Rating Scale.

Treatment was divided into the acute, continuation, and maintenance phases. Subjects with "clinically significant mood symptoms" began in the acute phase of treatment and were evaluated weekly by a psychiatrist and a master's-level clinician. Acute treatment continued until remission, defined as Ham-D-17 and YMRS scores ≤10 for 4 consecutive weeks. Subjects subsequently entered the continuation phase for 12 weeks during which evaluations occurred every 2 weeks. Subjects with Ham-D-17 and YMRS scores ≤10 for 12 consecutive weeks entered the maintenance phase of the study, which lasted for 1 year with study visits and mood ratings every 4 weeks. Subjects in the continuation or maintenance phases who developed an acute mood episode could reenter the acute phase and continue in the study for up to 2 years.

Medication adjustment followed protocols modeled after the Systematic Treatment Enhancement Program for Bipolar Disorder (STEP-BD) and included monotherapy with lithium or valproate, or combination therapy. The protocols are not detailed in the article. The authors disclosed that lithium doses ranged between 300 and 900 mg per day and were titrated up to a plasma level of 0.5 mEq/L–1.0 mEq/L. Valproate doses ranged between 500 and 1500 mg per day and were titrated to a plasma level of 40 mcg/ml–100 mcg/ml. One of the goals of the protocols was to minimize antipsychotic and antidepressant use. However, those medications were allowed if deemed clinically necessary by a study psychiatrist.

The intervention did not include manualized psychotherapy, but the treatment took place in a supportive clinic that regularly offered education about bipolar disorder, treatment adherence, sleep hygiene, and partnering with family members. The study did not include any measure of treatment adherence. However, patients who were "grossly noncompliant" were dismissed from the study.

Results Of the 31 patients who consented to the study, 4 participants withdrew consent due to the following reasons: family members' disapproval of research, discontent with investigators' recommendation to discontinue alcohol use, difficulty with transportation, and inconvenience of the study requirements. Two participants died from natural causes (one from cardiac arrest and one from respiratory failure), and two participants were terminated for treatment nonadherence.

The mean age of all participants was 71.9 years. There were 17 female participants recruited into the study. Regarding ethnicity, 28 were Caucasian, 2 were African American, and 1 was Asian. Twenty-three participants had bipolar I and eight participants had bipolar II. The median age of onset was 30 years. Seven participants developed bipolar disorder after the age of 50. The median follow-up period was 398 days (range, 20–735).

The mean modal dose of lithium (n = 17) was 657 mg/day (SD, 376; median, 600; range, 150–1500), and the mean modal serum level was 0.67 mEq/L (SD, 0.24; median, 0.7; range, 0.23–1.0). The mean modal dose of valproate (n = 11) was 806 mg/day (SD, 341; median, 750; range, 250–1500), and the mean modal serum level was 66.1 mcg/ml (SD, 14.8; median, 8.75; range, 2.5–30). Four subjects were treated with risperidone. Three subjects received a combination of lithium and olanzapine. One subject received a combination of lithium, valproate, and olanzapine. Seven subjects received a combination of a mood stabilizer, an atypical antipsychotic, and an antidepressant. In 24 subjects, antidepressant medications were initiated and continued. Subjects took an average of 2.4 mood stabilizers (SD, 1.6), 1.6 antidepressants (SD, 0.9), and 1.3 sedative-hypnotics (SD, 0.5) either sequentially or concurrently.

Upon entering the study, 11 subjects were in an acute episode. Over the entire study, 12 subjects were treated for mania or hypomania, 16 were treated for depression, and 4 were treated for a mixed episode. Twenty-nine participants achieved "recovery" with Ham-D-17 $\leq$ 10 and YMRS $\leq$7 on at least 1 assessment day. Three subjects (10%) were in remission throughout the study. The mean percentage of days well was 72.5% (SD, 23.4). The mean score on the total UKU Side Effect Rating Scale was 9.3 (SD, 3.3). The article did not include any description or analysis of subject-level data.

Conclusions Evidence from this prospective, open-label, pilot study indicated that it is feasible to recruit, assess, treat, and monitor older adults with bipolar disorder in a standardized treatment study. The results also suggest that lithium and valproate are beneficial and tolerable treatments for bipolar disorder in older adults. While the mean percentage of days well was 72.5%, only 10% of subjects experienced sustained recovery.

Strengths of the Study

1. This is a prospective trial.
2. It has few exclusion criteria.
3. This study demonstrated the feasibility of assessing standardized medication treatment protocols in older adults with bipolar disorder.
4. It highlights the morbidity of bipolar disorder in older adults and the need for more research.

Limitations of the Study

1. This study had a small sample size.
2. The study population lacked racial diversity.

3. There was no formal assessment of medication adherence.
4. There were no clear recommendations of how to optimize study protocols in a larger trial.

Take-Home Points This is a prospective, open-label, pilot study [2] that demonstrates the feasibility of studying standardized medication treatment protocols in older adults with bipolar disorder. It suggests that while lithium and valproate are beneficial and tolerable treatments, many older adults with bipolar disorder do not achieve sustained remission.

Practical Applications of the Take-Home Point Standardized treatment studies for older adults with bipolar disorder are feasible and necessary to improve clinical outcomes for these patients.

References

1. Bowden CL, Perlis RH, Thase ME, Ketter TA, Ostacher MM, Calabrese JR, Reilly-Harrington NA, Gonzalez JM, Singh V, Nierenberg AA, Sachs GS. Aims and results of the NIMH systematic treatment enhancement program for bipolar disorder (STEP-BD). CNS Neurosci Ther. 2012;18(3):243–9.
2. Kistin C, Silverstein M. Pilot studies: a critical but potentially misused component of interventional research. JAMA. 2015;314(15):1561–2.

Chapter 19
Differences in Clinical Features and Mental Health Service Use in Bipolar Disorder Across the Life Span

Colin M. Smith and Kristin McArthur

Authors of the Original Article Colin A. Depp, Ph.D.; Laurie A. Lindamer, Ph.D.; David P. Folsom, M.D.; Todd Gilmer, Ph.D.; Richard L. Hough, Ph.D.; Piedad Garcia, Ed.D.; Dilip V. Jeste, M.D.

Journal Publisher *The American Journal of Geriatric Psychiatry.*

Year of Publication 2005.

Type of Study A retrospective cross-sectional study.

Funding Sources The National Institute of Mental Health and Department of Veterans Affairs.

Objectives To determine the prevalence, clinical features, and mental health service use of older adults (60 years or older) treated in a large public mental health system [1].

Methods This study analyzed data from 2903 individuals in the San Diego County's Adult and Older-Adult Mental Health Services (AOAMHS) database from 1999 to 2003. Patients were included if they were diagnosed with bipolar I disorder, bipolar II disorder, bipolar disorder not otherwise specified, or cyclothymia (DSM-IV) [2] by a treating clinician and received at least one service from 2002 to

C. M. Smith
Duke University School of Medicine, Durham, NC, USA
e-mail: Colin.smith@duke.edu

K. McArthur (✉)
Psychiatry, Durham VA Medical Center, Durham, NC, USA
e-mail: Kristin.mcarthur@va.gov

R. R. Tampi et al. (eds.), *Essential Reviews in Geriatric Psychiatry*,
https://doi.org/10.1007/978-3-030-94960-0_19

2003. Exclusion criteria included patients who received a diagnosis of schizophrenia from 2002 to 2003 and those who resided in justice-related settings.

Demographic variables were age (categorized into a young adult group (age 18–39), middle-aged group (age 40–59), or elderly group (age 60 and older)), gender, ethnicity, language preference, education, marital status, and living situation. Clinical variables included the presence of any substance use disorder, cognitive use disorder, and Global Assessment of Functioning (GAF) scores averaged across admissions from all services received. Mental health service utilization was defined as the presence or absence of at least one visit to any mental health service (inpatient psychiatric hospitalization, crisis residential, emergency psychiatric unit, outpatient clinic, psychiatric emergency response team, or case management) from 2002 to 2003.

The investigators determined the prevalence of bipolar disorder across the three defined age groups from 1999 to 2000, 2000 to 2001, 2001 to 2002, and 2002 to 2003 and examined the demographic, clinical, and mental health service use variables in the 2002–2003 data set. The authors compared the demographic and clinical characteristics across the three age groups using two-tailed chi-square tests for categorical variables, analysis of variance for continuous variables, and Tukey's honestly significant difference tests in post hoc pairwise comparison of variables. They also used logistic regression analyses to determine the odds of using a particular mental health service while controlling for variables that significantly differed between elderly and younger groups (substance use disorder, independent living status, and GAF score).

Results Of 34,970 patients who received at least one mental health service during 2002–2003, 2903 (8.3%) were diagnosed with bipolar disorder. The elderly (age ≥ 60) accounted for only 9.2% of these cases (consistent from 1999 to 2003), while young and middle-aged adults comprised 46.1% and 44.7% of cases, respectively. The proportion of patients with bipolar disorder receiving care compared to the total number of patients receiving care from 2002 to 2003 was lower among the elderly (7.0%) when compared to middle-aged (8.7%) or younger groups (8.3%) ($\chi^2 = 35.7$; $P < 0.001$).

Elderly patients who received mental health services were less likely to have a substance use disorder (8.3%) when compared to young adults (37.6%) or middle-aged adults (27.8%) ($\chi^2 = 97.9$; $P < 0.001$). However, this same group was more likely to have a cognitive disorder (2.3%) when compared to younger groups (0.2%) ($\chi^2 = 24.1$; $P < 0.001$) and have lower GAF admission score (elderly, 39.6; young adult, 43; middle-aged adult, 42; $F^2 = 7.9$; $P < 0.001$).

Logistic regression found that when controlling for substance use and cognitive disorder diagnoses, independent living status, and GAF, elderly adults with bipolar disorder were less likely to use inpatient (adjusted odds ratio (aOR) = 0.26 (0.14–0.49), $P < 0.001$), outpatient (aOR = 0.43 (0.20–0.063), $P < 0.001$), and emergency psychiatric services (aOR = 0.46 (0.29–0.72), $P < 0.001$) when compared to younger adults. However, elderly adults with bipolar disorder were more than twice as likely (aOR = 2.07 (1.52–2.82), $P < 0.001$) to use case management services than their younger counterparts.

Conclusions Bipolar disorder is slightly less common among adults older than 60 years receiving public mental health services when compared to younger adults. Older adults with bipolar disorders are more likely to have cognitive disorder, functional impairment, and use case management services but are less likely to have substance use disorder and use acute care services.

Strengths of the Study

1. It has relatively large sample size of older adults with bipolar disorder when compared to previous studies.
2. Data is from large public mental health database, allowing comparisons across age groups.

Limitations of the Study

1. Cross-sectional study design limits ability to make inferences about changes over time.
2. Diagnoses were extracted from chart and not confirmed by structured clinical interview.
3. The use of a public mental health data set may miss older adults with private insurance.
4. The use of GAF scores for substance use and cognitive disorder diagnoses has unclear reliability and validity, as these were extracted from chart review.
5. Differences in GAF scores do not account for differences in service use by age.
6. Study population in San Diego is largely urban and limits ability to generalize to other populations.

Take-Home Points Despite limitations, this cross-sectional study with a relatively large sample size of adults in a public mental health system suggests that bipolar disorders are fairly common in adults older than 60 years of age. This population has unique clinical features and decreased acute psychiatric service utilization when compared to younger adults.

Practical Applications of the Take-Home Points Providers should recognize that bipolar disorders are fairly common among older adults and that comorbid cognitive disorders and reduced functioning may be more common in this population when compared to younger adults with bipolar disorder.

References

1. Depp CA, Lindamer LA, Folsom DP, Gilmer T, Hough RL, Garcia P, Jeste DV. Differences in clinical features and mental health service use in bipolar disorder across the lifespan. Am J Geriatr Psychiatry. 2005;13(4):290–8.
2. First M, Williams J, Spitzer R. Structured clinical interview for DSM-IV Axis I disorders. Washington, DC: American Psychiatric Association Press; 1997.

Chapter 20
Effect of Antidepressant Use on Admissions to Hospital Among Elderly Bipolar Patients

Christopher Morrow and Sophia Wang

Authors Ayal Schaffer, Muhammad Mamdani, Anthony Levitt, Nathan Herrmann.

Journal *International Journal of Geriatric Psychiatry.*

Year 2006.

Type of Study Population-based retrospective cohort design.

Funding Source None.

Objectives The purpose of this study was to determine the effect of antidepressant use among an older population of patients with bipolar disorder by examining the association between antidepressant prescriptions and hospitalizations for mania/mixed or depressive episodes in a large community-based sample [1].

Methods Patient Population: Using large administrative healthcare databases from Ontario, Canada, subjects aged 66 years or older were selected on the basis of having a primary or secondary hospital diagnosis of a manic, mixed, or bipolar depressive episode between January 1, 1992, and March 31, 2001. Subjects were also included if they received a prescription for lithium without a concurrent prescription for an antidepressant during the same time period.

C. Morrow
Division of Geriatric Psychiatry and Neuropsychiatry, Department of Psychiatry and Behavioral Sciences, Johns Hopkins School of Medicine, Baltimore, MD, USA
e-mail: cmorrow3@jhmi.edu

S. Wang (✉)
Indiana University School of Medicine, Department of Psychiatry, Indianapolis, IN, USA

Indiana Alzheimer's Disease Research Center, Indianapolis, IN, USA
e-mail: sophwang@iupui.edu

R. R. Tampi et al. (eds.), *Essential Reviews in Geriatric Psychiatry*,
https://doi.org/10.1007/978-3-030-94960-0_20

An antidepressant cohort consisting of 1072 individuals was defined from within the population of eligible bipolar subjects if a prescription for an antidepressant was received between April 1, 1997, and March 31, 2001. A control group of 3000 subjects was randomly selected from the eligible bipolar patient population who had not received a prescription for an antidepressant during the same time period. The primary outcome measure was admission to a hospital with a primary discharge diagnosis of a manic/mixed or depressive episode.

Statistical Methods Time-to-event analyses were conducted for hospital admissions with a primary diagnosis of a manic/mixed or depressive episode using Cox proportional hazard models with the control group as a reference. Covariates included demographic factors, psychiatric comorbidity, and medical comorbidities.

Results Demographics: The antidepressant cohort and control group did not appear to differ significantly with regard to age, sex, or income status. The antidepressant cohort did have a higher proportion of patients in long-term care facilities with 26% residing in long-term care when compared to 16% in the control group. The antidepressant cohort also showed a higher proportion of patients with recent psychiatric hospitalizations for mania/mixed episodes with 6.8% having a psychiatric hospitalization in the last 3 months compared to only 0.6% in the control group. In addition, lithium and valproic acid use were more common in the control group with 16.4% of controls being on either lithium or valproic acid when compared to only 8.1% of the antidepressant cohort.

Antidepressant Use Within the antidepressant cohort, selective serotonin reuptake inhibitors (SSRI) were the most commonly prescribed antidepressants comprising 68% of antidepressant prescriptions followed by tricyclic antidepressants (TCA) at 10%, serotonin and norepinephrine reuptake inhibitors (SNRI) at 10%, and other antidepressants (bupropion, moclobemide, nefazodone, and trazodone) compromising 12%. Sertraline was the most common antidepressant prescribed comprising 26% of antidepressant prescriptions.

Psychiatric Admissions During the study period, there were 113 admissions for a manic/mixed episode and 28 admissions for a depressive episode. The antidepressant cohort had fewer hospitalizations for mania/mixed episodes with 16 admissions when compared to 97 admissions in the control group. This difference was statistically significant with an adjusted rate ratio of 0.5 and a 95% confidence interval of 0.3–0.8.

The antidepressant cohort also had fewer admissions for depression with <5 admissions when compared to 24 admissions in the control group; however, this did not reach statistical significance with an adjusted rate ratio of 0.7 and a 95% confidence interval of 0.2–2.2. Admission numbers less than or equal to 5 were reported simply as <5 to ensure patient privacy.

Conclusions Evidence from this population-based retrospective cohort study suggests that elderly patients with bipolar disorder who are prescribed an antidepressant do not appear to be at higher risk of being hospitalized for mania/mixed episodes and may in fact be less likely to be hospitalized than elderly bipolar patients not prescribed an antidepressant.

Strengths of the Study This study used large administrative databases which tend to be highly reliable, accurate, and authentic sources of data. The study also captured all individuals aged 66 years or older in the Province of Ontario, Canada, who met eligibility criteria constituting a relatively large and diverse sample of patients with bipolar disorder. In addition, the control group was randomly selected from the population as a whole which further adds to the quality of the analysis. Furthermore, the study included a naturalistic design spanning several years which likely allowed the true course of patients' mood episodes to be observed. The statistical model also controlled for common demographic, psychiatric, and medical comorbidities decreasing the risk of confounding variables influencing the findings.

Limitations of the Study Since this is a retrospective cohort study, the conclusions are primarily hypothesis generating, and this cannot be used to make definitive conclusions about the use of antidepressants in older patients with bipolar disorder – a large randomized controlled trial would be necessary for this. It is also not clear that the results of this study generalize outside the population studied. Access to universal health care including prescription drugs and hospital admissions is not available in many countries outside of Canada which may limit the applicability of the findings in non-Canadian populations. Additional limitations include the use of the administrative databases to establish diagnoses as opposed to using structured clinical interviews. This may have led to the inclusion of patients without a true diagnosis of bipolar disorder. Furthermore, patients prescribed mood stabilizers other than lithium who had not received a recent admission diagnosis of a manic/mixed or depressive episode may not have been included in the population as only those on lithium monotherapy were included. There was also no indication as to whether those patients prescribed an antidepressant were also on a mood stabilizer which obscures the interpretation of the findings and makes it difficult to adapt them into clinical practice. In addition, only medication dispensing patterns were measured as opposed to true medication adherence. There were also no drug levels reported for patients on lithium or valproic acid which makes it difficult to ascertain the therapeutic impact of these drugs on the study population. Finally, only primary discharge diagnoses were used which may have led to missed hospitalizations where mania/mixed or depressive episodes were not the primary diagnosis.

Take-Home Points The use of antidepressants in patients with bipolar disorder has been a long-standing source of controversy in psychiatry with the risk of inducing a switch from depression to hypomania or mania being the primary concern. Observations that antidepressants may have the potential to precipitate abnormal mood elevation in certain patients occurred as early as the 1950s [2, 3]. More modern studies have confirmed these early observations and established a compelling body of evidence that antidepressant use, particularly without a mood stabilizer, is associated with an increased risk of mania in bipolar disorder [4–10].

Despite this body of evidence, however, there have been few studies examining the impact of antidepressant use in older populations with bipolar disorder. Recommendations for treatment of bipolar disorder in the aging population have largely been extrapolated from guidelines in the general adult population despite the fact that geriatric patients often have many unique characteristics including changes in physiology and pharmacokinetics. This study provides evidence that it may be safe to prescribe antidepressants to older patients with bipolar disorder and that rather than increasing their risk of mood instability, it may actually help prevent psychiatric hospitalizations for manic/mixed episodes. The reason for this observation is not entirely clear but may be due to differential neurobiology in the aging brain.

Practical Applications of the Take-Home Points The use of antidepressants in older populations of patients with bipolar disorder appears safe and is not associated with an increased risk of hospitalization for manic/mixed episodes. Further study is needed, however, to confirm this finding and to explore potential reasons underlying the differential risk of antidepressant use in older patients with bipolar disorder compared to younger patients.

References

1. Schaffer A, Mamdani M, Levitt A, Herrmann N. Effect of antidepressant use on admissions to hospital among elderly bipolar patients. Int J Geriatr Psychiatry. 2006;21(3):275–80.
2. Ball JR, Kiloh LG. A controlled trial of imipramine in treatment of depressive states. Br Med J. 1959;2(5159):1052–5.
3. Leyberg JT, Denmark JC. The treatment of depressive states with imipramine hydrochloride (tofranil). J Ment Sci. 1959;105:1123–6.
4. Viktorin A, Lichtenstein P, Thase ME, Larsson H, Lundholm C, Magnusson PK, et al. The risk of switch to mania in patients with bipolar disorder during treatment with an antidepressant alone and in combination with a mood stabilizer. Am J Psychiatry. 2014;171(10):1067–73.
5. Altshuler LL, Post RM, Leverich GS, Mikalauskas K, Rosoff A, Ackerman L. Antidepressant-induced mania and cycle acceleration: a controversy revisited. Am J Psychiatry. 1995;152(8):1130–8.
6. Boerlin HL, Gitlin MJ, Zoellner LA, Hammen CL. Bipolar depression and antidepressant-induced mania: a naturalistic study. J Clin Psychiatry. 1998;59(7):374–9.
7. Goldberg JF, Truman CJ. Antidepressant-induced mania: an overview of current controversies. Bipolar Disord. 2003;5(6):407–20.
8. Peet M. Induction of mania with selective serotonin re-uptake inhibitors and tricyclic antidepressants. Br J Psychiatry. 1994;164(4):549–50.

9. Prien RF, Klett CJ, Caffey EM. Lithium carbonate and imipramine in prevention of affective episodes. A comparison in recurrent affective illness. Arch Gen Psychiatry. 1973;29(3):420–5.
10. Truman CJ, Goldberg JF, Ghaemi SN, Baldassano CF, Wisniewski SR, Dennehy EB, et al. Self-reported history of manic/hypomanic switch associated with antidepressant use: data from the Systematic Treatment Enhancement Program for Bipolar Disorder (STEP-BD). J Clin Psychiatry. 2007;68(10):1472–9.

Chapter 21
GERI-BD: A Randomized Double-Blind Controlled Trial of Lithium and Divalproex in the Treatment of Mania in Older Patients with Bipolar Disorder

Mohamed A. Soliman and Susan W. Lehmann

Authors of the Original Article Robert C. Young, M.D.; Benoit H. Mulsant, M.D., M.S.; Martha Sajatovic, M.D.; Ariel G. Gildengers, M.D.; Laszlo Gyulai, M.D.; Rayan K. Al Jurdi, M.D.; John Beyer, M.D.; Jovier Evans, Ph.D.; Samprit Banerjee, Ph.D.; Rebecca Greenberg, M.S.; Patricia Marino, Ph.D.; Mark E. Kunik, M.D.; Peijun Chen, M.D., Ph.D.; Marna Barrett, Ph.D.; Herbert C. Schulberg, Ph.D.; Martha L. Bruce, Ph.D., M.P.H.; Charles F. Reynolds III, M.D.; George S. Alexopoulos, M.D., for the GERI-BD Study Group.

Journal Publisher *The American Journal of Psychiatry.*

Year of Publication 2017.

Type of Study Randomized placebo-controlled trial.

Funding Sources National Institutes of Health (NIH). Janssen Scientific Affairs provided risperidone to some sites in the study.

Objectives To determine the efficacy and the tolerability of lithium and divalproex for the treatment of acute late-life mania in patients aged 60 or older with bipolar I disorder from a double-blind, randomized, placebo-controlled trial [1].

M. A. Soliman
University of Michigan Department of Psychiatry, Ann Arbor, MI, USA
e-mail: mas873@cornell.edu

S. W. Lehmann (✉)
Johns Hopkins University School of Medicine, Baltimore, MD, USA
e-mail: slehman@jhmi.edu

R. R. Tampi et al. (eds.), *Essential Reviews in Geriatric Psychiatry*,
https://doi.org/10.1007/978-3-030-94960-0_21

Methods This study recruited 224 subjects who met eligibility criteria from 6 academic centers; 50% were initially inpatients, and 50% were outpatients.

Participants were 60 years or older (mean age 68); met DSM-IV criteria for bipolar I disorder with a current manic, mixed, or hypomanic episode as assessed by the SCID scale; and had a score ≥18 on the Young Mania Rating Scale (YMRS).

Exclusion criteria for this study were as follows: diagnosis of schizophrenia, schizoaffective disorder, or delusional disorder; diagnosis of delirium or dementia or other brain degenerative diseases; mood disorder due to a general medical condition (e.g., recent stroke, hyperthyroidism, porphyria, HIV, connective tissue diseases) or to a substance (e.g., steroids, L-dopa); active substance dependence or other substance-related safety issues; rapid cycling bipolar disorder; sensory impairment preventing participation in research assessments; high risk for suicide (in ambulatory patients); history of intolerance to lithium (at a concentration <1.0 mEq/L), divalproex (with a valproate concentration <100 μg/mL), lorazepam, or risperidone; any contraindications to lithium or divalproex; inability to communicate in English; and current episode that had failed to respond to at least 4 weeks of treatment with lithium (at a concentration ≥0.4 mEq/L) or divalproex (at a valproate concentration ≥40 μg/mL). The most frequent reasons for exclusion from the study were a low YMRS score or a major depressive episode.

Study participants were randomly assigned under double-blind conditions on a 1:1 basis to receive lithium or divalproex. Permuted-block randomization used random block sizes ranging from four to eight consecutive patients by the site.

Antidepressants and other non-study medications were tapered off to establish whether manic symptoms resolved with their discontinuation. Baseline assessments included the YMRS, Structured Clinical Interview for DSM Disorders (SCID), Montgomery-Asberg Depression Rating Scale (MADRS) and UKU Side Effect Rating Scale, physical examination, and laboratory studies.

Dosages were started 300 mg/day for lithium and 500 mg/day for divalproex and titrated to achieve target serum concentrations of 0.80–0.99 mEq/L of lithium or 80–99 μg/mL of valproate. Lithium or divalproex was given in over-encapsulated pills twice daily. During the course of the 9-week study, trough concentrations were determined 10–14 hours after the last dose on treatment days 4, 9, 15, and 21, at weeks 6 and 9, and more frequently if indicated and titration to the target ranges was carried out regardless of mood improvement. Dosing was reduced if serum concentrations exceeded the target range; if significant side effects occurred, e.g., tremor interfering with self-care, ataxic gait, excessive sedation, or heart rate <50 bpm; or if the blinded research psychiatrist had other concerns. It is to be noted that lithium and divalproex dosages were adjusted in patients who had to continue taking nonsteroidal anti-inflammatory agents or thiazide diuretics for comorbid medical conditions.

The investigators decided to allow the use of rescue or adjunctive medications. Lorazepam was used up to 3 mg/day during the first 3 weeks of treatment only when anxiety, agitation, or insomnia was significant and not responsive to behavioral interventions. Oral risperidone was used up to twice a day for up to 3 days in any week only in patients where anxiety, agitation, or insomnia did not respond to behavioral intervention and lorazepam. Oral risperidone, up to 4 mg/day, was used after week 3 for an inadequate response to lithium or divalproex, defined as a YMRS score ≥16 (lorazepam was tapered off).

The research medication was discontinued, and the participant terminated the study if adverse effects of lithium or divalproex persisted despite a dosage reduction. These included inability to tolerate at least 0.40 mEq/L of lithium or 40 μg/mL of valproate, delirium, platelet count below 80,000, elevation in serum glutamic oxaloacetic transaminase (SGOT), serum glutamic-pyruvic transaminase (SGPT), or amylase twofold or more above the upper limit of normal or diabetes insipidus. Participants also terminated the study if they were nonadherent to study procedures or medications, withdrew consent, had a serious adverse event, had an increase in YMRS score >40% above baseline, or developed major depression and had a score ≥18 on the 21-item Hamilton Depression Rating Scale on 2 successive assessments or needed antidepressant treatment.

The primary clinical tolerability measure in this study was the sleepiness/sedation item of the UKU Side Effect Rating Scale; the primary pharmacologic tolerability measure was the proportion of participants in each group who achieved serum concentrations within the target range, and the primary efficacy measure was the change in YMRS score. The analysis for primary outcome measures was based on the intent-to-treat principle with a generalized linear mixed model for continuous and binary or multinomial longitudinal responses. The site was included as a covariate in the model. Post hoc tests were conducted for each outcome on the chosen mixed model to test group differences at weeks 3 and 9.

Results The 224 randomized participants did not differ in their demographic and clinical characteristics between the two treatment groups. In the lithium treatment group, 55 out of 112 completed the study; in the divalproex treatment group, 63 out of 112 subjects completed the study.

Attrition rates were similar between lithium and divalproex groups (14% and 18% at week 3 and 51% and 44% at week 9, respectively). Similarly, the reasons for attrition did not differ significantly between groups: refusal/nonadherence, 28.1% and 42.9% in the lithium and divalproex groups, respectively; inability to tolerate the protocol, 38.6% and 26.5%; clinical worsening/lack of efficacy, 24.6% and 18.4%; and administrative/others, 8.8% and 12.2% in the lithium and divalproex groups, respectively.

There was no significant difference between the treatment groups in the primary tolerability measure, i.e., change in sleepiness/sedation. Comparable proportions of participants in the lithium and divalproex groups achieved target concentrations at week 3 (35.1% and 32.6%, respectively) and week 9 (57.1% and 56.3%, respectively). Odds of needing rescue lorazepam or adjunctive risperidone did not differ significantly between groups (60.7% and 50.9% in the lithium and divalproex groups, respectively; odds ratio (OR) = 1.49; 95% CI = 0.88, 2.5). After day 28, twice as many subjects receiving divalproex as those on lithium required daily lorazepam (20% vs. 10%). Of note, participants randomized to lithium tended to experience more tremors.

Lithium, however, was associated with stronger reduction in YMRS scores by 1.57 at week 3 ($d = 0.18$, 97.5% CI = −0.05, 0.60) and 3.90 at week 9 ($d = 0.54$, 97.5% CI = 0.32, 1.15). Subjects with a baseline YMRS score >30 in the lithium group had a greater reduction in YMRS score than in the divalproex group at week 3 and week 9. No difference in YMRS score reductions was seen between the two groups in participants who had a baseline YMRS score <30. Among all participants, the reduction of at least 50% in YMRS score was not statistically significant between the two groups at week 3 (62.5% for lithium group and 57.1% for divalproex group, adjusted odds ratio (aOR) = 0.78, $P = 0.37$) and at week 9 (78.6% for lithium group and 73.2% for divalproex group, aOR = 0.72, $P = 0.31$). The cumulative rates of remission, defined as a YMRS score ≤9, were not statistically significant between the lithium and the divalproex groups at week 3 (45.5% for lithium group and 43.8% for divalproex group; aOR = 0.91, $P = 0.74$) and at week 9 (69.6% for lithium group and 63.4% for divalproex group; aOR = 0.73, $P = 0.29$). Neither lithium nor divalproex was associated with increased ratings for depressive symptoms during this study.

Conclusions Evidence from this 9-week randomized, double-blind, and placebo-controlled study indicates that both lithium and divalproex were adequately tolerated and efficacious for the treatment of mania in patients aged 60 and older with bipolar I disorder. Lithium was associated with a greater reduction in mania severity rating scores on the YMRS over the 9 weeks.

Strengths of the Study

1. Study design is randomized, double-blind, and placebo-controlled.
2. The study assessed based on Jadad score indicates that this was a high-quality study with a score of 5 out of 5.

Questions Yes (1) No (0)	Was the study described as random?	Was the randomization scheme described and appropriate?	Was the study described as double-blind?	Was the method of double-blinding appropriate? (Were both the patient and the assessor appropriately blinded?)	Was there a description of dropouts and withdrawals?	Total score Range of score quality 0–2, low 3–5, high
Score	1	1	1	1	1	5

3. The study sample included only older adults (≥60 years).
4. The use of reasonably large and random block size reduced the potential for bias that could occur if treatment assignments became known or predictable, which is a common problem with fixed block size RCTs.

5. Despite the very high attrition rate in this study, the rates were similar to those reported in studies of younger patients with mania [2].
6. The study findings are in line with recent literature that found that lithium monotherapy was associated with remission in 42% of older participants (STEP-BD) study [3].
7. The reported greater efficacy for lithium compared to divalproex is congruent with the findings in the BALANCE study, where lithium was associated with statistically lower relapse rates [4].
8. The study used lower dosages and lower serum level targets (<1 mEq/L for lithium and <100 μg/mL for divalproex) than the ones conventionally used in studies (0.80–1.20 mEq/L for lithium and 80–120 μg/mL for valproate). Yet, the rates of response were not inferior [5]. This is of special consideration given that optimal serum concentrations for older adults with bipolar disorder have not been delineated.
9. The authors adjusted for several confounding factors that could have accounted for the similar attrition rates between lithium and divalproex. These included analysis of the time of attrition and distribution of reasons for attrition, which were similar between the two groups.
10. The authors adjusted for age and medical burden as potential confounding factors behind the observed similar rates of completing the study between the two groups. Using the Cumulative Illness Rating Scale-Geriatric, the rates of 9-week study completion did not differ between treatment groups based on age or medical burden.

Limitations of the Study

1. There was a 52% completion rate for the study – only 118 participants completed the study out of 224 participants.
2. The study inclusion criteria excluded participants with a current diagnosis of schizophrenia or schizoaffective disorder. It also excluded participants with a diagnosis of dementia, or substance use disorder.
3. A relatively large number of potential participants were excluded (1830 out of 2403) because of safety concerns.
4. No placebo group was included. This would have controlled for confounding factors related to observed improvements other than the study medications.
5. The study had a limited duration of 9 weeks. The findings might not be generalizable regarding the long-term tolerability and efficacy of lithium or divalproex in elders with bipolar disorder.
6. Thirty-four percent of subjects (74 out of 224) included in the final analysis had a psychotic mood state during the 9-week treatment. The reduction of YMRS score in these groups could be partly attributed to adjunctive risperidone treatment rather than lithium or divalproex alone.
7. Eighty-seven percent of the participants were Caucasian, 11% were African American, and 2% were Asian. This might not be representative of the normal distribution of bipolar I among the different races in the country.

Take-Home Points This high-quality randomized, double-blind, and placebo-controlled study found that both lithium and divalproex at conservative serum concentrations were substantially effective for mania in patients age 60 and older and had similar tolerability and efficacy outcomes. Lithium more effectively reduced the severity of reported manic symptoms over 9 weeks. This study is the first randomized controlled trial of the treatment of late-life mania. So far, it is the only head-to-head trial comparing any two agents in the treatment of mania in the geriatric population.

Practical Applications of the Take-Home Points Both lithium and divalproex could be used as first-line agents in the treatment of older patients with mania. Either agent as monotherapy should be considered before combination treatment with antipsychotics such as quetiapine or olanzapine, which are associated with premature mortality in older patients [6]. Lithium's anti-suicidal and potentially neuroprotective properties should also be taken into consideration when selecting a first-line agent for older patients with bipolar disorder [7].

References

1. Young RC, Mulsant BH, Sajatovic M, Gildengers AG, Gyulai L, Al Jurdi RK, Beyer J, Evans J, Banerjee S, Greenberg R, Marino P, Kunik ME, Chen P, Barrett M, Schulberg HC, Bruce ML, Reynolds CF 3rd, Alexopoulos GS, GERI-BD Study Group. GERI-BD: a randomized double-blind controlled trial of lithium and divalproex in the treatment of mania in older patients with bipolar disorder. Am J Psychiatry. 2017;174(11):1086–93.
2. Hirschfeld RM, Bowden CL, Vigna NV, Wozniak P, Collins M. A randomized, placebo-controlled, multicenter study of divalproex sodium extended-release in the acute treatment of mania. J Clin Psychiatry. 2010;71(4):426–32.
3. Al Jurdi RK, Marangell LB, Petersen NJ, Martinez M, Gyulai L, Sajatovic M. Prescription patterns of psychotropic medications in elderly compared with younger participants who achieved a "recovered" status in the systematic treatment enhancement program for bipolar disorder. Am J Geriatr Psychiatry. 2008;16(11):922–33.
4. BALANCE Investigators and Collaborators, Geddes JR, Goodwin GM, Rendell J, Azorin JM, Cipriani A, Ostacher MJ, Morriss R, Alder N, Juszczak E. Lithium plus valproate combination therapy versus monotherapy for relapse prevention in bipolar I disorder (BALANCE): a randomised open-label trial. Lancet. 2010;375(9712):385–95.
5. Bowden CL, Brugger AM, Swann AC, Calabrese JR, Janicak PG, Petty F, Dilsaver SC, Davis JM, Rush AJ, Small JG, et al. Efficacy of divalproex vs lithium and placebo in the treatment of mania. The Depakote Mania Study Group. JAMA. 1994;271(12):918–24.
6. Ray WA, Chung CP, Murray KT, Hall K, Stein CM. Atypical antipsychotic drugs and the risk of sudden cardiac death. N Engl J Med. 2009;360(3):225–35.
7. Cipriani A, Hawton K, Stockton S, Geddes JR. Lithium in the prevention of suicide in mood disorders: updated systematic review and meta-analysis. BMJ. 2013;346:f3646.

Chapter 22
History of Bipolar Disorder and the Risk of Dementia: A Systematic Review and Meta-Analysis

Vahid Pasovic, Adan Aslam Khan, Andrew Wong, and Esther Akinyemi

Authors of the Original Article Breno S Diniz, Antonio L Teixeira, Fei Cao, Ariel Gildengers, Jair C Soares, Meryl A Butters, Charles F Reynolds 3rd.

Journal Publisher *The American Journal of Geriatric Psychiatry.*

Year of Publication 2017.

Type of Study Systemic review and meta-analysis.

Funding Sources Supported in part by NIMH (P50 AG005133, P30 MH090333) and the UPMC Endowment in Geriatric Psychiatry.

Objectives To evaluate whether a history of BD increases the risk of dementia in older adults [1].

Methods The authors used the Preferred Reporting Items for Systematic Reviews and Meta-Analyses (PRISMA) guidelines for conducting and reporting this systematic review. They searched PubMed and Scopus databases for potentially relevant studies of BD and dementia risk. Literature search was conducted in June 2016 using bipolar disorder and dementia as broad terms with the search criteria limited to papers published in the English language after January 1, 1980. The references of the selected papers were also searched for additional studies.

Study selection and data extraction for statistical analysis were carried out via two independent authors' review with a third author serving as a tiebreaker in cases of disagreement. Potential abstracts/papers for inclusion were assessed for quality

V. Pasovic · A. A. Khan · A. Wong · E. Akinyemi (✉)
Henry Ford Health System, Detroit, MI, USA
e-mail: vpasovi1@hfhs.org; EAkinye2@hfhs.org

R. R. Tampi et al. (eds.), *Essential Reviews in Geriatric Psychiatry*,
https://doi.org/10.1007/978-3-030-94960-0_22

using the Newcastle-Ottawa Scale (NOS) [2] with studies for data extraction selected based on three pre-defined criteria following review of references. These criteria included cohort, case-control, or case registry study; identification of BD and control/comparison group; and report of dementia cases in the BD and control groups. A pooled risk of dementia in BD subjects when compared to control subjects was calculated by extracting the number of individuals with dementia from each study and in each diagnostic group. This was organized in a 2×2 Table (BD with dementia, BD without dementia, control with dementia, control without dementia).

The study authors used comprehensive meta-analysis software v2 for Windows. DerSimonian and Laird random effects method were used to calculate pooled odds ratio of dementia in patients with BD given the evidence of high heterogeneity among included studies in the analysis. Sensitivity analysis was conducted using the leave-one-out method to evaluate whether each individual study significantly influenced the pooled odds ratio. Visual inspection of funnel plot and classic fail-safe N analysis was used to evaluate for publication bias.

Results A total of 1656 papers were selected for review. Of these 1640 were excluded for the following reasons: literature reviews (529), letters or case reports (379), and papers in which dementia risk was not the main outcome (732). Of the 16 full-text articles assessed for eligibility, 10 were excluded for the following reasons: inappropriate methodology (8) or overlapping sample (2). This resulted in a total of 6 studies included in the meta-analysis consisting of a pooled total of 194,055 subjects (3026 individuals with a history of BD and 191,029 individuals without a history of BD).

The prevalence rate of BD in the pooled sample was 1.5%. This rate is similar to what is usually observed among population-based epidemiological studies. The investigators noted significant heterogeneity among the various studies ($P < 0.001$; $I^2 = 93\%$). The pooled odds ratio (OR) of dementia in individuals with BD was 2.36 and 95% CI 1.36–4.09. No single study appeared to significantly influence the analysis. There was no significant publication bias noted on the classic fail-safe N analysis ($z = 11.6$; $P < 0.001$).

Conclusions The investigators concluded that a history of BD is associated with significantly increased risk of dementia diagnosis among older adults.

Strengths of the Study

1. The investigators followed the PRISMA guidelines in conducting and reporting this systemic review.
2. The investigators controlled for outliers with potential proportional effect on findings using the "leave-one-out" method of statistical analysis.
3. The study had a large sample size.
4. There was evaluation for publication bias using visual inspection of funnel plot and classic fail-safe N analysis.

Limitations of the Study

1. The investigators included registry-based studies of moderate methodological quality in the data extraction.
2. Rigorous control was not exercised in the collection of data including how the diagnoses of BD and dementia were made.
3. There were different definitions used for BD and dementia.
4. There was a lack of information about potential confounders.
5. Interpretation of results was limited by inability to carry out analysis with specific dementia diagnosis.
6. The investigators did not control for important variables that could potentially impact the risk for developing dementia including the number of manic or depressive episodes, the age of onset of BD, and the presence of medical and/or psychiatric comorbidities.
7. The investigators did not control for exposure to mood-stabilizing agents including lithium which appears to have a neuroprotective effect by modulating beta-amyloid and tau protein metabolism.

Take-Home Points This study provides robust evidence that BD increases the risk for dementia among older adults. It is prudent to screen for cognitive disorders among individuals with BD.

Practical Applications of the Take-Home Point Efforts should be made to optimize cognition in patients with BD. This could include the use of medications that are considered to have neuroprotective effects including lithium. Additionally, the care of patients with bipolar disorder should include routine screening for cognitive impairment.

References

1. Diniz BS, Teixeira AL, Cao F, Gildengers A, Soares JC, Butters MA, Reynolds CF 3rd. History of bipolar disorder and the risk of dementia: a systematic review and meta-analysis. Am J Geriatr Psychiatry. 2017;25(4):357–62.
2. Stang A. Critical evaluation of the Newcastle-Ottawa scale for the assessment of the quality of nonrandomized studies in meta-analyses. Eur J Epidemiol. 2010;25(9):603–5.

Part IV
Delirium

Chapter 23
A Multicomponent Intervention to Prevent Delirium in Hospitalized Older Patients

Adan Aslam Khan, Andrew Wong, Vahid Pasovic, and Esther Akinyemi

Authors of the Original Article Sharon K. Inouye, M.D., M.P.H.; Sidney T. Bogardus, Jr., M.D.; Peter A. Charpentier, M.P.H.; Linda Leo-Summers, M.P.H.; Denise Acampora, M.P.H.; Theodore R. Holford, Ph.D.; and Leo M. Cooney, Jr., M.D.

Journal Publisher *The New England Journal of Medicine.*

Year of Publication 1999.

Type of Study Controlled clinical trial.

Funding Sources Supported by grants from the National Institute on Aging, the Commonwealth Fund, the Retirement Research Foundation, The Community Foundation for Greater New Haven, and the Patrick and Catherine Weldon Donaghue Medical Research Foundation.

Objectives
1. To compare the effectiveness of a multicomponent strategy with usual plan of care in preventing delirium in hospitalized older adults.
2. To determine the adherence level to the intervention protocol.
3. To measure the intervention's effect on the targeted risk factors [1].

Methods In this study, a controlled clinical trial was conducted to compare patients admitted to one intervention group or two usual-care (control) groups on a general medicine inpatient service. A pilot study confirmed that random assignment was not feasible due to the large number of participants in all the medical units; therefore,

A. A. Khan · A. Wong · V. Pasovic · E. Akinyemi (✉)
Henry Ford Health System, Detroit, MI, USA
e-mail: vpasovi1@hfhs.org; EAkinye2@hfhs.org

R. R. Tampi et al. (eds.), *Essential Reviews in Geriatric Psychiatry*,
https://doi.org/10.1007/978-3-030-94960-0_23

individuals were matched by a computer algorithm using a prospective, individual matching strategy [2]. This computerized algorithm matched patients based on the following characteristics on admission: age, sex, and baseline risk of delirium (intermediate or high). Baseline risk of delirium was defined by a predictive model including four risk factors: visual impairment, severe illness, cognitive impairment, and a high blood urea nitrogen to creatinine ratio. The presence of one or two risk factors indicated intermediate risk, and the presence of three or four risk factors indicated high risk.

All participants who met eligibility criteria were enrolled in the intervention unit and identified in the usual-care units. The eligibility criteria included admission to one of the three general medical units, at least 70 years old, no delirium at time of admission, and at intermediate or high risk of delirium at baseline. Patients were excluded for inability to participate in interviews (1265 patients) due to profound dementia (154), language barrier (92), profound aphasia (38), intubation or respiratory isolation (14), coma or terminal illness (69), hospital stay of 48 hours or less (219), or prior enrolment in study (324). Other exclusion reasons included unavailability of patient or interviewers (due to examinations/procedures) (355), inability to find matching patient (67), or refusal of enrolment by patient, family, or physician (250). Of the 2434 potentially eligible patients, 852 were included in the final study sample and were matched as 426 pairs receiving the study intervention or usual care.

Assessments were conducted by research staff who were not involved in the intervention and were blinded to the nature of the study or patient group assignments. Screening interviews and baseline assessments for patients were conducted within 48 hours after admission. The screening interview included assessments using the Mini-Mental State Examination (MMSE), the Digit Span Test, the Confusion Assessment Method (CAM), the Katz's Activities of Daily Living, and the standard Jaeger test for vision. Chart review was also conducted to determine the Acute Physiology, Age, and Chronic Health Evaluation (APACHE II) score. Baseline assessments included collecting demographic data, assessment of instrumental activities of daily living, the whisper test for hearing, and assessment of sleep. At the time of admission, a family member was interviewed to describe the patient's cognitive functioning before admission and recent cognitive changes and to complete the modified Blessed Dementia Rating scale. The ratio of blood urea nitrogen to creatinine was also obtained, with a value greater than or equal to 18 mg/dL as a marker for dehydration. Structured daily interviews were conducted until day of discharge consisting of the MMSE, the Digit Span Test, and CAM rating. Risk factors for delirium were reassessed on hospital day 5 (or on day of discharge if before day 5). After discharge, a review of medical records was conducted for evidence of delirium, final diagnoses, laboratory results, medications, and discharge destination.

A trained multidisciplinary team implemented the intervention strategy, called the Elder Life Program. This team consisted of a geriatric nurse specialist, two Elder Life specialists, a certified therapeutic-recreation specialist, a physical therapy consultant, a geriatrician, and trained volunteers. Six risk factors for delirium were targeted in the intervention group: cognitive impairment, sleep deprivation, immobility, visual impairment, hearing impairment, and dehydration. These factors were selected based on evidence of their contribution to delirium, and feasibility of hospital mitigation strategies. Standardized intervention protocols were established with a targeted outcome for reassessment. The usual-care group received standard hospital services provided in other general medical units.

The primary outcome was delirium, defined by the CAM criteria as an "acute onset and a fluctuating course of symptoms of delirium, inattention, and either disorganized thinking or an altered level of consciousness" based on daily assessments made during interviews. For the primary analysis of the effectiveness of intervention, delirium was either present or absent. Only one episode of delirium per patient was counted. Other measured variables included the total number of days of delirium, number of episodes of delirium, recurrence, and severity of these episodes. Intervention adherence was recorded daily as daily adherence (patient received all parts of signed protocol), partial adherence (patient received some but not all parts of the protocol), and nonadherence (patient received none of the parts of the assigned protocol).

Admission characteristics were compared between patients and matched pairs by matched statistical analysis using either t-tests (for continuous variables) or McNemar's test (for binary variables). Results were confirmed with unmatched analyses. The effectiveness of the intervention was analyzed using intention to treat analyses. Analysis of the effectiveness of intervention in reducing the incidence of delirium was conducted using the conditional logistic regression method. All baseline characteristics were examined in bivariate analysis to identify potential confounders. The cumulative incidence of delirium was compared between the study groups using the Kaplan-Meier analysis and the log-rank test. The severity, duration, and rate of recurrence of delirium were compared between study groups. Rates of adherence were calculated according to patient-day in the intervention group; eligible days were those when patient was expected to receive interventions. At the time of reassessment, changes in risk factors or outcomes were compared between groups using unmatched statistical analyses. All statistical tests were two-tailed; P values of less than 0.05 were considered statistically significant.

Results The characteristics of the intervention and usual-care groups did not differ significantly. The number of risk factors for delirium was similar in the two groups. The severity scores and rates of recurrence of delirium did not differ between the two groups. Of note, 25 percent had dementia with MMSE scores of 20 or less.

The overall adherence to the intervention protocol was 87%. Reasons for nonadherence included refusal by patient, lack of availability of the patient due to having procedures elsewhere, medical contraindications, and lack of availability of intervention staff members. Six patients in the intervention group (1.4%) and seven patients in the usual-care group (1.6%) died during hospitalization ($P = 0.78$). Complete information of delirium was available for these individuals.

The delirium-related outcomes during hospitalization differed between the two study groups. The rate of incidence of delirium was significantly lower in the intervention group than in the usual-care group (9.9% vs. 15.0%, $P = 0.02$). The matched odds ratio of 0.60 (95% CI, 0.39–0.92) supports a risk reduction associated with the intervention; the cumulative incidence of delirium was lower in the intervention group.

The total days of delirium were significantly lower in the intervention group (105 vs. 161, $P = 0.02$). The total number of episodes of delirium was also lower in the intervention group (62 vs. 90, $P = 0.03$), although this was primarily from the effects of intervention on the first episode of delirium (rather than on recurrent episodes). Using matched subgroup analyses, it was noted that in the group at a baseline intermediate risk of delirium, the intervention significantly reduced the rate of incidence of delirium (OR, 0.52; 95% CI, 0.29–0.92). In the group at a high risk of delirium at baseline, the intervention was associated with a reduced incidence, but this was not statistically significant (OR, 0.73; 95% CI, 0.38–1.38). No adverse effects were associated with the intervention protocols.

On reassessment at day 5 (or at discharge, if earlier), there were more improvement and fewer risk factors in the intervention group (64% vs. 55%, $P = 0.02$). In the intervention group, there were an improvement in the orientation score (7.2 ± 0.2 vs. 6.8 ± 0.2, $P = 0.06$) and a reduction in the rate of use of sedative drugs for sleep in the intervention group (35% vs. 46%, $P = 0.001$). Though the authors indicate that there is a trend toward improvement in the intervention group compared to the usual-care group for the Activities of Daily Living score, the whisper test score, and vision, these results were not statistically significant.

The total cost of intervention was $139,506 or an average of $327 per patient. This includes the staff time spent in intervention activities, equipment, supplies, and consultant costs. The cost of intervention per case of delirium prevented (22 fewer cases in the intervention group) was $6341.

Conclusions This study supports a multicomponent, targeted intervention strategy (the Elder Life Program), for preventing delirium in medically hospitalized older adults. There was a reduction in the initial development and total number of days of delirium in patients with an intermediate risk of delirium at baseline. However, after the first episode, the intervention strategies were less efficient and less effective. These findings support the importance of primary prevention in delirium management.

Strengths of the Study

Jadad Scoring Criteria [3].

Questions Yes (1) No (0)	**Was the study described as random?**	**Was the randomization scheme described and appropriate?**	**Was the study described as double-blind?**	**Was the method of double blinding appropriate? (were both the patient and the assessor appropriately blinded?)**	**Was there a description of dropouts and withdrawals?**	**Total score Range of score quality 0–2, low 3–5, high**
Score	0	0	0	0	1	1

1. Daily assessments were conducted of patients using a standardized, validated instrument.
2. There was no loss to follow-up in the study.

3. Tracking of adherence to the intervention protocols was detailed.
4. There was a realistic nature of the intervention protocols and it had feasibility of application to other settings.

Limitations of the Study

1. Twenty-five percent of patients had dementia.
2. The study was unable to implement random assignment.
3. There is possible decrease in the overall rates of delirium in the usual-care group due to "contamination effect." For example, staff members in usual-care units may have been informed of intervention protocols verbally. Additionally, there may have been utilization of intervention protocols in usual-care groups by physicians, who rotated on all floors and may have carried them over.
4. This study is not a randomized or double-blind study, as is reflected in the Jadad score of 1. There were appropriate measures however to mitigate the lack of randomization, and grading staff were blinded to reduce bias.

Take-Home Points Multicomponent interventions for treatment of delirium may result in better outcomes. Preventing delirium early an intervention may result in lower total number of episodes of delirium.

Practical Applications of the Take-Home Points Implementing a multicomponent intervention protocol for prevention of delirium results in decreased incidence and duration of delirium among hospitalized older adults and reduced risk factors for episodes of delirium.

References

1. Inouye SK, Bogardus ST Jr, Charpentier PA, Leo-Summers L, Acampora D, Holford TR, Cooney LM Jr. A multicomponent intervention to prevent delirium in hospitalized older patients. N Engl J Med. 1999;340(9):669–76.
2. Holford TR, Bracken MB, Eskenazi B. Log-linear models for the analysis of matched cohort studies. Am J Epidemiol. 1989;130(6):1247–53.
3. Jadad AR, Moore RA, Carroll D, Jenkinson C, Reynolds DJ, Gavaghan DJ, McQuay HJ. Assessing the quality of reports of randomized clinical trials: is blinding necessary? Control Clin Trials. 1996;17(1):1–12.

Chapter 24
Delirium in Elderly Patients and the Risk of Post-Discharge Mortality, Institutionalization, and Dementia: A Meta-Analysis

Sarah Kim and Tracey Holsinger

Authors of the Original Article Joost Witlox, Lisa S M Eurelings, Jos F M de Jonghe, Kees J Kalisvaart, Piet Eikelenboom, Willem A van Gool.

Journal Publisher *Journal of the American Medical Association.*

Year of Publication 2010.

Type of Study Meta-analysis.

Funding Sources None.

Objective To determine the association between delirium in elderly patients and long-term adverse outcomes including mortality, institutionalization, and dementia [1].

Methods The investigators conducted a comprehensive literature search on MEDLINE, Embase, PsycINFO, and CINAHL databases for studies published between January 1981 and April 2010. Search keywords for delirium (*delirium, confusion, acute confusional state, acute confusional syndrome*) were cross-referenced to citations pertinent to outcome (*mortality, prognos**, *predict**, *course*). Studies meeting the following criteria were considered eligible: mean or median

S. Kim
Duke University Department of Psychiatry and Behavioral Sciences, Durham, NC, USA
e-mail: kyung.kim@duke.edu

T. Holsinger (✉)
Duke University Department of Psychiatry and Behavioral Sciences, Durham, NC, USA

Durham VA Medical Center, Durham, NC, USA
e-mail: Tracey.holsinger@duke.edu

R. R. Tampi et al. (eds.), *Essential Reviews in Geriatric Psychiatry*,
https://doi.org/10.1007/978-3-030-94960-0_24

age of the study population of 65 years or older, delirium as a study variable, presentation of quantitative data (i.e., event rates, odds ratios, or hazard ratios), hospital or post-acute care setting, and follow-up at 3 months or later. Exclusion criteria were as follows: delirium patients only without controls, homogeneous populations of terminally ill patients such as end-stage cancer, and homogeneous populations of patients with central nervous system disease such as stroke or Parkinson disease.

For primary analyses, the investigators gathered statistically adjusted odds ratios (ORs) and hazard ratios (HRs) with corresponding 95% confidence intervals (CIs). Statistical control was used for covariates which could impact the association between delirium and long-term poor outcomes such as age, sex, comorbid illness or illness severity, and baseline dementia. Then secondary analyses were performed on a much larger, unadjusted sample to examine the robustness of results from the primary analyses. In secondary analyses, the investigators extracted the number of events relative to the total number of study participants in the delirium groups and control groups. Then event rates that considered only post-discharge mortality and incident cases of institutionalization were preferentially extracted, as the investigators were interested in the longer-term outcome *after* delirium. Event rates for mortality were corrected for death during the index hospitalization, event rates for hospitalization were corrected for baseline rates of institutionalization, and event rates for dementia were corrected for baseline rates of dementia. Furthermore, the unadjusted ORs were stratified according to age, country of origin, length of follow-up, and whether the participants who were institutionalized or had dementia at baseline were included.

Mortality, institutionalization, and dementia were examined as separate outcomes, and each study contributed only 1 effect size per analysis. Random effects models rather than fixed-effects models were used for analyses, and the *I*-square statistic was used to account for heterogeneity among studies. Publication bias was evaluated by using two funnel-plot-based methods. Sensitivity analysis was performed for studies using different methods for the diagnosis of both baseline dementia and incident dementia.

Results From the database search, 2939 articles were identified, of which 2777 were excluded based on review of title or abstract. From 162 potentially relevant articles, 120 were excluded after a full review. The 42 included articles along with 9 articles identified from reference lists were further screened on inclusion criteria. Nine articles failed to satisfy quality criteria (retrospective studies, no validated delirium ascertainment), and 42 high-quality articles were finally included in this meta-analysis.

For primary analyses, 12 studies provided 7 HRs and 7 ORs for the primary analysis of the association between delirium and mortality. Seven studies provided 9 ORs for the primary analysis of the association between delirium and institutionalization. Two studies provided adjusted ORs for the association between delirium and dementia. For secondary analyses, 38 studies provided 40 ORs on mortality, 18 studies provided 20 ORs on institutionalization, and 6 studies provided 6 ORs on dementia.

Mortality
For primary analysis, after a mean follow-up of 22.7 (15.5) months (range, 3–48 months), 271 of 714 patients with delirium (38%) died compared with 616 of 2243 controls (27.5%) (HR = 1.95 [95% CI, 1.51–2.52]; I^2 = 44.0%). Secondary analysis confirmed the significance of the results of the primary analysis. After a mean follow-up of 11.4 (14) months (range, 3–38 months), 183 of 483 patients with delirium (37.9%) died, showing a significant association with mortality, compared to 316 of 1583 controls (20.0%) (OR = 1.71 [95% CI, 1.27–2.30]; I^2 = 0%).

Institutionalization
After a mean follow-up of 14.6 (12) months (range, 3–38 months), 176 of 527 patients with delirium (33.4%) had a higher risk of institutionalization, compared to 219 of 2052 controls (10.7%) (OR = 2.41 [95% CI, 1.77–3.29]; I^2 = 0%).

Dementia
Only two studies were included in the primary analysis of adequately adjusted ORs. Thirty-five of the 56 patients with delirium (62.5%) had a follow-up diagnosis of dementia compared with 15 of 185 controls (8.1%) after 3.2 and 5.0 years of follow-up (OR = 12.52 [95% CI, 1.86–84.2]; I^2 = 52.4%).

Conclusions Evidence from this meta-analysis indicates that delirium in elderly patients is associated with an increased risk of death, institutionalization, and dementia, independent of confounding covariates such as age, sex, comorbid illness, illness severity, and presence of dementia at baseline.

Strengths of the Study
1. The investigators performed two separate analyses, a primary analysis controlled for selective covariates and a secondary analysis on a larger, unadjusted sample to confirm the results of the primary analyses.
2. The meta-analysis examined both HR and OR for the outcome of mortality.
3. The adverse outcomes were divided into individual categories to help limit potential heterogeneity.

Limitations of the Study
1. All studies included in this meta-analysis were observational studies.
2. The studies included in this meta-analysis were pooled irrespective of the definition of delirium.
3. Only two studies met criteria to examine the association between delirium and dementia.
4. Etiology and duration of delirium, which could have an impact on the long-term adverse outcomes, were not taken into account.
5. A neurodegenerative process may have been already in process regardless of the ascertainment of the diagnosis of dementia in the vulnerable population.

Take-Home Points Despite some limitations, this meta-analysis performed a thorough review of high-quality studies to determine the association between delirium in elderly patients and the adverse long-term outcomes of mortality, institutionalization, and dementia. Given the innate essence of *delirium*, it is challenging not only to control confounding factors but also to ascertain a distinction between delirium and dementia. The results from the meta-analysis indicate an increased risk of mortality, institutionalization, and dementia in elderly patients with delirium when compared to controls.

Practical Applications of the Take-Home Points Delirium is a common and serious complication in elderly patients. Not only can it lead to the long-term adverse outcomes shown in this study, it is also associated with complication of medical illness, prolonged hospital stay, and morbidity in addition to mortality. More clinical focus on the prevention of delirium could help prevent serious outcomes.

Reference

1. Witlox J, Eurelings LS, de Jonghe JF, Kalisvaart KJ, Eikelenboom P, van Gool WA. Delirium in elderly patients and the risk of postdischarge mortality, institutionalization, and dementia: a meta-analysis. JAMA. 2010;304(4):443–51.

Chapter 25
Effectiveness of Multicomponent Nonpharmacological Delirium Interventions: A Meta-Analysis

Vahid Pasovic, Adan Aslam Khan, Andrew Wong, and Esther Akinyemi

Authors of the Original Article Tammy T Hshieh, Jirong Yue, Esther Oh, Margaret Puelle, Sarah Dowal, Thomas Travison, Sharon K Inouye.

Journal Publisher *JAMA Internal Medicine.*

Year of Publication 2015.

Type of Study Systemic review and meta-analysis.

Funding Sources The National Institute on Aging.

Objectives To evaluate the available evidence on multicomponent nonpharmacological delirium interventions in reducing the incidence of delirium and preventing associated poor outcomes [1].

Methods This study followed Preferred Reporting Items for Systematic Reviews and Meta-Analyses (PRISMA) guidelines in conducting a comprehensive systemic literature review of PubMed, Google Scholar, ScienceDirect, and the Cochrane database of systemic reviews to identify studies related to delirium prevention. The studies included were published from January 1999 to December 2013 and identified using the following search terms: delirium prevention, targeted multicomponent intervention, multicomponent intervention, nonpharmacological intervention, and Hospital Elder Life Program.

Studies were selected based on pre-defined two-level inclusion criteria as well as exclusion criteria. The articles were initially screened based on the first-level

V. Pasovic · A. A. Khan · A. Wong · E. Akinyemi (✉)
Henry Ford Health System, Detroit, MI, USA
e-mail: vpasovi1@hfhs.org; EAkinye2@hfhs.org

R. R. Tampi et al. (eds.), *Essential Reviews in Geriatric Psychiatry*,
https://doi.org/10.1007/978-3-030-94960-0_25

Table 25.1 Study inclusion and exclusion criteria

First-level inclusion criteria	1. Original articles with human subjects 2. Articles published in English 3. Articles with samples of individuals with a median or mean age of 65 years or older using relevant topics (given search terms)
Exclusion criteria	1. Qualitative studies 2. Case series 3. Commentaries 4. Reviews 5. Guidelines/recommendations 6. Study protocols and cost-effective analyses 7. Studies that did not have relevant outcome measures or control group. 8. Studies involving terminally ill patients
Second-level inclusion criteria	1. Multicomponent, nonpharmacological interventions 2. Delirium incidence 3. Use of validated delirium instruments for ascertainment

inclusion criteria and exclusion criteria. The remaining articles were subsequently evaluated and excluded if they failed to meet the second-level inclusion criteria (Table 25.1).

Initial search yielded 2334 articles, which was narrowed down to 46 based on the initial inclusion and exclusion criteria. Fourteen original articles were included in the final meta-analysis following the second-level inclusion criteria. Of the 14 selected studies, 12 consisted of unique intervention trials with 2 additional studies addressing different outcomes in different study subgroups (function and cognition post-discharge and falls). The primary outcomes were incidents of delirium and falls. Incidence of delirium was defined as new-onset delirium during hospitalization as measured by two validated delirium instruments, the Confusion Assessment Method (CAM) and Delirium Observation Screening (DOS). Incidence of falls was defined as the total number of falls per 1000 patient-days. Secondary outcomes included the length of stay (total number of days the patient was in the hospital from initial arrival in the emergency department to date of discharge), institutionalization (new placement in senior residential or nursing home facility upon discharge), and function/cognitive decline. The cognitive status was measured by the difference in Mini-Mental State Examination (MMSE) scores between admission and discharge, and the functional status was measured by changes in either Activities of Daily Living Scale/Lawton scale, Barthel Index, or admission and 6 months' post-discharge functional scores in one study.

Study quality of the papers included in the meta-analysis was assessed using the six domains of the Cochrane Collaboration's tool for assessing risk of bias. Data collection was conducted by developing a standardized date extraction protocol based on input from experts in delirium, multicomponent interventions, geriatrics, and systemic reviews/meta-analysis with two reviewers independently extracting and cross-checking data and two additional reviewers conducting spot-checks to confirm accuracy. For each primary and secondary outcome measured, data extracted included means with standard deviations, number of occurrences/total number of sample, odds ratios or relative risks, and associated 95% confidence intervals with corresponding authors contacted up to three times when essential data were not reported.

Statistical analysis was conducted using Review Manager (RevMan) software. Studies were grouped into either randomized/matched trials (RMTs) and non-RMTs. Blinded RCTs were included due to the small number of RCTs precluding separate meta-analysis. Odds ratio and 95% confidence intervals for proportions and rates were estimated according to intention-to-treat principles with number needed to treat (NNT) calculated for statistically significant effects using the inverse of pooled absolute risk. Continuous data was assessed by using means with standard deviations, mean differences, and standardized mean differences. Chi-square statistic Q was used to assess heterogeneity for study results considered for inclusion into meta-analysis with $p < 0.1$ as the threshold indicator for heterogeneity of effects. Lastly, the proportion of total variation due to heterogeneity across studies was estimated using I^2. For low heterogeneity ($I^2 < 25\%$), fixed-effect models for meta-analysis were used, whereas random-effects model was applied for moderate heterogeneity (I^2 25–75%). For high heterogeneity ($I^2 > 75\%$), meta-analysis was not considered appropriate for interpretation. Linear regression analysis was used to assess the association between study quality and effectiveness of interventions in addition to dividing studies based on Cochrane score into lower (<3) and higher (4 or greater) subgroups with independent med analysis conducted for each subgroup.

Results The 14 articles included in the meta-analysis consisted of 6 RMTs and 8 non-RMT (3 of which had non-matched concurrent controls and 5 with historical controls). There were 4267 patients across 12 sites (acute medical and surgical wards in academic and community hospitals) with an average age of 79.7 years.

The incidence of delirium was measured by 11 studies ($N = 3751$) with the multicomponent nonpharmacological intervention group exhibiting 53% lower odds of delirium incidence (OR 0.47, 95% CI 0.42–0.79) and NNT of 14.3 (95% CI 11.1–20.0). Stratified by study type, the 4 RMTs ($N = 977$ intervention patients) showed 44% lower odds (RR 0.56, 95% CI 0.42–0.76) with NNT of 20.0 (95% CI 12.5–33.3), and the 7 non-RMTs ($N = 752$ intervention patients) showed 63% lower odds (OR 0.37, 95% 0.27–0.53) with NNT of 11.1 (95% CI 8.3–16.7).

The number of falls per patient-days was examined by 4 studies ($N = 1038$) with the intervention arm exhibiting 62% lower odds of falling (OR 0.385, 95% CI 0.25–0.60). There were 4.26 falls prevented per 1000 patient-days (2.79 falls per patient-days in the intervention arm vs 7.05 falls per 1000 patient-days in the control arm). When stratified by study type, 2 RMT studies ($N = 245$) showed a statistically significant reduction in falls (OR 0.36, 95% CI 0.22–0.61) representing 8.53 falls prevented per 1000 patient-days with the 2 non-RMT ($N = 274$) showing a trend of lower odds of falling although not statistically significant (OR 0.46, 95% CI 0.19–1.10), representing 2.3 falls prevented per 1000 patient-days.

Length of stay was examined by 9 studies ($N = 3358$) which showed a mean reduction of −0.16 days with a trend toward significance (95% CI -0.97–0.64). When stratified by study type, the 4 RMTs ($N = 977$) showed reduction in length of stay by −0.33 (95% CI −1.38–0.72) with the 5 non-RMTs ($N = 561$) showing an increased length of stay by 0.01 days (95% CI −1.72–1.73). Neither findings in the stratified subgroups were found to be statistically significant.

Rate of institutionalization post-hospital discharge was examined by 4 studies ($N = 1176$) with intervention arm showing 5% reduction (OR 0.95, 95% CI 0.71–1.26) in odds of discharge to long-term care. When stratified by study type, the 2 RMTs ($N = 120$) showed OR of 0.94 in the intervention arm (95% CI 0.69–1.30) and OR of 0.79 (95% CI 0.25–2.51) in the 2 non-RMTs ($N = 132$). Neither the pooled data nor stratified subgroup findings achieved statistical significance.

Functional change was examined by 4 high heterogeneity ($I = 96\%$, $p < 0.00001$) studies (1 high-quality RMT, 3 non-RMTs, $N = 1068$) which showed a standard main difference for functional improvement of 0.57 in the interventional arm using random-effects models that did not achieve statistical significance (95% CI −0.03–1.18).

Cognitive change was examined by 3 high heterogeneity ($I = 83\%$, $p = 0.02$) studies (1 high-quality RMT, 3 non-RMTs, $N = 1610$) which showed cognitive improvement of 0.97 in the interventional arm using random-effects models that did not achieve statistical significance (95% CI −0.46–2.41).

Examining the relationship between quality rating and effectiveness revealed that study quality ratings were not highly correlated with effectiveness. This was indicated by the decrease attributable to intervention per unit increase on Cochrane measure in preventing incident delirium or falls of 4% ($R = 0.025$) and 10% ($R = 0.438$), respectively. Results were unchanged when stratified into lower- and higher-quality study subgroups with the incidence among higher-quality studies showing odds ratio of 0.53 (95% CI 0.39–0.71) compared to 0.38 (95% CI 0.23–0.64) among lower-quality studies with $p = 0.28$.

Conclusions Multicomponent nonpharmacological delirium prevention interventions are effective in reducing delirium incidence and preventing falls in older patients admitted to acute medical or surgical units with the trend toward reducing cost of care, decreasing length of stay, and avoiding institutionalization.

Strengths of the Study

1. There was a comprehensive search strategy and a systemic review model leading to improved power for meta-analysis of study.
2. There was adherence to clear, predetermined selection criteria.
3. The assessment of study quality based on Cochrane Collaboration's Risk of Bias guidelines that controlled for potential sources of bias and limited heterogeneity.
4. The study utilized heterogeneity analysis to account for confounding factors/variables influencing outcomes of interest.
5. The authors made effort to contact authors when essential data was not reported.

Limitations of the Study

1. There was exclusion of terminally ill patients limiting generalizability given prevalence of delirium in terminally ill patients.
2. Final number of included studies was small with limited sample size, and only 1/3 of interventions were randomized controlled trials (29%, 4 of 14).
3. The unit-wide nature of many nonpharmacological prevention interventions made blinding difficult to achieve, restricting strength of conclusions made due to limited data available for synthesis.
4. Interpretation of pooled estimates is limited by moderate to high degree of heterogeneity for all studies examining length of stay, functional and cognitive decline, and non-RMTs examining institutionalization.

Take-Home Points Multicomponent nonpharmacological delirium prevention interventions are effective in reducing the incidence of both delirium and falls in older persons receiving care on acute medical or surgical units. This leads to a reduction in hospital-based complications and improvement of cost-effectiveness of care.

Practical Applications of the Take-Home Points Nonpharmacological delirium prevention interventions are effective and economical and can be readily implemented on acute medical and surgical units to decrease the incidence of delirium and prevent falls.

Reference

1. Hshieh TT, Yue J, Oh E, Puelle M, Dowal S, Travison T, Inouye SK. Effectiveness of multicomponent nonpharmacological delirium interventions: a meta-analysis. JAMA Intern Med. 2015;175(4):512–20.

Chapter 26
Antipsychotic Medication for Prevention and Treatment of Delirium in Hospitalized Adults: A Systematic Review and Meta-Analysis

Pallavi Joshi and Rajesh R. Tampi

Authors of the Original Article Neufeld KJ, Yue J, Robinson TN, Inouye SK, Needham DM.

Journal Publisher *Journal of the American Geriatrics Society*

Year of Publication 2016.

Type of Study Systematic review and meta-analysis

Funding Sources John A. Hartford Foundation, National Institute on Aging, Milton and Shirley F. Levy Family Chair

Objectives To evaluate the efficacy and safety of antipsychotics for the prevention and treatment of delirium from a systematic review and meta-analysis [1].

Methods The investigators conducted a systematic review in accordance with the Institute of Medicine guidelines of PubMed, Embase, and CINAHL electronic databases for the period from January 1, 1988, to November 26, 2013, using specific search terms. In addition, data from ClinicalTrials.gov regarding completed studies was evaluated. Furthermore, the investigators reviewed the reference list of published review articles and systematic reviews for additional studies.

P. Joshi
University of Arizona College of Medicine, Phoenix, AZ, USA

R. R. Tampi (✉)
Creighton University School of Medicine, Omaha, NE, USA
e-mail: rajesh.tampi@yale.edu

R. R. Tampi et al. (eds.), *Essential Reviews in Geriatric Psychiatry*,
https://doi.org/10.1007/978-3-030-94960-0_26

The investigators included published and unpublished randomized controlled trials (RCTs) in addition to prospective or historical cohort, case-control, and other observational studies. They included studies that evaluated the prevention or treatment of delirium in an adult medical or surgical inpatient settings. The exclusion criteria were non-English publications, narrative review articles, editorials, commentaries, letters, dissertations, and studies that focused exclusively on pediatric, alcohol or substance withdrawal, schizophrenia, dementia, stroke, neurosurgery or trauma patient populations, or nursing home, and other nonhospital settings. The investigators also excluded studies if the delirium identification was not conducted using a validated tool.

Two investigators independently reviewed each title and abstract to determine whether the study was eligible for inclusion in the review. They also reviewed the full article if there was any uncertainty regarding its eligibility for inclusion. Four separate trained reviewers created evidence tables using a standardized form. The Cochrane risk of bias assessment was completed for each eligible article by at least two independent reviewers. If there was any discrepancy, it was adjudicated by one specific author. This investigator also independently reviewed a random 10% subsample of all articles to ascertain the accuracy of the abstractions and risk of bias assessment ratings. Three specific investigators evaluated the individual risk of bias ratings to select the final articles with low risk of bias for inclusion in the review.

The investigators performed a meta-analysis when two or more studies using similar interventions were identified. They presented dichotomous outcomes as odds ratios (OR) with 95% confidence intervals (95% CIs). The continuous outcomes were analyzed using mean difference (MD) or standardized mean difference (SMD) when different scales were used across studies. If specific data was not identified in the published papers, the authors were contacted by the investigators to obtain this information. The heterogeneity in the studies was assessed using the chi-square and I^2 statistics, with $P < 0.1$ and $I^2 > 50\%$ being considered as substantial heterogeneity. When there was high heterogeneity, the investigators used a random effects model for meta-analysis; otherwise they used a fixed-effect model.

Results The results were reported in accordance with the Preferred reporting items for systematic reviews and meta-analyses (PRISMA) guidelines.

The investigators included a total of 19 studies in this review. There were 7 studies that evaluated the prevention of postoperative delirium and 12 studies that evaluated delirium treatment among a mixed samples of hospitalized adults. The seven studies that evaluated postoperative delirium prevention include trials where the treatment was started in the perioperative period (average age 61 to 87 years). Six of these were RCTs investigating an antipsychotic versus placebo (four with haloperidol, two with risperidone, and one with olanzapine). The dosages ranged from 1.0 to 7.5 mg equivalents of haloperidol per day, administered either orally or intravenously. The delirium treatment studies included individuals with an average age range of 39 to 84 years. Five of the studies focused on an ICU population. Ten of the

12 studies were RCTs. Five of the studies compared antipsychotics (haloperidol and atypical antipsychotics) to placebo or no treatment, and seven of the studies provided comparisons between antipsychotic agents.

Three prevention and three treatment studies were found to be of low risk for bias. There was no evidence systematic bias in reporting mortality outcome.

Seven postoperative prevention studies were used for meta-analysis on the effect of antipsychotic medication on incident delirium (n = 1970). The authors did not find a significant effect of antipsychotics in preventing postoperative delirium when compared to placebo (OR = 0.56; 95% CI 0.23, 1.34; $I^2 = 93\%$). Antipsychotic use was also not associated with decreased duration of delirium in the 7 studies reporting this finding (n = 581; MD −0.65 days; 95% CI −1.59, 0.29; $I^2 = 80\%$). The authors did not find a decrease in severity of delirium with antipsychotic use in 464 patients in 8 studies (SMD −0.11; 95% CI −0.43, 0.22; $I^2 = 61\%$).

The meta-analysis did not find a decrease in hospital length of stay in 1454 patients in 8 studies (MD = −0.01 days; 95% CI, −0.16, 0.14; $I^2 = 42\%$) or in ICU length of stay in 1400 patients in 7 studies (MD = −0.46 days; 95% CI, −1.15, 0.24; $I^2 = 91\%$).

The authors did not find a significant association of antipsychotics with mortality up to 30 days following a hospital stay in 1439 patients in 10 studies (OR = 0.90; 95% CI 0.62, 1.29; $I^2 = 0\%$). Adverse events were not included in the meta-analysis due to the heterogeneity of outcomes.

Conclusions This systematic review and meta-analysis of 19 studies indicates that the use of antipsychotics does not decrease delirium severity, duration, or hospital length of stay when compared to placebo.

Strengths of the Study

1. The meta-analysis included 1970 participants in the delirium prevention analysis, 581 in the delirium duration analysis, 464 in the delirium severity analysis, 1454 patients in the hospital length of stay analysis, 1400 in the ICU length of stay analysis, and 1439 in the mortality analysis.
2. Fifteen studies included in the meta-analysis had an average age ≥60 years.

Limitations of the Study

1. Included studies did not focus specifically on older postoperative adults.
2. There was substantial variability in outcome measures and study methodology.
3. Few postoperative studies evaluated mortality and functional outcomes.
4. The included studies did not evaluate the effects of antipsychotics on agitation or distress in adults with delirium.

Take-Home Points This systematic review and meta-analysis of 19 studies indicates that antipsychotics do not decrease delirium severity, duration, or hospital length of stay when compared to placebo. However, symptomatic effects of antipsychotics, including changes in agitation or distress, were not assessed.

Practical Applications of the Take-Home Points Current evidence does not support use of antipsychotics in the prevention or treatment of postoperative delirium in older adults, although the use of these agents was not associated with increased mortality up to 30 days post-hospital stay.

Reference

1. Neufeld KJ, Yue J, Robinson TN, Inouye SK, Needham DM. Antipsychotic medication for prevention and treatment of delirium in hospitalized adults: a systematic review and meta-analysis. J Am Geriatr Soc. 2016;64(4):705–14.

Chapter 27
Interventions for Preventing Delirium in Older People in Institutional Long-Term Care

Matthew Erisman and Marianne Klugheit

Authors of the Original Article Rebecca Woodhouse, Jennifer K Burton, Namrata Rana, Yan Ling Pang, Jennie E Lister, Najma Siddiqi.

Journal Publisher *Cochrane Database of Systemic Reviews.*

Year of Publication 2019.

Type of Study Cochrane systemic review.

Funding Sources No internal funding sources. The National Institute for Health Research (NIHR) via Cochrane Infrastructure funding to Cochrane Dementia and Cognitive Impairment Group.

Objectives To assess the effectiveness of interventions for preventing delirium in older people in institutional long-term care settings [1].

Methods The investigators searched ALOIS and the Cochrane Dementia and Cognitive Improvement Group (CDCIG)'s specialized register of dementia trials up until February 27, 2019. Additionally, they searched Cochrane Central Register of Controlled Trials (CENTRAL), major healthcare databases, trial registers, and gray literature sources (unpublished) to complete search.

M. Erisman
University of Arizona Department of Psychiatry, Tucson, AZ, USA
e-mail: matthew.erisman@bannerhealth.com

M. Klugheit (✉)
Southern AZ VA Health Care System, Tucson, AZ, USA

R. R. Tampi et al. (eds.), *Essential Reviews in Geriatric Psychiatry*,
https://doi.org/10.1007/978-3-030-94960-0_27

The investigators selected randomized controlled trials (RCTs) and cluster RCTs of single and multicomponent non-pharmacological and pharmacological interventions for preventing delirium among older adults (≥65 years) who live permanently in long-term care settings.

The investigators used standard methodological procedures outlined by the Cochrane Library. The primary outcomes that were addressed included prevalence, incidence, severity of delirium, and mortality. The secondary outcomes included falls, hospital admissions, other adverse events, cognitive function, new diagnosis of dementia, activities of daily living, quality of life, and cost-related outcomes. The review used risk ratios (RR) as measures of treatment effect for dichotomous outcomes, hazard ratios (HR) for time-to-event outcomes, and mean difference (MD) for continuous outcomes. For each outcome, the review assessed the overall certainty of the evidence using GRADE methods (subjective ratings of certainty based on critical read).

Results The investigators included a total of 3 trials with 3851 participants in the review. All three trials were cluster RCTs. Two trials were of complex, single-component, non-pharmacological interventions, and one trial was a feasibility trial of a complex, multicomponent, non-pharmacological intervention. It was not possible to statistically combine (pool) the data from the studies due to significant heterogeneity among the studies.

The first study was a cluster RCT of a 4-week hydration management intervention [2]. The trial was funded by the National Institute of Nursing Research. This study recruited 98 participants across 7 nursing homes in the USA. The intervention was a hydration management program where an individual's fluid intake goal was calculated according to participant's bodyweight. A total of 75% of the fluid intake goal was delivered with meals and the remaining 25% was provided during non-meal times. The nursing staff were instructed on the treatment regimen, and a research assistant calculated the fluid goal and measured fluid intake randomly to ensure compliance with the protocol. The control arm participants had no individual fluid intake goal. Follow-up was at 4 weeks post-randomization. The effect of hydration-based intervention on incidence of delirium could not be calculated because of very low certainty of evidence (RR = 0.85, 95% confidence interval (CI) 0.18 to 4.00). This trial did not report data on prevalence or severity of delirium or for any of the secondary outcomes.

The second study was a cluster RCT of the Geriatric Risk Assessment MedGuide (GRAM) software program which included 3538 residents across 25 care homes in the USA. Medicare- and Medicaid-certified nursing homes with contracts with Omnicare pharmacies with 50 or more geriatric beds and few short-stay residents were eligible for inclusion [3]. This trial was funded by the Agency for Healthcare Research and Quality and the National Institutes of Health Center for Research Resources. The investigators used GRAM to identify medications that may contribute to delirium and falls risk for individual residents. The pharmacy automatically generated a GRAM report within 24 hours of nursing home admission, and for those individuals who were identified as being on medication contributing to risk of delirium or falls, an automatic report was sent to the pharmacist to coincide with a monthly visit to the nursing home. This resulted in a medication review being undertaken at the visit by the pharmacist. This was followed by a proactive monitoring plan that was initiated by the care-home staff to assess for medication side effects. The control nursing homes did not receive the triggered pharmacist visit or the proactive monitoring plan. The outcomes were recorded electronically by the participating care-home staff over a 12-month period. In the trial resident months were used rather than individuals as its unit of outcome measurement. The results only applied to new admissions during 2004. This trial did not report of the prevalence of delirium. The incidence of delirium appeared to be lower in the intervention group when compared to the control group (12-month HR = 0.42, CI 0.34 to 0.51). This trial did not report on the severity of delirium. Their intervention appeared to produce little or no effect mortality (HR 0.88, CI 0.66 to 1.17). The intervention appeared to have little or no effect of the intervention on hospital admissions (HR 0.89, CI 0.72 to 1.10) or falls (HR 1.03, CI 0.92 to 1.15). There were a 3% absolute reduction in use of opiates and anticonvulsant medications and an approximate 4% reduction in tranquillizers in the intervention group but not in the control groups.

The third study was a cluster randomized, controlled feasibility trial of a 16-month educational package that was delivered to 14 independent sector care homes in 1 metropolitan district in the UK [4]. This trial was funded by the National Institute for Health Research. The trial included a total of 215 care-home residents. In this study a specialist delirium practitioner delivered three 20-minute interactive educational sessions to care-home staff. A facilitated monthly staff working group was also organized to identify targets for delirium prevention and to develop solutions for each of the care homes. In addition, a delirium champion was trained at each home to deliver the educational sessions and facilitate the working groups. The control care homes continued with usual care. These care homes were offered the intervention package at the end of the trial. All delirium assessments were conducted by the investigators 16 months post-randomization, over a 1-month period. In addition, other outcomes were collected electronically from care-home records in a 6-month period starting 10 months post-randomization. Hospitalization data were collected during this period from routinely collected hospital data. In this trial, it was not possible to determine an effect of intervention on delirium prevalence, although the prevalence appeared to be lower in the intervention group (RR = 0.57, 95% CI 0.15 to 2.19). It was also not possible to determine the effect of intervention on delirium incidence (RR = 0.62, 95% CI 0.16 to 2.39). The intervention group had a delirium incidence rate of 4.9 and 95% CI of 0.7 to 15, and the control group had a delirium incidence rate of 7.9 and 95% CI of 1.4 to 22 per 100 resident months. The severity of delirium was not reported. There was probably little of no effect of the Stop Delirium! In this trial, there was little or no effect of the intervention on mortality (RR = 0.82, 95% CI 0.50 to 1.34). The intervention appeared to reduce hospital admissions when compared to controls (RR = 0.67, 95% CI 0.57 to 0.79). There was no difference in the quality of life measure, EQ-5D (MD = 0.04, 95% CI -0.09 to 0.17), between the intervention and control groups. The total cost of delivering the intervention was 138 Great Britain pound (GBP) per resident. The hospital resources used for the intervention homes were lower (estimated costs, 3281 GBP) when compared to the control homes (estimated costs, 7210 GBP). The monthly cost per resident in the intervention homes was 219.72 GBP when compared with 253.01 GBP in control homes.

Conclusions

1. Hydration-based intervention in long-term care (LTC) facilities did not reduce the incidence of delirium. In addition, the results were imprecise and there were serious design flaws in the study.
2. Using a computerized system to identify medications that may contribute to increased risk of delirium risk and trigger a pharmacist-led medication review appeared to reduce the incidence of delirium among older adults living in LTC facilities, but did not reduce the rates of hospital admissions, mortality, or falls among these individuals.
3. The educational intervention to identify risk factors for delirium along with staff-driven meetings to develop solutions within individual care homes did not appear to reduce the incidence or prevalence of delirium, and the results were imprecise. There was no effect on mortality, but the intervention appeared to reduce hospital admissions. There were design flaws in the study.

Strengths of the Study

1. A methodical approach was used to conduct the systematic review.
2. There was control of investigator bias.
3. The investigators queried specific issues and focused on individuals living at LTC.
4. The systematic review was graded as being of good quality based on the AMSTAR checklist with all ten of the ten criteria for systematic review being met [5].

Limitations of the Study

1. There were only three studies that met the inclusion criteria with little overlap between the studies.
2. The results from the studies could not be pooled due to significant heterogeneity between the studies.
3. Significant design flaws and imprecise results prevent the results being clinically useful.
4. The use of subjective GRADE system introduces investigator bias, although this was minimized by preventing investigators involved in the component studies and being part of this review from being involved in the interpretation of the studies using the GRADE system.

Take-Home Points

This systematic review indicates that an automated software-based medication review for medications that contribute to delirium which then triggers action by a pharmacist is the only intervention that reduced the incidence of delirium among individuals living at long-term care facilities. None of the other interventions reported reduce the incidence or prevalence of delirium and mortality from delirium in the LTC setting. Additional well-conducted RCTs are needed to determine effective interventions that prevent delirium among individuals living at long-term care facilities.

Practical Applications of the Take-Home Points
If LTC facilities can implement a software-based intervention to identify medications that could contribute to delirium risk and which then triggers a pharmacist-led medication review, it might reduce the incidence of delirium among individuals living at these facilities. All other interventions studied do not currently have adequate evidence to determine their impact on the incidence and prevalence of delirium and mortality from delirium.

References

1. Woodhouse R, Burton JK, Rana N, Pang YL, Lister JE, Siddiqi N. Interventions for preventing delirium in older people in institutional long-term care. Cochrane Database Syst Rev. 2019;4(4):CD009537.
2. Mentes JC, Culp K. Reducing hydration-linked events in nursing home residents. Clin Nurs Res. 2003;12(3):210–28.
3. Lapane KL, Hughes CM, Daiello LA, Cameron KA, Feinberg J. Effect of a pharmacist-led multicomponent intervention focusing on the medication monitoring phase to prevent potential adverse drug events in nursing homes. J Am Geriatr Soc. 2011;59(7):1238–45.
4. Siddiqi N, Cheater F, Collinson M, et al. The PiTSTOP study: a feasibility cluster randomized trial of delirium prevention in care homes for older people. Age Ageing. 2016;45(5):652–61.
5. Shea BJ, Reeves BC, Wells G, et al. AMSTAR 2: a critical appraisal tool for systematic reviews that include randomised or non-randomised studies of healthcare interventions, or both. BMJ. 2017;358:j4008.

Part V
Depressive Disorders

Chapter 28
Nortriptyline and Interpersonal Psychotherapy as Maintenance Therapies for Recurrent Major Depression: A Randomized Controlled Trial in Patients Older than 59 Years

Maureen Waweru and Seetha Chandrasekhara

Authors of the Original Article Charles F Reynolds 3rd, Ellen Frank, James M Perel, Stanley D Imber, Cleon Cornes, Mark D Miller, Sati Mazumdar, Patricia R Houck, Mary Amanda Dew, Jacqueline A Stack, Bruce G Pollock, David J Kupfer

Journal Publisher *Journal of the American Medical Association*

Year of Publication 1999

Type of Study Randomized controlled study

Funding Sources National Institute of Mental Health (NIMH)

Objectives The objective of the study was to compare the efficacy of nortriptyline and interpersonal therapy (IPT) separately and as a combination in the treatment of recurrent major depression in adults older than 59 years [1].

Methods A total of 687 older adults with recurrent, nonpsychotic, non-dysthymic, unipolar depression at a university-based geropsychiatric clinic were screened over a 7-year period. Of the 187 recruited, 180 individuals began treatment. Study participants were required to be 60 years or older, meet diagnostic criteria (per the Schedule for Affective Disorder and Schizophrenia—Lifetime Version structured interview) for recurrent nonpsychotic unipolar major depression, be in at least their

---

M. Waweru
Hospital at University of Pennsylvania, Philadelphia, PA, USA

S. Chandrasekhara (✉)
Lewis Katz School of Medicine at Temple University, Philadelphia, PA, USA
e-mail: Seetha.Chandrasekhara@tuhs.temple.edu

R. R. Tampi et al. (eds.), *Essential Reviews in Geriatric Psychiatry*,
https://doi.org/10.1007/978-3-030-94960-0_28

second lifetime episode, have had an interepisode wellness interval no longer than 3 years, have Hamilton Depression Rating Scale (HAM-D) score ≥17 and a Mini-Mental State Examination (MMSE) score ≥27, and be able to provide written consent. Participants excluded from the study had an age less than 60 years ($n = 12$), a single episode of major depression ($n = 119$), a wellness interval of 3 years or more ($n = 63$), medical contraindications to nortriptyline ($n = 43$), co-occurring dysthymia and major depression ($n = 23$), delusional depression ($n = 24$), or other psychiatric diagnoses ($n = 135$). Those excluded were referred to another clinic. Of the included participants, 48.7% were clinically referred, 42.6% were recruited through media and community presentations, and 8.7% learned about it by word of mouth.

During the acute phase, participants received open treatment of a combination of nortriptyline and weekly IPT to achieve remission (HAM-D ≤10). Of the 180 participants, 92 (51.1%) received adjunctive pharmacotherapy with lithium or perphenazine during this phase. Following the acute phase, participants were maintained on their current nortriptyline dose but with frequency of IPT reduced to every other week for a 16-week period. Twenty-eight of 159 participants did not show stable remission after the two phases (acute and continuation) and were considered treatment resistant. Participants with stable mood for the previous phase were randomly assigned to one of four maintenance therapy conditions below (180 participants were randomized and 13 relapsed during transition to maintenance). In the placebo maintenance condition, nortriptyline was slowly discontinued over 6 weeks under double-blind conditions. The participants stayed in maintenance therapy for 3 years or until recurrence of a major depressive episode. Placebo and nortriptyline tablets were identical in size and weight:

1. Medication only clinic with nortriptyline hydrochloride (80–120 ng/ml)
2. Medication only clinic with placebo
3. Monthly maintenance with IPT and nortriptyline
4. Monthly maintenance with IPT and placebo

Individual randomization was stratified by the therapist and blocked in units of four participants. The allocation schedule was determined by a computer-generated randomized subroutine permutation procedure (Fortran program). The treatment team, outcome assessors, and data analyst were blind to the treatment assignment. Each participant was seen monthly during maintenance treatment by the same two clinicians who treated them during the acute and continuation treatment, a nonphysician clinician and a coinvestigator. Those in the medication clinic option were only asked about symptoms and side effects. All visits included vitals, blood samples, and clinical ratings (HAM-D, Beck Depression Inventory, Global Assessment Scale, and Asberg Side Effect Rating Scale). This data was reviewed non-blinded in order to make nortriptyline dose adjustments. IPT was conducted by experienced clinicians with previous training and ongoing supervision by four investigators. Integrity and compliance of medication visits and IPT were evaluated using audio recorded sessions. Recurrence of a major depressive episode was determined by a structured interview first by a research nurse and confirmed independently by a senior psychiatrist. No protocol deviations were noted.

A Kaplan-Meier survival analysis was used to test for survival differences in maintenance treatment groups. The pairwise comparison used a Cox proportional hazards model to control for possible covariates using the placebo group as a reference.

Results Of the 187 individuals who entered the trial, 107 participants who had fully recovered began maintenance treatment, and recurrence data from these subjects was analyzed. Five participants were still active at the time of the outcome analyses, and their data was censored. The study used survival analysis to show a significant effect for active treatment over placebo in preventing recurrence of major depressive episodes ($P < 0.001$) and showed that 80% of participants in the combined treatment condition remained free of symptoms.

The study found that each of the active treatment conditions was significantly better than placebo in preventing recurrence: nortriptyline and IPT ($P < 0.001$); medication clinic with nortriptyline ($P < 0.001$); and IPT with placebo ($P = 0.03$). They also found that combination treatment was superior to IPT and placebo ($P = 0.003$) and showed a superior efficacy over medication clinic with nortriptyline ($P = 0.06$). Medication clinic vs. IPT and placebo did not differ ($P = 0.16$).

The study found that most recurrences occurred in the first year of treatment. They also found that of the 17 recurrences in participants taking nortriptyline, 9 were associated with nonadherence. Additionally, during the first year of maintenance treatment, older age was associated with a higher and more rapid rate of recurrence, and only combined treatment with nortriptyline and IPT effectively prevented recurrence in participants 70 years or older. However, in participants aged 60–69 years, each of the monotherapies and combined therapy was equally effective in preventing recurrences during the first year. Higher age at the study entry was associated with recurrence ($p = 0.05$). Attrition due to other causes (not recurrence) was low with 6/58 participants from the nortriptyline group due to medical problems that later excluded them from continued medication use. In the placebo group, 4/61 participants left against medical advice compared to 1/58 taking nortriptyline. One participant committed suicide 1 year after leaving the study against medical advice.

Conclusions The results from this study indicate efficacy in treatment of recurrent major depression in the elderly population (>60 years) with nortriptyline monotherapy or in combination with IPT when compared to placebo. A combination of both nortriptyline and IPT has also been shown to effectively prevent recurrences during the first year of maintenance therapy in adults 70 years or older.

Strengths of the Study

1. This was a randomized controlled trial.
2. There was inclusion of both pharmacotherapy and interpersonal therapy treatment.

3. There was adequate length of study that allowed assessment of efficacy in treatment and recurrence of symptoms.
4. This was a high-quality study with a Jadad score of 5 [2].

Questions Yes (1) No (0)	Was the study described as random?	Was the randomization scheme described and appropriate?	Was the study described as double-blind?	Was the method of double blinding appropriate? (Were both the patient and the assessor appropriately blinded?)	Was there a description of dropouts and withdrawals?	Total score Range of score quality 0–2, low 3–5, high
Score	1	1	1	1	1	5

Limitations of the Study

1. The sample studied may not represent the general population of older adults with chronic depression as the participants were recruited from a single academic outpatient clinic in a metropolitan area, and does not include participants from other settings.
2. There is no clear indication if participants with multiple medical comorbidities were included or excluded in the study.
3. The study does not elaborate on the cause of situational depression, which may affect the therapy approach.
4. There was no mention of a history of insomnia in the study participants.
5. Tricyclic antidepressants are known for having side effects that affect older adults including anticholinergic effects, cardiac risks, and fall risks that may impact adherence to treatment. The study does not explain how side effects impacted adherence.
6. The study population was predominantly white, female, and with an education level higher than the 12th grade, raising concerns about its generalizability.
7. The study does not give details on the severity of depression among the participants (about 15.5% of participants had previous suicide attempts) or on use of other psychotropic medication.
8. The sample size that was randomized was small.

Take-Home Points There is clear significant effect for continued combined treatment (nortriptyline and IPT) over monotherapy (nortriptyline alone) in the prevention of relapse of depression, especially in the first year of treatment when risk of recurrence is high. The results obtained in this study show that nortriptyline (range of 80–120 mg/ml) alone or in combination with IPT prevents or delays recurrences of major depression in older adults aged over 59 years. The study also showed that combined treatment of nortriptyline with IPT prevented relapse during the first year of maintenance treatment in participants 70 years or older.

Practical Applications of the Take-Home Points Depression in older adults is complicated by both medical and psychosocial challenges that make it very difficult to treat. Therefore, medication management and therapy are efficacious in treating depression, especially in combination.

References

1. Reynolds CF 3rd, Frank E, Perel JM, Imber SD, Cornes C, Miller MD, Mazumdar S, Houck PR, Dew MA, Stack JA, Pollock BG, Kupfer DJ. Nortriptyline and interpersonal psychotherapy as maintenance therapies for recurrent major depression: a randomized controlled trial in patients older than 59 years. JAMA. 1999;281(1):39–45.
2. Jadad AR, Moore RA, Carroll D, Jenkinson C, Reynolds DJ, Gavaghan DJ, McQuay HJ. Assessing the quality of reports of randomized clinical trials: is blinding necessary? Control Clin Trials. 1996;17:1–12.

Chapter 29
Continuation Treatment of Delusional Depression in Older Adults

Maureen Waweru and Seetha Chandrasekhara

Authors of the Original Article Barnett S Meyers, Sibel A Klimstra, Michelle Gabriele, Mimi Hamilton, Tatsu Kakuma, Fughik Tirumalasetti, George S Alexopoulos

Journal Publisher *The American Journal of Geriatric Psychiatry*

Year of Publication 2001

Type of Study Randomized controlled study

Funding Sources National Institute of Mental Health

Objectives The objective of the study was to compare the risks and benefits of combination continuation pharmacotherapy (antidepressant and antipsychotic) with those of antidepressant monotherapy among older adults who achieved remission from delusional depression after electroconvulsive therapy (ECT) [1].

Methods For this trial, 111 inpatient admissions were screened with 76 (69%) meeting baseline inclusion criteria. Of those excluded, 8 individuals had other diagnosis (dementia, schizoaffective disorder, or bipolar disorder), and 27 individuals did not have a diagnosis of delusion. Of the 76 participants who screened positive at baseline, 58 (76%) began ECT. Of these, 44 participants (76%) achieved a post-

M. Waweru
Hospital at University of Pennsylvania, Philadelphia, PA, USA

S. Chandrasekhara (✉)
Lewis Katz School of Medicine at Temple University, Philadelphia, PA, USA
e-mail: Seetha.Chandrasekhara@tuhs.temple.edu

R. R. Tampi et al. (eds.), *Essential Reviews in Geriatric Psychiatry*,
https://doi.org/10.1007/978-3-030-94960-0_29

ECT Hamilton Depression Rating Scale (HAM-D) score of <10. Ten of the 44 participants who initially remitted were not included because the second HAM-D score exceeded 10. A total of 34 participants were considered suitable for study entry, and 29 individuals from this group (85.3%) with an average age of 72.2 +/− 8.5 years consented to enter the randomized continuation trial. One participant from the combination-therapy group withdrew from the study after suffering a fall prior to the post-randomization assessment.

Inclusion criteria were individuals age 50 years or older, a pre-ECT score >21 and post-ECT score on the HAM-D, and achieving a score >24 on the Mini-Mental Sate Exam (MMSE) within 1 week of remission. Included participants also met DSM-IV criteria for psychotic depression and had scores >3 using the Delusional Rating Scale from the Schedule for Affective Disorders and Schizophrenia (SADS) and scores >2 on the Subjective Feeling of Certainty, Acting on Belief, and Accommodation subscales of the Conviction item on the Rating Scale for Delusions. Participants with hallucinations who had a delusion and did not meet criteria for schizophrenia and schizoaffective disorder were still included.

Exclusion criteria included individuals with an unstable medical illness that could influence treatment, use of medications known to cause psychiatric or extrapyramidal symptoms, a history of cognitive impairment preceding the onset of depression, those who met criteria for tardive dyskinesia, and any person unable to provide consent or who did not sustain a HAM-D score <10 during the week after ECT.

The primary hypothesis was that participants with combination therapy would have fewer relapses compared to monotherapy. A secondary hypothesis was that participants who received combination antipsychotic therapy had higher risks of extrapyramidal side effects and falls. The researchers calculated that 42 participants in each group would yield >80% power for determining statistical significance between the treatment groups.

Included participants were enrolled from inpatient psychiatric admissions at New York Presbyterian Hospital – Westchester Division between June 1994 and December 1998 and met DSM-IV criteria for psychotic depression. Participants provided written informed consents. Major depression was assessed using the Structured Clinical Interview for Diagnosis (SCID-P). These participants were then assessed for delusions using the Delusional Rating Scale from the Schedule for Affective Disorders and Schizophrenia (SADS) to determine whether the patient was convinced of an irrational idea (scale score >3). The researchers developed the Rating Scale for Delusions, adapted from the Dimension of Delusional Beliefs Scale to confirm the presence of delusional ideation. Scores >2 on the Subjective Feeling of Certainty, Acting on Belief, and Accommodation subscales of the Conviction item on the Rating Scale for Delusions were needed.

Nortriptyline was started at 25 mg/day for 2 to 3 days, followed by 50 mg for 5 days. Nortriptyline was preferred, but sertraline (dose, 50 mg/day–100 mg/day) was also included for participants with contraindications to nortriptyline or a previous failed trial. Nortriptyline plasma levels were obtained 5 to 7 days after the

50 mg/day dose was reached to ensure that concentrations were within the target range of 50 ng/ml–150 ng/ml. Those with contraindications to nortriptyline were given sertraline at a target dose of 50 mg/day–100 mg/day. Perphenazine or placebo was initiated up to 7 days later with a target dose of three to four tablets a day (12 mg–16 mg/perphenazine or placebo).

Participants were rated weekly for the first 4 weeks after randomization, then twice monthly for 2 months, and then monthly until 26 weeks after randomization. The researchers defined relapse by the DSM-IV criteria for major depression or the development of delusional ideation. The continuation phase of the study was complete at 26 weeks, and perphenazine was tapered over 8 weeks, at which point participants entered a 24-month maintenance study.

The researchers assessed extrapyramidal side effects at each visit using a modified five-item version of the Simpson-Angus Scale (SAS) to assess gait, shoulder shaking, elbow rigidity, leg pendulousness, and tremor. The SAS, Barnes Akathisia Scale, and the Abnormal Involuntary Movement Scale (AIMS) were also administered at each visit. Schooler and Kane criteria for tardive dyskinesia (TD) were used, and TD was defined as a score of 1 on two AIMS items or two or more on a single item. The researchers also monitored number of falls at each visit.

Researchers included randomized participants with at least one post-randomization assessment for data analyses. The between-group comparisons used chi-square analyses or Fisher's exact test, if the cell sizes were more than five and the continuous data were compared using Student's t-test. Between-group comparisons of continuous data that were not normally distributed use the Mann-Whitney U test. Kaplan-Meier survival analyses were carried out to compare the two treatment groups for time to relapse.

Results The study found no significant differences in clinical characteristics between the 15 combination-treatment and 13 monotherapy participants included in efficacy analyses.

Of the 28 participants, a total of 7 (25%) suffered a relapse during the 26-week trial; 5 (33%) were from the combination-therapy group, and 2 (15.4%) were from the monotherapy group (Fisher's exact test $P = 0.40$). The Kaplan-Meier survival curves for combination and monotherapy groups were statistically comparable (log-rank X2 = 2.1; $P = 0.2$). Participants who relapsed and those who remained well for predictor factors were similar in age (71.3 +/− 7.7 years vs. 71.9 +/− 8.8 years; $t = 0.19$; $P = 0.87$); baseline HAM-D scores (27.6 +/− 5.3 vs. 27.3 +/− 7.9; $t = 0.07$; $P = 0.94$); and MMSE scores (26.1 +/− 4.0 vs. 27.3 +/− 3.5; $t = 0.73$; $P = 0.47$). Participants who relapsed had higher initial continuation-phase HAM-D scores (4.7 +/− 6 vs. 2.7 +/− 3.0; $t = 1.56$; $P = 0.09$), but these differences were not statistically significant.

The study also found that six of the seven participants who relapsed met criteria for major depression without concurrent psychotic symptoms and one participant who relapsed had major depression with guilt and paranoid delusions. Of those participants randomized to take sertraline, two received monotherapy treatment with 50 mg/day of sertraline, and one received combination therapy with a sertraline dose of 75 mg/day. The sertraline combination-therapy participant relapsed, but the two monotherapy participants did not.

The study found that combination-therapy participants had significantly more extrapyramidal side effects ($t = 3.69$; $P = 0.001$) and a greater number of falls ($P = 0.05$). Six from the combination-therapy group but none from the monotherapy group ($P = 0.01$) experienced TD. Of the six participants who suffered from TD, three were emergent cases that required consideration for treatment discontinuation. However, TD developed 26 and 34 weeks after perphenazine discontinuation in two other cases, respectively. In three of the six participants, TD resolved between 7 and 18 months of its onset. TD persisted in the other three participants at follow-up at 1 week, 5 months, and 24 months after completion of the study.

The average dose of perphenazine in combination participants was 10.3 +/− 3.0 compared with 11.0 +/− 1.9 mg/day of placebo perphenazine. Among the 25 nortriptyline participants, those randomized to combination therapy required significantly lower nortriptyline doses (53.5 +/− 16.3 mg/day vs. 70.1 +/− 13.4 mg/day; $t = 2.72$; $P = 0.01$) and had higher nortriptyline levels per dose ($t = 3.36$; $P = 0.0001$).

Conclusion The findings of this study indicated that combination treatment resulted in greater relapses than monotherapy treatment and had significantly higher rates of extrapyramidal side effects, tardive dyskinesia, and falls.

Strengths of the Study

1. Study design was randomized, double-blind, and placebo-controlled.
2. The quality of study assessed on the basis of Jadad score indicates that this was a high-quality study with a score of 4 out of 5 [2].

Questions Yes (1) No (0)	Was the study described as random?	Was the randomization scheme described and appropriate?	Was the study described as double-blind?	Was the method of double blinding appropriate? (Were both the patient and the assessor appropriately blinded?)	Was there a description of dropouts and withdrawals?	Total score Range of score quality 0–2, low3–5, high
Score	1	1	1	1	0	4

3. The study found no significant differences in clinical characteristics between the 15 combination-treatment and 13 monotherapy participants included in efficacy analyses.
4. The results were consistent with previous studies on treatment of psychotic depression in late life [3].

Limitations of the Study

1. The study had a small sample size that also did not meet power (less than 42 participants in each group).
2. The study does not elaborate on the reason for dropouts.
3. Potential factors such as anticholinergic side effects of tricyclic antidepressants among older adults may have contributed to the attrition rate.
4. Risk factors contributing to high relapse rates, especially in the combination-therapy group, were not investigated due to sample size.

Take-Home Points

Major depression with psychotic features in older adults has a poor prognosis, but ECT is the only modality that has shown modest response rates. This study did not show significant difference in efficacy between combination pharmacotherapy (antipsychotic and tricyclic antidepressant) and monotherapy (tricyclic antidepressant). The study also indicates that combination therapy has higher rates of relapses than monotherapy and is associated with higher extrapyramidal side effects, tardive dyskinesia, and falls.

Practical Applications of the Take-Home Points

The study of adequate treatment for major depression with psychotic features among older adults is challenging given its poor prognosis and high risk for harmful pharmacologic side effects in this population. One of the strengths of the study is their choice in using nortriptyline, a tricyclic antidepressant that is better tolerated in older adults, and the use of low doses of perphenazine decreasing the potential for extrapyramidal side effects. Further studies are needed to investigate pharmacologic treatments that are better tolerated with fewer side effects and modest improvement in symptoms.

References

1. Meyers BS, Klimstra SA, Gabriele M, Hamilton M, Kakuma T, Tirumalasetti F, Alexopoulos GS. Continuation treatment of delusional depression in older adults. Am J Geriatr Psychiatry. 2001;9(4):415–22.
2. Jadad AR, Moore RA, Carroll D, Jenkinson C, Reynolds DJ, Gavaghan DJ, McQuay HJ. Assessing the quality of reports of randomized clinical trials: is blinding necessary? Control Clin Trials. 1996;17:1–12.
3. Mulsant BH, Sweet RA, Rosen J, Pollock BG, Zubenko GS, Flynn T, Begley AE, Mazumdar S, Reynolds CF 3rd. A double-blind randomized comparison of nortriptyline plus perphenazine versus nortriptyline plus placebo in the treatment of psychotic depression in late life. J Clin Psychiatry. 2001;62(8):597–604.

Chapter 30
Reducing Suicidal Ideation and Depressive Symptoms in Depressed Older Primary Care Patients: A Randomized Controlled Trial

Jenny Nguyen and Seetha Chandrasekhara

Authors of the Original Article Martha L Bruce, Thomas R Ten Have, Charles F Reynolds 3rd, Ira I Katz, Herbert C Schulberg, Benoit H Mulsant, Gregory K Brown, Gail J McAvay, Jane L Pearson, George S Alexopoulos

Journal Publisher *Journal of the American Medical Association*

Year of Publication 2004

Type of Study Randomized controlled trial

Funding Sources The National Institute of Mental Health; Advanced Centers for Intervention and Services Research of Cornell University, the University of Pennsylvania, and the University of Pittsburgh; John A. Hartford Foundation; Forest Laboratories

Objectives To determine the effect of a primary care intervention on suicidal ideation and depression in older adults [1]

Methods The Prevention of Suicide in Primary Care Elderly: Collaborative Trial (PROSPECT) intervention focused on two major components of care: physician knowledge and treatment management using a clinical algorithm and depression care managers, respectively. The algorithm recommended a first-line trial of a selective serotonin reuptake inhibitor (SSRI), specifically citalopram. Other antidepressants could be prescribed, if clinically indicated. If participants declined medication,

---

J. Nguyen · S. Chandrasekhara (✉)
Lewis Katz School of Medicine at Temple University, Philadelphia, PA, USA
e-mail: Seetha.Chandrasekhara@tuhs.temple.edu

R. R. Tampi et al. (eds.), *Essential Reviews in Geriatric Psychiatry*,
https://doi.org/10.1007/978-3-030-94960-0_30

interpersonal psychotherapy from the care manager was recommended. Research funds covered costs of interpersonal psychotherapy and citalopram only.

Fifteen practice-based, depression care managers (social workers, nurses, psychologists) worked with physicians to help recognize depression, offer guideline-based treatment recommendations, monitor clinical status, and provide appropriate follow-up. They had psychiatric backup, weekly supervision, and monthly interpersonal therapy cross-site supervision. Care managers were introduced to participants following the baseline interview. They interacted with participants in person or by telephone to monitor depressive symptoms, adverse effects, and treatment adherence at scheduled intervals, or when clinically necessary. In both groups, physicians were informed by letter about participants reporting suicidal ideation.

Older adults age 60 or older were selected from a participant pool from 20 randomly selected primary care practices across the greater New York City area, Philadelphia, and Pittsburgh. Practices were paired up within each region by setting (urban, suburban, rural), academic affiliation, size, and racial distribution regarding its potential participants. Practices were randomly assigned within the pairs to provide participants with the PROSPECT intervention or usual care.

A representative sample of primary care participants with the DSM-IV criteria for major or minor depression persisting for at least 1 month was achieved via a two-stage sampling process. A random sample of participants over the age of 60 was screened by telephone for depressive symptoms using the Center for Epidemiologic Studies Depression Scale (CES-D) following oral consent and stratified into either the 60–74 years old group or a group of those 75 or older. A total of 1888 patients with a CES-D >20, those with a history of prior depressive episodes or treatment, and a 5% random sample of participants with lower scores were invited to participate. The 1238 who consented were interviewed in person and administered the Structured Clinical Interview for DSM-IV. Exclusion criteria included those without a diagnosis of depression and those who missed follow-up assessments.

The severity of depression was assessed with the 24-item Hamilton depression scale (HAM-D), suicidal ideation was rated with the Scale for Suicide Ideation (SSI), anxiety was quantified with the Clinical Anxiety Scale, and hopelessness was assessed with the Beck Hopelessness Scale. Cognitive impairment was rated with the Mini-Mental State Examination, and limitations in functioning due to physical problems/emotional difficulties were assessed using the Medical Outcomes Study 12-item Short-Form Health Survey. Antidepressant treatment intensity was quantified using the Composite Antidepressant Treatment Intensity Scale.

Participants were followed for 18 months with telephone assessments at 4, 8, and 18 months, and an in-person interview 12 months after entry. The research assistants were unable to be blinded to the treatment assignments. Those meeting modified criteria for major depression or significant minor depression (four depressive symptoms and HAM-D ≥10 over 4 weeks) were included. A total of 598 participants (320 from the intervention group, 278 from usual care) were included for analyses.

Over 12 months, there was a dropout of 30.9% (99/320) for the intervention group and 31.3% (87/278) for the usual care group. The influence of the dropout rates was assessed by comparing the results from the study analyses to a shared parameter model, which yielded similar results and did not differ more than 5%. The statistical analysis consisted of descriptive and intent-to-treat (ITT) models, and differences for both continuous and binary outcomes were based on longitudinal random models for participant, practice, or practice-pair clusters.

Results This study showed that first remission occurred earlier and was more common among participants receiving the intervention than among those who received usual care. There were no statistically significant differences in age, gender, race, education, depression severity, anxiety, cognitive impairment, disability, or antidepressant treatment at baseline between participants included in analysis and those excluded because of missed follow-up assessments. The intervention group had a larger assignment of Hispanic participants compared with usual care (22.8% vs. 6.3%, $P = 0.06$). Intervention participants were also significantly more likely than usual care patients to report depression treatment at each follow-up period. At 4 months, 89.2% of intervention patients reported treatment of their depression, while only 52.5% of usual care patients did ($P < 0.001$). They also had higher rates of medication-only and psychotherapy-only treatments ($P < 0.001$ for both).

The study first evaluated the impact of the intervention on the prevalence of suicidal ideation over time. There was a larger proportion of suicidal ideation being reported by participants of the intervention group compared to those in usual care (29.4% vs. 20.1%, $P = 0.01$). At 4 months and beyond, there was no longer a significant difference between the groups. There was a greater decline in raw rates of suicidal ideation (12.9% intervention vs. 3.0% usual care; $P = 0.01$). After adjusting for differences of the longitudinal ITT change from baseline (all depressed participants $P = 0.01$, major depression $P = 0.006$, minor depression $P = 0.98$), only those participants with minor depression did not show significance in suicidal ideation. There was no statistical significance between the intervention and depression diagnosis interaction on suicidal ideation ($P = 0.64$).

Second, the clinical course of the study groups was compared using three depression scales. The first analyses involved depression severity as measured by the HAM-D. At 4 months, the HAM-D score had a greater decrease in the intervention group compared to the usual care group (7.4 vs. 3.9; $P < 0.001$). A significant decrease in the intervention group scores was consistent at 8 months (8.2 vs. 6.2; $P < 0.001$) and 12 months (8.8 vs. 7.2; $P = 0.006$). This showed significance in the overall longitudinal HAM-D scores from baseline ($P < 0.001$). Intervention effects remained significant for those with major depression ($P < 0.03$) across the study periods. No significant effects were demonstrated across time for those with minor depression ($P = 0.39$). Statistical significance was shown between group and change in depression severity ($P = 0.008$).

The second outcome measured response to treatment of depression. The study's definition of response was a minimum 50% decrease of HAM-D scores from baseline. More intervention participants had responses compared to usual care at 4 months (42.7% vs. 29.1%; $P = 0.001$), 8 months (46.2% vs. 35.5%; $P = 0.02$), and 12 months (52.1% vs. 42.0%; $P = 0.02$). The overall longitudinal change from baseline was significant ($P = 0.003$). There was a statistically significant effect from the intervention on those with major depression only. Again, no statistical significance was demonstrated between the group and diagnosis interaction ($P = 0.30$).

Remission from depression, as defined by HAM-D <10, was the third outcome measured. Remission rates at 4 months were significantly higher in the intervention group compared to usual care (48.2% vs. 34.2%; $P < 0.001$), but were no longer significant at 8 months ($P = 0.08$) or 12 months ($P = 0.26$). However, the longitudinal trend was significant ($P < 0.001$). As with the other outcomes, those participants with major depression only have more significant findings. The study then redefined remission as HAM-D <7, but the data continued to demonstrate similar findings.

Two sets of post hoc analyses stratified both depression diagnosis and suicidality to assess the effect of the intervention. Those with baseline suicidal ideation showed resolution by 4 months in 66.7% of intervention patients compared to 58.7% of usual care patients ($P = 0.34$). There was a statistically significant difference at 8 months (70.7% vs. 43.9%, $P = 0.005$), but it was no longer significant at 12 months ($P = 0.89$). The change in significance over time was due to the majority of both groups no longer expressing suicidal ideation.

Greater decreases in HAM-D scores were recorded for the intervention group compared with usual care regardless of reported suicidal ideation at baseline. There was a significant decrease in all depressed participants ($P < 0.001$) and those with major depression ($P < 0.001$). However, participants with minor depression did not have a large reporting of suicidality, so the intervention's effect on their depressive symptoms was not significant ($P = 0.72$). For those with minor depression and suicidal ideation ($N = 23$) though, the intervention showed a significantly greater decrease in depression severity ($P = 0.03$).

Conclusions The intervention showed effectiveness in reducing suicidal ideation at 4 months. The impact of the intervention on depressive symptoms was greater for those with major depression and minor depression with suicidality. It has its challenges, but it is a potential prevention strategy to reduce suicide among older adults in the community.

Strengths of the Study

1. It had a randomized controlled trial design.
2. This study had a Jadad score of 3, indicating that it was a high-quality study [2].

Questions Yes (1) No (0)	Was the study described as random?	Was the randomization scheme described and appropriate?	Was the study described as double-blind?	Was the method of double blinding appropriate? (Were both the patient and the assessor appropriately blinded?)	Was there a description of dropouts and withdrawals?	Total score Range of score quality 0–2, low3–5, high
Score	1	1	0	0	1	3

3. The algorithm suggested starting doses of 30 mg for citalopram to reduce undertreatment.
4. This was reflective of real-world practice because it was conducted in a variety of practices, mostly nonacademic and small and serving heterogeneous populations.
5. Sampling and screening procedures led to more heterogeneity of participants, making it more relevant to real-world practice.
6. It included participants with mild cognitive impairment, medical comorbidity, concurrent medical treatments, or suicidality.
7. It used formal depression screening and diagnostic procedures to standardize findings.
8. Real-life conditions were mimicked.
9. It had increased feasibility to implement this in large medical practices.
10. There was standardized training and supervision for health professionals who provided participants with the intervention.
11. This study exhibited a long duration of follow-up which went to 18 months.
12. They used ITT analyses in order to help correct for bias.

Limitations of the Study

1. There was a higher baseline prevalence of suicidal ideation reported in the intervention practices compared with usual care.
2. There was a lack of information on the discrete medical problems of participants.
3. Raters were blinded.
4. Only the cost of citalopram and interpersonal psychotherapy were covered.

Take-Home Points

Primary care intervention programs are effective in reducing suicidal ideation, regardless of depression severity, in older adults.

Practical Applications of the Take-Home Points

Routine depression screening in primary care has the potential to improve outcomes when followed with appropriate treatment and care management. Collaborative care by trained care managers and primary care physicians should be more widely implemented.

References

1. Bruce ML, Ten Have TR, Reynolds CF 3rd, Katz II, Schulberg HC, Mulsant BH, Brown GK, McAvay GJ, Pearson JL, Alexopoulos GS. Reducing suicidal ideation and depressive symptoms in depressed older primary care patients: a randomized controlled trial. JAMA. 2004;291(9):1081–91.
2. Jadad AR, Moore RA, Carroll D, Jenkinson C, Reynolds DJ, Gavaghan DJ, McQuay HJ. Assessing the quality of reports of randomized clinical trials: is blinding necessary? Control Clin Trials. 1996;17(1):1–12.

Chapter 31
Remission in Depressed Geriatric Primary Care Patients: A Report from the PROSPECT Study

Jenny Nguyen and Seetha Chandrasekhara

Authors of the original article George S Alexopoulos, Ira R Katz, Martha L Bruce, Moonseong Heo, Thomas Ten Have, Patrick Raue, Hillary R Bogner, Herbert C Schulberg, Benoit H Mulsant, Charles F Reynolds III, PROSPECT Group

Journal publisher *American Journal of Psychiatry*

Year of publication 2005

Type of study Randomized controlled trial

Funding sources National Institute of Mental Health (NIMH), Hartford Foundation, Forest Pharmaceuticals

Objectives To compare the time to first remission for depressed older adults in primary care practices that implemented a care management model compared to a usual care model, and to identify risk factors for non-remission that can guide referrals and treatment planning [1].

Methods This study analyzed data from the Prevention of Suicide in Primary Care Elderly: Collaborative Trial (PROSPECT). Older adults age 60 or older were selected from a pool of 9072 randomly selected primary care participants from 20 practices from the greater New York City area, Philadelphia, and Pittsburgh. Practices were paired up within each region by setting (urban, suburban, rural), academic affiliation, size, and racial distribution of its patients. They were randomly

J. Nguyen · S. Chandrasekhara (✉)
Lewis Katz School of Medicine at Temple University, Philadelphia, PA, USA
e-mail: Seetha.Chandrasekhara@tuhs.temple.edu

R. R. Tampi et al. (eds.), *Essential Reviews in Geriatric Psychiatry*,
https://doi.org/10.1007/978-3-030-94960-0_31

assigned within the pairs to provide participants with the PROSPECT intervention or usual care.

A representative sample of primary care participants with DSM-IV criteria for major or minor depression persisting for at least 1 month was achieved via a two-stage sampling process. A random sample of patients from the participating practices was screened by telephone for depressive symptoms using the Center for Epidemiologic Studies Depression Scale (CES-D Scale) following oral consent and stratified into either the 60–74-year-old group or a group of those 75 or older. 1888 patients with a CES-D Scale score above 20, those with a history of depression, and a 5% random sample of patients with lower scores were invited to participate. Patients with lower scores were included to assess "false-negative" cases for depression screening.

Inclusion criteria were individuals age 60 years or older who were able to provide informed consent, had a Mini-Mental State Exam (MMSE) score of 18 or greater, and spoke English. Those that were not included due to a CES-D score of 20 or lower and not previously included with the random sample were also recruited if they answered affirmatively to supplemental questions indicating previous depressive episodes or treatment. Suicidal ideation was not an eligibility criterion. Those without a diagnosis of depression or who missed follow-up assessments were excluded [2]. A primary outcome of the PROSPECT study was the time to remission, defined as the first occurrence of a patient achieving a HAM-D score <10 before any missed assessment session, starting with their enrollment into the study or no instance of remission before the first missed appointment. A score of 10 was chosen as a threshold because somatic symptoms originating from medical illness may lead to them still having points. Secondary analysis used a definition of remission that was a HAM-D score <7.

Participants who consented were interviewed in person following a protocol. They were administered the Structured Clinical Interview for DSM-IV, severity of depression was assessed with the HAM-D, suicidal ideation was rated with the Scale for Suicide Ideation, anxiety was quantified with the Clinical Anxiety Scale, and hopelessness was assessed with the Beck Hopelessness Scale. Cognitive impairment was rated with the MMSE, and limitations in functioning due to physical problems and emotional difficulties were assessed using the Medical Outcomes Study 12-item Short-Form Health Survey. The intensity of antidepressant pharmacotherapy at entry was quantified using the Composite Antidepressant Treatment Intensity Scale.

The PROSPECT intervention consisted of 15 trained care managers who gave algorithm-based recommendations to physicians based on the Agency for Health Care Policy and Research Guidelines. These care managers also monitored psychopathology, treatment adherence, response, and side effects, as well as provided follow-up care at predetermined intervals or when clinically necessary. The first step of the algorithm recommended citalopram at a target daily dose of 30 mg in order to minimize the likelihood of undertreatment. If participants declined medication, they were offered interpersonal psychotherapy from the care managers; 12.1% of participants in the intervention group chose interpersonal psychotherapy alone. The cost of citalopram and interpersonal psychotherapy were covered, but other antidepressants or types of psychotherapy were not covered by research costs. "Usual care" practices were notified in writing of participants' depression diagnosis. The investigators contacted physicians when the Risk Management Guideline indicated suicide risk in individual participants. Physicians also received educational materials (video and printed) on geriatric depression and treatment guidelines to help increase recognition of geriatric depression. Participants were followed for 18 months with telephone assessments at 4, 8, and 18 months and an in-person interview 12 months after entry. The research assistants were unable to be blinded to the treatment assignments.

Baseline demographics and clinical characteristics were compared using a t-test for continuous variables and the chi-square for binary variables. The Kaplan-Meier survival analysis was used to determine significance of differences in the primary study outcome. Predictors to remission were identified using a mixed effects regression model which adjusted for the research assessment months. Small number of large primary care clusters used a statistical inference and goodness of fit was measured by statistical deviance. A hierarchal backward elimination method was used to identify groups where the intervention was more effective than usual care.

Results The initial sample included 16,708 older adult participants with 9072 being screened for depression with the CES-D. Of those, 1888 were invited to participate with 1238 providing consent at the in-person interview. 267 participants met criteria for major depression and had a HAM-D ≥18 at entry. For the analysis, 215 participants met the inclusion criteria and also were evaluated at the 4-month follow-up visit. There was no statistical significance (age, gender, race, education, severity of depression, anxiety, cognitive impairment, disability, or intensity of antidepressant treatment) at baseline between those included in the analysis and those excluded due to missed follow-up sessions.

For the primary outcome (HAM-D<10), the intervention group showed a higher cumulative probability of remission ($P < 0.05$) and higher likelihood of remission for patients demonstrating depression in a previous follow-up session. For secondary outcomes (HAM-D <7), the data was not significant when comparing the two groups ($P = 0.30$).

Remission occurrence across the 3 site regions (total of 20 practices) differed ($P < 0.01$), but was determined to not be due to site-by-treatment assignment interaction when the primary outcome was analyzed. With the secondary outcome, the rates of remission differed again across the site regions ($P = 0.03$) without any site-by-treatment assignment interaction. The goodness of fit for predicting remission between a HAM-D score of 10 and 7 was similar ($P < 0.99$).

Demographic variables were not significantly associated with remission occurrence. However, clinical variables such as depression severity [odds ratio (OR) = 0.93, $P < 0.01$], suicidal ideation (OR = 0.89, $P < 0.05$), physical (OR = 1.03, $P < 0.05$)/emotional (OR=1.04, $P < 0.01$) functioning limitations, and adverse life events (OR = 1.65, $P < 0.05$) were significantly associated with occurrence of remission.

Limitations in emotional and physical functions, hopelessness, and anxiety were less likely to achieve remission regardless of treatment option. Those with hopelessness were less likely to achieve remission with usual care and had no significant influence for the intervention group. Anxiety did influence remission rates ($P < 0.04$). However, for those with high levels of anxiety, similar remission rates were achieved across groups. The remission rate with usual care eventually reached the level achieved with the intervention.

Conclusions It is critical to have longitudinal assessments of depression, anxiety, hopelessness, and emotional and physical functional limitations in older primary care adults struggling with depression. Those who received the intervention experienced first remission earlier and more commonly than those who received usual care. Those with prominent symptoms or impairment in the described areas may benefit from care management or mental health care because they are at risk for remaining disabled and depressed.

Strengths of the study

1. A representative sample of depressed, older primary care adults.
2. Feasibility to provide participants with care management in large medical practices with ability for reimbursement.
3. There was a long duration of follow-up which went to 18 months.
4. Starting doses of 30 mg for citalopram which reduced the likelihood of under-treatment and prolonged titration periods.

Questions Yes (1) No (0)	Was the study described as random?	Was the randomization scheme described and appropriate?	Was the study described as double-blind?	Was the method of double blinding appropriate? (Were both the patient and the assessor appropriately blinded?)	Was there a description of dropouts and withdrawals?	Total score Range of score quality 0–2 Low 3–5 High
Score	1	1	0	0	0	2

Limitations of the study

1. There was a lack of information on the discrete medical problems of participants and impact on remission.
2. The raters were not blinded.
3. There was infrequent follow-up care.
4. The cost of citalopram and interpersonal psychotherapy were covered, but not other options. This may not reflect potential financial barriers in the real world that can affect continuation of treatment.

5. There was a lack of information regarding specific antidepressant treatments received by each group over the course of 18 months.
6. It scored a 2 on the Jadad scale as the majority of the outlined protocol was located in a different paper with limited information provided in this particular article [3].

Take-home points Participants who received an intervention through trained care managers experienced first remission earlier and more commonly than those who received usual care. The intervention was more effective in those with low baseline anxiety levels, but had little benefit for patients with more severe anxiety.

Practical applications of the take-home point Primary care settings can be a strategic target in the management of late-life depression with collaborative care. Treatment of older adults with major depression and physical and emotional function limitations should be more aggressive with antidepressants and potential referral to a mental health professional, if the symptoms persist.

References

1. Alexopoulos GS, Katz IR, Bruce ML, Heo M, Ten Have T, Raue P, Bogner HR, Schulberg HC, Mulsant BH, Reynolds CF III, PROSPECT Group. Remission in depressed geriatric primary care patients: a report from the PROSPECT study. Am J Psychiatry. 2005;162(4):718–24.
2. Bruce ML, Ten Have TR, Reynolds CF III, Katz IR, Schulberg HC, Mulsant BH, Brown GK, McAvay GJ, Pearson JL, Alexopoulos GS. Reducing suicidal ideation and depressive symptoms in depressed older primary care patients: a randomized controlled trial. JAMA. 2004;291:1081–91.
3. Jadad AR, Moore RA, Carroll D, Jenkinson C, Reynolds DJ, Gavaghan DJ, McQuay HJ. Assessing the quality of reports of randomized clinical trials: is blinding necessary? Control Clin Trials. 1996;17:1–12.

Chapter 32
Executive Dysfunction and the Course of Geriatric Depression

Clay Gueits, Padmapriya Marpuri, and Rajesh R. Tampi

Authors of the original article George S. Alexopoulos, Dimitris N. Kiosses, Moonseong Heo, Christopher F. Murphy, Bindu Shanmugham, and Faith Gunning-Dixon

Journal published *Biological Psychiatry*

Year of publication 2005

Type of study Controlled treatment study

Funding sources National Institute of Mental Health grants RO1 MH65653, RO1 MH42819, RO1 MH51842, and P30 MH68638, Forest Pharmaceuticals, the Sanchez Foundation, and Dr. I Foundation (GSA)

C. Gueits
Psychiatry Resident, Einstein Medical Center, Philadelphia, PA, USA
e-mail: gueitscl@einstein.edu

P. Marpuri (✉)
Attending Geriatric Psychiatrist, Frontier Psychiatry, Billings, MT, USA

R. R. Tampi
Creighton University School of Medicine, Omaha, NE, USA
e-mail: rajesh.tampi@yale.edu

R. R. Tampi et al. (eds.), *Essential Reviews in Geriatric Psychiatry*,
https://doi.org/10.1007/978-3-030-94960-0_32

Objectives In this study the investigators examined the relationship between executive impairment and the course of depressive symptoms among older adults with major depressive disorder [1].

Methods Individuals >60 years were recruited from a University-based geriatric psychiatry clinic. For inclusion in the study, individuals were required to meet the Research Diagnostic Criteria and the DSM-IV criteria for unipolar major depression and have a score of >17 on the 24-item Hamilton Depression Rating Scale (HAM-D). Exclusion criteria included a diagnosis of major depressive disorder with psychotic features, a history of psychiatric disorders prior to diagnosis of major depression (except personality disorders), severe or acute medical illness within 3 months of the beginning of the study, neurological disorders (dementia or delirium, history of head trauma, Parkinson's disease, and multiple sclerosis), medical conditions associated with depression, taking drugs causing depression, or a Mini-Mental State Examination score of <24. The inclusion and exclusion criteria yielded a group of individuals >60 years with unipolar major depression without psychosis or a diagnosis of dementia.

Diagnoses were made using the Schedule for Affective Disorders and Schizophrenia (SADS) and parts of the Structured Clinical Interview for DSM-IV (SCID) administered at participants at baseline by trained raters. Depressive symptoms were measured using the HAM-D and baseline cognitive impairment was rated using the Mattis Dementia Rating Scale (DRS). The DRS measures impairment in several cognitive domains including initiation and perseveration (IP). Executive functions were tested using the IP domain of the DRS and the Stroop Color-Word test. At study entry, medical burden was evaluated using the Cumulative Illness Rating Scale, modified version for geriatrics (CIRS-G).

Patients underwent a 1-week drug washout period and placebo lead-in phase followed by baseline evaluation. Study participants were then given citalopram 20 mg daily and the dose was increased by 10 mg to target dose of 40 mg citalopram daily in 1 week. Citalopram was given as once a day dose either at night or in the morning. Participants were then seen by a research psychiatrist weekly. Each visit consisted of a review of symptoms, explanations regarding the need for treatment, and encouraging the participants to be adherent to treatment. Participants were assessed using the HAM-D on the 2nd, 4th, 6th, and 8th week after starting treatment with citalopram. A pill count to assess medication adherence was also conducted at the same time.

Participants were then divided into groups consisting of responders (≥50% change in HAM-D score from baseline) and non-responders during treatment. Comparisons between the two groups were performed using the Wilcoxon-Mann-Whitney test.

To analyze the effect of executive dysfunction on changes in depressive symptoms with citalopram treatment, the researchers used mixed-effects linear models to identify the point that differentiated the progression of HAM-D scores over the 8-week citalopram treatment period. They also used quadratic trends to identify nonlinear relationships of the HAM-D scores to IP and Stroop scores over time. The researchers then used the Akaike information criterion (AIC) to identify the quartile of participants with the highest degree of differentiation.

Results A total of 112 participants (mean age 73.17±6.5 years) including 58 women and 54 men were enrolled in the study. All participants met the criteria for moderate major depression according to DSM-IV criteria and were found to have high medical burden. They were treated with citalopram for 8 weeks with an average maximum daily dose of 35.29 mg [standard deviation (SD) = 8.39]. A total of 16 participants had left by the end of the study. Age, medical burden, cognitive impairment, and severity of depression at baseline were similarly distributed among participants who complete the trial and among those individuals who left the study early.

The responders and non-responders had similar severity of depression at baseline and received citalopram treatment of similar intensity, but the non-responder group was older, had fewer years of formal education, had greater medical burden, and had greater baseline cognitive impairment (poor performance in the IP domain) than the responder group.

After accounting for age, education, and medical burden, the mixed-effects models with quadratic time trend demonstrated that baseline IP was predictive of the course of depressive symptoms as measured by HAM-D over time. The investigators found that impairment in the DRS cognitive domain of IP below the median (≤35) was associated with higher HAM-D scores over time with less improvement on citalopram: t-value of 2.47 ($P<0.015$) at 4 weeks, t-value of 2.90 at 6 weeks ($P<0.0047$), and t-value of 2.68 at 8 weeks ($P<0.009$). The mean t-value was 2.20 with a P value of 0.03. They did not find any significant association with impairment in other cognitive domains rated by the DRS and the course of depressive symptoms.

The investigators also found that lower baseline Stroop-Color Word scores (≤22) were predictive of limited changes in depressive symptoms as measured by the HAM-D. The t-value at 2 weeks was 2.57 ($P<0.017$), t-value at 4 weeks was 3.17 ($p<0.002$), and t-value at 6 weeks was 2.72 ($P<0.0079$) with a mean t-value of 2.10 and $P<0.038$.

Conclusions In this study, abnormal scores in initiation and perseveration (measured by DRS) and response inhibition (measured by Stroop-Color Word Test) predicted a poor response to treatment with citalopram among older adults with major depression. Hence, older adults with major depression who have executive dysfunction require close monitoring as they may be at risk of non-response to a selective serotonin reuptake inhibitor (SSRI).

Strengths of the study

1. This study used assessment tools with proven validity and reliability including SCID, DRS, HAM-D, and Stroop-Color Word Test.
2. This was the first controlled treatment study that demonstrated a relationship between abnormal executive functioning and the course of symptoms of major depression.

Limitations of the study

1. The study has limited power as there were only 112 participants enrolled in the study.
2. The short washout period of 1 week could have contributed to psychiatric symptoms in addition to baseline functional impairment.
3. Behavioral abnormalities associated with executive dysfunction including psychomotor retardation and apathy may have interfered with the longitudinal assessment of depressive symptoms.
4. The IP and Stroop tests used in this study provide a limited assessment of executive functions. More comprehensive tests of executive functions may be needed to replicate the findings of this study.
5. There was no placebo arm for the study.

Take-home points Older adults with major depression who have executive dysfunction may not respond adequately to treatment with SSRIs. It is important to closely monitor these patients due to their increased risk of treatment failure.

Practical applications of the take-home points Due to the greater risk of non-response to antidepressant treatment among older adults with major depression and executive dysfunction, clinicians will need to carefully monitor the progress of these individuals. These individuals may need combination treatment with both pharmacotherapy and psychotherapy to attain adequate response to treatment.

Reference

1. Alexopoulos GS, Kiosses DN, Heo M, Murphy CF, Shanmugham B, Gunning-Dixon F. Executive dysfunction and the course of geriatric depression. Biol Psychiatry. 2005;58(3):204–10.

Chapter 33
Maintenance Treatment of Major Depression in Old Age

Sarah Kim and Tracey Holsinger

Name of the article Maintenance Treatment of Major Depression in Old Age

Authors of the original article Charles F Reynolds III, Mary Amanda Dew, Bruce G Pollock, Benoit H Mulsant, Ellen Frank, Mark D Miller, Patricia R Houck, Sati Mazumdar, Meryl A Butters, Jacqueline A Stack, Mary Ann Schlernitzauer, Ellen M Whyte, Ariel Gildengers, Jordan Karp, Eric Lenze, Katalin Szanto, Salem Bensasi, David J Kupfer

Journal published *New England Journal of Medicine*

Year of publication 2006

Type of study Randomized, double-blind, placebo-controlled trial

Funding sources National Institute of Mental Health (NIMH), National Center for Minority Health and Health Disparities, and GlaxoSmithKline

Objective To determine the efficacy of paroxetine and monthly interpersonal psychotherapy in maintenance treatment of major depression in elderly patients [1].

S. Kim
Duke University Department of Psychiatry and Behavioral Sciences, Durham, NC, USA
e-mail: kyung.kim@duke.edu

T. Holsinger (✉)
Duke University Department of Psychiatry and Behavioral Sciences, Durham, NC, USA

Durham VA Medical Center, Durham, NC, USA
e-mail: Tracey.holsinger@duke.edu

R. R. Tampi et al. (eds.), *Essential Reviews in Geriatric Psychiatry*,
https://doi.org/10.1007/978-3-030-94960-0_33

Methods This study recruited 210 participants from the initial screening of 363 patients, ≥70 years in age, who meet the diagnostic criteria for current major depression (non-psychotic and non-bipolar) according to *Diagnostic and Statistical Manual of Mental Disorders, fourth edition* (DSM-IV), from March 1, 1999, to February 28, 2003. The participants, who were treated at a university clinic for depressed older adults, also had a score of at least 15 on the 17-item Hamilton Rating Scale for Depression and a score of at least 17 out of 30 on the Folstein Mini-Mental State Examination (MMSE).

Of the 210 patients recruited, 195 began a course of short-term treatment, which consisted of paroxetine started at 10 mg per day and titrated over an 8-week period to a maximum of 40 mg per day along with weekly psychotherapy. From the 195 participants, 151 patients who had a clinical response (Hamilton score of 0 to 10 for 3 consecutive weeks) from this initial short-term treatment moved on to a 16-week course of continued treatment: paroxetine maintained at the same dose and frequency of psychotherapy decreased to once every 2 weeks. Of note, 69 patients were receiving augmented pharmacotherapy (bupropion, nortriptyline, or lithium), which was continued during this phase of the continued treatment.

A total of 116 participants completed the continued treatment phase with a full or partial recovery (109 full recovery, 7 partial recovery). This group was randomly assigned to one of four maintenance treatments: paroxetine plus monthly interpersonal psychotherapy (28 participants), placebo plus monthly interpersonal psychotherapy (35 participants), paroxetine plus monthly clinical-management sessions (35 participants), and placebo plus monthly clinical-management sessions (18 participants). For participants assigned to maintenance placebo, paroxetine dose was slowly tapered over a period of 6 weeks. From the 69 patients mentioned above who were receiving augmentation treatment during the initial phase, 38 completed the continued treatment. Nineteen were randomly assigned to paroxetine and 19 to placebo; the augmenting agent along with paroxetine was tapered in this latter placebo group. The authors report that the paroxetine, placebo, and augmentation pharmacotherapy tablets were identical in size, weight, and appearance. Clinical-management sessions and interpersonal psychotherapy sessions were 30-minute visits and 45-minute visits, respectively. The same clinicians conducted clinical-management and psychotherapy sessions, which were all audiotaped to be rated in blinded fashion. The maintenance treatment continued for 2 years or until the recurrence of a major depressive episode, again as defined by DSM-IV criteria and a Hamilton score of at least 15.

For statistical analysis, the investigators used Kaplan-Meier survival analysis with log-rank chi-square statistics to test for differences in recurrence rates of depression among the four different groups. The survival analysis was stratified according to the number of episodes of major depression, level of cognitive impairment, and the use of augmented pharmacotherapy. Secondly, the Cox proportional-hazards models were used to test for the effect of covariates clinically relevant for the recurrence of depression; the number and severity of concomitant medical illnesses defined by scores on the Cumulative Illness Rating Scale for Geriatrics

(CIRS-G); anxiety, as defined by scores on the Brief Symptom Inventory Anxiety Subscale; cognitive impairment, as defined by scores on the Mattis Dementia Rating Scale; and subjective sleep quality as defined by scores on the Pittsburgh Sleep Quality Index. The investigators also used Cox models to test for moderation effect of maintenance treatment on recurrence of depression, as evidenced by interaction of treatment with each clinical covariate.

Results Eight of the 28 participants (35%) in the paroxetine plus interpersonal psychotherapy group had recurrence of major depression during the maintenance treatment. Twenty-one of the 35 participants (68%) in the placebo plus interpersonal psychotherapy group had recurrence of depression. Twelve of the 35 participants (37%) in the paroxetine plus clinical-management group had recurrence. Ten of the 18 participants (58%) in the placebo plus clinical-management group had recurrence.

The Cochran-Mantel-Haenszel statistic for recurrence among the four groups stratified according to the use of augmented pharmacotherapy was also significant ($P = 0.03$). The recurrence rates were higher among participants who had been receiving augmented pharmacotherapy (74%) than among those who did not (29%, $P<0.001$).

For the hypothesized pairwise contrasts, paroxetine plus psychotherapy was superior to placebo plus psychotherapy ($P = 0.03$) and to placebo plus clinical management ($P = 0.05$) in prevention of recurrence of depression. Of note, paroxetine plus clinical management was significantly more effective than placebo plus psychotherapy ($P = 0.03$) and also more effective than placebo plus clinical management ($P = 0.06$). The number of participants needed to be treated with paroxetine to prevent one recurrence was 4 (95% confidence interval (CI), 2.3–10.9). After the adjustment for the effect of psychotherapy, the relative risk of recurrence among participants receiving placebo was 2.4, as compared with those receiving paroxetine (95% CI, 1.4–4.2).

In the Cox models examining covariates, more severe anxiety ($P = 0.04$), more numerous and severe concomitant medical illnesses ($P = 0.02$), and poorer sleep quality ($P = 0.001$) all predicted a shorter period without an episode of depression. There was a significant association between medical burden (as measured by CIRS-G) and drug assignment ($P = 0.03$), indicating a moderating effect of the number and severity of comorbid medical illnesses on the long-term outcome. Moreover, paroxetine was more effective in preventing recurrent depression in participants with fewer and less severe concomitant medical illnesses such as hypertension or cardiac disease ($P = 0.03$).

Conclusions Patients 70 years of age or older with an episode of major depression, who had an initial response to combined treatment of paroxetine plus interpersonal psychotherapy (either full or partial recovery), were less likely to develop a recurrent episode of depression if they transitioned to maintenance treatment with paroxetine. Monthly maintenance interpersonal psychotherapy had no significant effect on prevention of recurrent depression.

Strengths of the study

1. There is limited data on maintenance treatment of depression in the elderly. This longitudinal study focused on maintenance treatment and prevention of recurrence.
2. Stepwise method beginning with initial short-term treatment, followed by continued treatment and maintenance treatment.
3. Identification of potential confounding factors for depression in elderly population.
4. The study assessed on the basis of Jadad score indicates that this was a high-quality study with a score of 5 out of 5 [2].

Questions Yes (1) No (0)	Was the study described as random?	Was the randomization scheme described and appropriate?	Was the study described as double-blind?	Was the method of double blinding appropriate? (Were both the patient and the assessor appropriately blinded?)	Was there a description of dropouts and withdrawals?	Total score Range of score quality 0–2 Low 3–5 High
Score	1	1	1	1	1	5

Limitations of the study

1. The recurrence rate was reported as the number of patients who developed a recurrent episode of depression over the total number of participants in the group not accounting for the subjects who dropped out.
2. Cognitive impairment can have an impact on occurrence, recurrence, duration, and severity of depression in the elderly. It can also impact the efficacy of a structure, manual-based psychotherapy in the elderly. These older adults had high MMSE scores at the start of the maintenance phase. MMSE is a fairly insensitive screening for cognitive impairment especially in relatively well-educated samples.
3. Time to recurrent event not identified in the maintenance treatment.
4. Duration and severity of the recurrent episode not examined.
5. Study completion rate of 77.5%.
6. No individual data provided on each cohort with a different augmented pharmacotherapy (bupropion, nortriptyline, lithium).

Take-home points Few data exist on management of depression and prevention of recurrent depressive episode in elderly population. Data on efficacy of psychotherapy in elderly population is also limited. This longitudinal study examined the efficacy of both a selective serotonin reuptake inhibitor (SSRI) and manual-based interpersonal psychotherapy in maintenance treatment of geriatric depression. The findings suggest not only the use of an SSRI but also the continuation of SSRI as a maintenance pharmacotherapy for at least 2 years of duration to prevent the recurrence of depression in elderly patients.

Practical applications of the take-home points Many clinicians may hesitate to initiate and continue antidepressant medication in elderly patients for various reasons including concerns for adverse events. Although the existence of comorbid medical illness can impact the tolerability of antidepressants, integrated long-term disease management strategies for both depression and other concomitant medical illnesses can help treat and prevent recurrence of geriatric depression.

References

1. Reynolds CF 3rd, Dew MA, Pollock BG, Mulsant BH, Frank E, Miller MD, Houck PR, Mazumdar S, Butters MA, Stack JA, Schlernitzauer MA, Whyte EM, Gildengers A, Karp J, Lenze E, Szanto K, Bensasi S, Kupfer DJ. Maintenance treatment of major depression in old age. N Engl J Med. 2006;354(11):1130–8.
2. Jadad AR, Moore RA, Carroll D, Jenkinson C, Reynolds DJ, Gavaghan DJ, McQuay HJ. Assessing the quality of reports of randomized clinical trials: is blinding necessary? Control Clin Trials. 1996;17(1):1–12.

Chapter 34
Placebo-Controlled Study of Relapse Prevention with Risperidone Augmentation in Older Patients with Resistant Depression

Audrey Eichenberger, Izabella Dutra de Abreu, Daniela Vela, Megan Tusken, and Mary "Molly" Camp

Authors of the original article George S Alexopoulos , Carla M Canuso, Georges M Gharabawi, Cynthia A Bossie, Andrew Greenspan, Ibrahim Turkoz, Charles Reynolds III

Journal Publisher *American Journal of Geriatric Psychiatry*

Year of publication 2008

Type of study Multicenter open-label longitudinal study with randomized placebo-controlled double-blind maintenance phase

Funding sources Janssen, LLP

Objectives
1. To evaluate the effect of risperidone augmentation of citalopram for relapse prevention in older patients with antidepressant-resistant depression.
2. To compare the efficacy and safety of continuation treatment with combined citalopram and risperidone with those of citalopram alone in older depressed patients with drug-resistant depression who improved after acute treatment with the combination of citalopram and risperidone [1].

Methods The subjects selected for this analysis were inpatients or outpatients, aged ≥55 years, meeting the Diagnostic and Statistical Manual of Mental Disorders,

A. Eichenberger · I. D. de Abreu · D. Vela · M. Tusken · M. M. Camp (✉)
UT Southwestern Medical Center at Dallas, Dallas, TX, USA
e-mail: Audrey.Eichenberger@PHHS.org; Izabella.DeAbreu@UTSouthwestern.edu; Daniela.Vela@UTSouthwestern.edu; Megan.Tusken@PHHS.org; Molly.Camp@UTSouthwestern.edu

R. R. Tampi et al. (eds.), *Essential Reviews in Geriatric Psychiatry*,
https://doi.org/10.1007/978-3-030-94960-0_34

Fourth Edition (DSM-IV) diagnostic criteria for major depressive disorder, single or multiple episode, with or without psychotic features, and with a 17-item Hamilton Depression Rating Scale (HAM-D) total score ≥20 and a Mini-Mental State Examination score >23. Subjects were required to have a history of resistance to standard antidepressant treatment, defined as failure to respond to at least one but no more than three antidepressants during the current episode, administered at adequate doses for a minimum of 6 consecutive weeks.

Patients included within the study received citalopram monotherapy (20–40 mg) for 4–6 weeks to confirm nonresponse (<50% reduction in HAM-D scores). Full nonresponse to citalopram was described as <25% reduction in HAM-D scores at endpoint. Those individuals who were non-responders to a trial of citalopram were then treated with open-label combination treatment of citalopram and risperidone. The dose of citalopram was kept at the dose received at the endpoint of the initial phase. The risperidone augmentation dose was targeted at 0.5 mg/day (0.25–1 mg/day). Among this group of individuals, those who achieved remission (HAM-D score ≤7 or Clinical Global Impressions severity score 1 or 2) after 4–6 weeks then entered a 24-week double-blind maintenance phase during which they received citalopram augmented with risperidone or placebo.

The efficacy measures during the open-label phases were the HAM-D and the Montgomery-Åsberg Depression Rating Scale (MADRS), whereas the primary measure of efficacy during the double-blind maintenance phase was the time to relapse. The safety evaluations included the Simpson-Angus Scale, Barnes Akathisia Scale, Abnormal Involuntary Movement Scale, and the reports of adverse events.

Results Phase 1 was completed by 101 patients, and 93 patients met the criterion for citalopram nonresponse (<50% reduction in HAM-D scores) and entered open-label risperidone augmentation. Of the 89 patients who completed risperidone augmentation, 63 achieved symptom resolution and entered the 6-month double-blind maintenance phase: 32 received risperidone augmentation and 31 received placebo augmentation. The difference in improvement rates observed during the two open-label phases was significant ($P<0.001$). The median time to relapse (Kaplan-Meier estimates) was 105 days in the risperidone group and 57 days in the placebo group ($P = 0.069$). Overall, 18 of 32 (56%) from the risperidone group and 20 of 31 (65%) from the placebo group relapsed. The numbers needed to treat to prevent relapse over 3–6 months indicated that risperidone augmentation would result in 1 less relapse for approximately 6–9 patients treated. Among the 40 individuals who were fully nonresponsive to citalopram in the initial phase, the median time to relapse was 142 days in the risperidone plus citalopram group and 35 days in the placebo plus citalopram group ($P = 0.068$). In the risperidone plus citalopram group, the relapse rate was 53% (8 of 15) and it was 68% (17 of 25) in the placebo plus citalopram group.

Treatments were well tolerated in the study with the most common adverse events reported in the open-label phases being headache, insomnia, and diarrhea during citalopram monotherapy and dizziness and dry mouth during risperidone augmentation. In the double-blind maintenance phase, the only adverse event reported in more than two patients of either group was headache. There were no deaths or cerebrovascular events reported among the participants in this phase.

Conclusions This study indicates that risperidone augmentation may be an effective treatment strategy when treating older patients with a history of antidepressant-resistant major depression.

Strengths of the study

1. The characteristics of the patients included within the study are similar to those of previous studies of older patients with treatment-resistant depression.
2. Except for those with severe and unstable cardiovascular, kidney, liver, or neurological diseases, patients with comorbid medical illnesses were included within the study. Therefore, findings may be more generalizable to the majority of patients with medical comorbidities.
3. To meet inclusion criteria, patients needed a Mini-Mental State Examination score >23. This helped exclude for dementia, which could be a confounding factor.
4. The double-blinded nature of the maintenance face helps to reduce observer bias.

Limitations of the study

1. Subjects aged ≥55 years were included within the study and only about one-third of the patients were aged ≥65 years. Thus, the majority of patients included within the study may not fall into the age group that typically qualifies as "geriatric."
2. The single time-point criterion for relapse may be too stringent for an illness with a chronically fluctuating course.
3. The citalopram monotherapy phase may have been too short to establish whether improvement in depression during risperidone augmentation was in response to the addition of risperidone or further exposure to citalopram.
4. The lack of a stabilization phase in patients who met criteria for remission may have permitted entry into the double-blind phase of patients with an unstable remission.
5. The continuation phase of this study was short and cannot establish the long-term safety of risperidone augmentation of antidepressants in older patients.
6. A controlled study is needed to confirm the post hoc findings, involving the analysis of patients considered fully nonresponsive to open-label citalopram monotherapy and a linear regression model comparing the improvement rates in MADRS scores during the open-label citalopram monotherapy and risperidone augmentation phases.

Take-home points

1. The delay in time to relapse among the patients who received continuation treatment with risperidone and citalopram when compared to those who received placebo and citalopram was not statistically significant, but perhaps clinically meaningful.

2. The findings indicate a possible role for risperidone augmentation in the population of older adults with antidepressant-resistant nonpsychotic depression.
3. Overall, relatively short-term treatment augmentation with risperidone was safe and well tolerated and was not accompanied by movement disorders or significant extrapyramidal signs or changes in body weight.

Practical application of the take-home points

1. Risperidone augmentation of citalopram is a therapeutic strategy to stabilize older individuals with antidepressant-resistant depression.
2. The long-term safety of risperidone augmentation in older adults with antidepressant-resistant major depression has not been established.
3. The study might help clinicians to establish an evidence-based algorithm to address antidepressant-resistant depression.
4. Brief periods of augmentation might be sufficient to help those patients suffering from depression who are not responding to a selective serotonin reuptake inhibitor (SSRI).

Reference

1. Alexopoulos GS, Canuso CM, Gharabawi GM, Bossie CA, Greenspan A, Turkoz I, Reynolds C 3rd. Placebo-controlled study of relapse prevention with risperidone augmentation in older patients with resistant depression. Am J Geriatr Psychiatry. 2008;16(1):21–30.

Chapter 35
Efficacy of Second-Generation Antidepressants in Late-Life Depression: A Meta-analysis of the Evidence

Martin Witkin, Padmapriya Marpuri, and Rajesh R. Tampi

Authors of the original article J. Craig Nelson, MD; Kevin Delucchi, PhD; Lon S. Schneider, MD

Journal published *American Journal of Geriatric Psychiatry*

Year of publication 2008

Type of study Meta-analysis

Funding sources None

Objectives This systematic review and meta-analysis evaluated the efficacy of second-generation antidepressants in the treatment of late-life major depression [1].

M. Witkin
PGY-4 Psychiatry Resident, Einstein Medical Center, Philadelphia, PA, USA
e-mail: witkinma@einstein.edu

P. Marpuri (✉)
Attending Geriatric Psychiatrist, Frontier Psychiatry, Billings, MT, USA

R. R. Tampi
Creighton University School of Medicine, Omaha, NE, USA
e-mail: rajesh.tampi@yale.edu

R. R. Tampi et al. (eds.), *Essential Reviews in Geriatric Psychiatry*,
https://doi.org/10.1007/978-3-030-94960-0_35

Methods The investigators searched the Cochrane Controlled Trials Register (2006, Issue 3) using specific terms: elder, geriatr, senil, older, old age, late-life, aged, 80-and-over, depress antidepressants, fluoxetine, sertraline, paroxetine, citalopram, escitalopram, venlafaxine, duloxetine, mirtazapine, bupropion, nefazodone, and trazodone. In addition, they searched MEDLINE (1966 to August 2006) and proceedings from geriatric psychiatric and psychiatric professional society meetings since 2000. The investigators also searched previous reviews and queried pharmaceutical manufacturers for additional information when needed.

The investigators included the trials if they met the following criteria: if they were acute phase trials, had a parallel group design, were double-blinded, and were placebo controlled with random assignment to an orally administered second-generation antidepressants (i.e., non-tricyclics) that was marketed in the United States. In addition, the participants should have nonpsychotic, unipolar major depression that was not associated with a specific medical disorder. Furthermore, the participants had to be living in the community and were ≥60 years in age. Also, the information regarding the number of participants who were randomized, their outcomes, and dropout rates should be obtainable. These trials need not have been published or peer reviewed and could be reported in the form of a manuscript, technical trial report, or poster. The trials to be included in the review were identified by two of the authors based on the abovementioned criteria. The quality of the studies was assessed using the Jadad scores [2].

The investigators collected the following clinical outcomes: response rates, remission rates, and change scores on the Hamilton Depression Rating Scale (HAM-D) or Montgomery-Asberg Depression Rating Scale (MADRS) using the intent-to-treat (ITT) samples using the last observation carried forward among participants with at least one posttreatment rating. They defined response as ≥50% improvement from baseline on the HAM-D or the MADRS. The investigators used remission as defined by the individual study.

Among trials that used flexible dose of the same medication, the investigators combined the drug groups to make one contrast that was then compared to placebo. In fixed-dose trials that compared two doses of the same medication, they compared each dosage group to placebo. For an active comparator, the investigators compared each drug within that trial to the placebo group. The abstracted data was carefully checked for any discrepancy. Investigators or sponsors of the study were contacted for necessary information that was not included in the publication or presentation. For studies where the standard deviation (SD) of the change scores was not available, the investigators estimated it from standard error (SE) and sample sizes or imputed it using the largest SD reported in other trials.

The investigators used the Peto fixed-effects model to statistically combine the number of responders, remitters, and dropouts and the number of individuals who were randomized into each drug and placebo group for each trial. Odds ratios (ORs) and absolute risk differences (RDs) with their 95% confidence intervals (CIs), test of significance (Wald z), number (*N*) of contrasts, and *P* values were used to indicate the effects of treatment. A potential retrieval bias was identified using a funnel plot in which the standard error (SE) of the log OR against the log OR was used. To test the heterogeneity among the contrasts, χ^2 tests and the I^2 statistic derived from the χ^2 values were used.

Results The investigators identified a total of five trials from the Cochrane search and six trials from the MEDLINE search that met inclusion criteria. An additional four placebo-controlled studies were identified from a search of the abstracts, posters, and slide presentations from medical conferences.

The investigators identified a total of 10 trials with 13 contrasts: fluoxetine 3, escitalopram 2, sertraline 1, paroxetine 3, citalopram 1, venlafaxine 1, duloxetine 1, and bupropion 1, that met the inclusion criteria. The trials were 6–12 weeks in duration and included 178–752 participants per trial. The mean age of participants ranged from 68 to 80 years. The mean proportion of women in the trials ranged from 46% to 76%. Specific psychotherapy comparison was not used in any of the trials. All trials were sponsored by the manufacturer of antidepressants. All the trials were noted to be of good to excellent methodological quality based on the Jadad scores of 4 or 5.

A total of 6 of the 10 trials reported that there was a statistically significant advantage for using the drug when compared to placebo on response rates. The overall response rate in the trials for antidepressants when compared to placebo was 35% to 69% versus 19% to 47%, respectively. The overall OR by meta-analysis for response with antidepressants when compared to placebo was 1.40 (95% CI 1.24 to 1.57, $z = 5.45$, $N = 13$, $P<0.001$). The RD by meta-analysis was 0.08 (95% CI, 0.05–0.11, $z = 5.51$, $N = 13$, $P<0.001$). The pooled response rate for antidepressants when compared to placebo was 44.4% versus 34.7%.

The remission rates for antidepressants when compared to placebo ranged from 21% to 44% versus 13% to 42%, respectively. The overall OR by meta-analysis for remission with antidepressants when compared to placebo was 1.27 (95% CI 1.12 to 1.44, $z = 3.67$, $N = 13$, $P<0.001$). The RD by meta-analysis was 0.05 (95% CI 0.02 to 0.08, $z = 3.71$, $N = 13$, $P<0.001$). The pooled remission rate for antidepressants when compared to placebo was 32.6% versus 26.5%.

In 8 of the trials (10 contrasts) that reported the HAMD scores, changes in scores were greater in the antidepressant group when compared to the placebo group, WMD = 1.40 (95% CI 0.89–1.90, $z = 5.39$, $N = 10$, $P<0.001$) and heterogeneity: $\chi^2 = 19.27$, $df = 9$, $P = 0.02$, I^2=53.3%.

The discontinuation rates for antidepressants when compared to placebo ranged from 17% to 36% and 11% to 30%, respectively. The OR by meta-analysis for discontinuation due to antidepressants when compared to placebo was 1.22 (95% CI 1.06 to 1.40, $z = 2.80$, $N = 13$, $P = 0.005$; $\chi^2 = 23.15$, $df = 12$, $P = 0.03$, $I^2 = 48.2\%$). The pooled mean discontinuation rate for antidepressants when compared to placebo was 24% versus 20%, respectively. The RD by meta-analysis was 0.03 (95% CI 0.01 to 0.06, $P = 0.005$).

The discontinuation rates due to adverse effects for antidepressants when compared to placebo ranged from 8% to 27% versus 1% to 11% for placebo. The OR for discontinuations due to adverse effects for antidepressants when compared to placebo was 1.84 (95% CI 1.51 to 2.24, z = 6.02, N = 13, P<0.001; χ^2 = 30.82, df = 12, P = 0.002, I^2 = 61.1%). The pooled mean adverse event dropout rates for antidepressants when compared to placebo were 12% versus 7%. The RD by meta-analysis was 0.05 (95% CI 0.03 to 0.07, z = 6.10, N = 13, P<0.001).

Data from 8 trials (10 contrasts) that included an SSRI antidepressant as one of the treatment arms indicated that the OR by meta-analysis for response rates for antidepressants when compared to placebo was 1.36 (95% CI 1.19 to 1.56, z = 4.55, N = 10, P<0.001; χ^2 = 25.45, df = 9, P = 0.003, I^2 = 64.6%). The ORs for the SSRIs and the non-SSRIs had overlapping CIs indicating similar effects between these drugs.

There were a total of 6 trials that were of 6–8 weeks' duration and 4 trials that were of 10–12 weeks' duration. The OR for response by meta-analysis for the 10- to 12-week trials was 1.73 (95% CI 1.42 to 2.09, z = 5.51, N = 5, P<0.001). The OR for response by meta-analysis for the 6- to 8-week trials was 1.22 (95% CI 1.05 to 1.42, z = 2.60, N = 8, P = 0.01). The difference in the ORs between the 10- to 12-week trials and the 6- to 8-week trials was significant (χ = 7.42, df = 1, P<0.01). The pooled mean response rates for antidepressants when compared to placebo were 55% versus 41% in the 10- to 12-week trials and were 38% versus 31% in the 6- to 8-week trials. The RDs by meta-analysis for antidepressants when compared to placebo were 0.14 (95% CI 0.09–0.18, z = 5.57, N = 5, P<0.001) for the 10- to 12-week trials and 0.05 (95% CI 0.01–0.08, z = 2.63, N = 8, P = 0.009) for the 6- to 8-week trials, respectively.

A funnel plot indicated a symmetrical distribution about the mean indicating that there was no evidence for publication bias.

Conclusions This meta-analysis indicates that second-generation antidepressants are more effective than placebo in treating nonpsychotic unipolar major depressive disorder among community-dwelling individuals ≥60 years in age. The effect of these drugs was modest and there was no superiority demonstrated for any particular drug. Longer duration trials appear to produce better response and remission rates when compared to shorter duration trials.

Strengths of the study

1. The investigators conducted a meta-analysis that was rigorous in both design and execution.
2. The investigators used the Jadad scale to assess the quality of the included studies.
3. The results of the study are clear and easy to interpret.

Limitations of the study

1. All the trials included in the study were conducted by the manufacturers of antidepressants which can induce selection bias.
2. The investigators also included trials that had not yet been published and their results not having been peer reviewed.

3. The investigators only included second-generation antidepressants that were available in the United States.
4. The investigators only included clinical trials with medically stable community-dwelling individuals who were ≥60 years in age.
5. The investigators only included 10 trials with 13 contrasts in their analysis.
6. There were no trials of monoamine oxidase inhibitors (MAOIs), trazodone, mirtazapine, or nefazodone that met the selection criteria.

Take-home points Second-generation antidepressants are more effective than placebo in treating nonpsychotic unipolar major depressive disorder among community-dwelling individuals ≥60 years in age. No one drug or drug class in particular is superior to the other in treating this condition among older adults, but longer duration trials appear to confer additional benefits when compared to shorter-term trials.

Practical applications of the take-home points When older adults present with unipolar nonpsychotic major depressive disorder, treatment with second-generation antidepressants is both efficacious and safe. There is no evidence to suggest a superiority of one drug or drug class over the other in treating this condition, but longer duration trials appear to produce additional benefits.

References

1. Nelson JC, Delucchi K, Schneider LS. Efficacy of second generation antidepressants in late-life depression: a meta-analysis of the evidence. Am J Geriatr Psychiatry. 2008;16(7):558–67.
2. Jadad AR, Moore RA, Carroll D, Jenkinson C, Reynolds DJ, Gavaghan DJ, McQuay HJ. Assessing the quality of reports of randomized clinical trials: is blinding necessary? Control Clin Trials. 1996;17(1):1–12.

Chapter 36
A Double-Blind Randomized Controlled Trial of Olanzapine Plus Sertraline Versus Olanzapine Plus Placebo for Psychotic Depression: The Study of Pharmacotherapy of Psychotic Depression (STOP-PD)

Pallavi Joshi and Rajesh R. Tampi

Authors of the original article Barnett S Meyers, Alastair J Flint, Anthony J Rothschild, Benoit H Mulsant, Ellen M Whyte, Catherine Peasley-Miklus, Eros Papademetriou, Andrew C Leon, Moonseong Heo, STOP-PD Group

Journal publisher *Archives of General Psychiatry*

Year of publication 2009

Type of study Randomized placebo-controlled trial

Funding sources US Public Health Service, National Center for Research Resources, National Institute of Mental Health (NIMH)

Objectives To compare the remission rates of major depression with psychotic features in individuals treated with a combination of olanzapine plus sertraline with those treated with olanzapine monotherapy, and to compare response by age [1].

Methods This study recruited a total of 259 adults over 18 years in age (142 adults ≥60 years in age) from the community to participate in a 12-week randomized, double-blind, and placebo-controlled trial of olanzapine plus sertraline compared

P. Joshi
University of Arizona College of Medicine, Phoenix, AZ, USA

R. R. Tampi (✉)
Creighton University School of Medicine, Omaha, NE, USA
e-mail: rajesh.tampi@yale.edu

R. R. Tampi et al. (eds.), *Essential Reviews in Geriatric Psychiatry*,
https://doi.org/10.1007/978-3-030-94960-0_36

with olanzapine monotherapy for major depression with psychotic features. To be eligible, participants were required to meet the DSM-IV-TR criteria for unipolar major depression with psychotic features. Inclusion criteria required the presence of at least one delusional belief, a score of 2 or higher on one of the conviction items of the Delusional Assessment Scale, and a score of 3 or higher on the delusion severity rating item of the Schedule for Affective Disorders and Schizophrenia (SADS). Participants were required to score 21 or higher on the 17-item Hamilton Depression Scale (HAM-D), indicating moderate-severe depression.

Exclusion criteria for this study were as follows: a diagnosis of dementia, presence of another Axis I psychotic or mood disorder, current body dysmorphic disorder or obsessive-compulsive disorder, or substance abuse during the preceding 3 months, unstable medical illness, neurological illness that might affect neuromuscular function, and ongoing need for medications that may cause depression or psychosis. Participants were excluded if immediate electroconvulsive therapy (ECT) was indicated because of their refusal to eat or drink or imminent risk for suicide. Participants with current suicidal ideation without intent were enrolled as inpatients. Participants receiving 15 mg or more of olanzapine per day for a minimum of 4 weeks during the current episode or those benefiting from their current psychotropic regimen were also excluded. The investigators allowed participants with known hyperlipidemia or diabetes mellitus to enroll if their metabolic conditions were stable.

In this 12-week study, the participants were evaluated every week for the first 6 weeks and every other week thereafter. The participants were randomly assigned to receive sertraline plus olanzapine or olanzapine plus placebo on the basis of a computer program that used stratified permuted block randomization. Additionally, the medication was provided in a double-blind fashion. Participants were started on olanzapine 5 mg a day and sertraline 50 mg a day or placebo, with dose increases every 3 days as tolerated. Frail older participants were started on 2.5 mg of olanzapine and 25 mg of sertraline or placebo. Doses were increased to 10 mg of olanzapine per day and 100 mg of sertraline or placebo before the end of week 1, and 15 mg of olanzapine per day and 150 mg of sertraline or placebo per day by the end of week 2, with further increases allowed to a maximum of 20 mg of olanzapine per day and 200 mg of sertraline per day as tolerated beginning in week 3.

The primary outcome measures in this study were scores on the HAM-D. Remission was defined as HAM-D score $\leq$10 at two consecutive assessments and SADS delusional item score=1 at the second assessment. Participants who achieved a HAM-D score $\leq$10 without delusions for the first time at week 12 were assessed again at week 13. Investigators were allowed to withdraw participants with insufficient clinical response, defined as having both a Clinical Global Improvement (CGI) Improvement scale score of $\leq$2 and a CGI-S score of $\geq$4. The side effects from the medications were measured using the Udvalg for Kliniske Undersøgelser (UKU) Side Effect Rating Scale.

The investigators used data from the last available visit to determine response (intent-to-treat principle) for participants who dropped out of the study. The two-tailed chi-square tests and linear modeling were used to compare the rates of response and side effects between the two groups.

Results

From a total of 375 individuals who signed the consent forms to participate in the study, a total of 259 individuals enrolled in the study. A total of 65 participants did not meet criteria, 26 withdrew consent prior to randomization, and 11 were excluded for medical reasons.

A total of 129 participants were assigned to the combination therapy group when compared to 130 participants in the monotherapy group. The groups were stratified by age (<60 or ≥60 years). The demographic characteristics and baseline clinical measures were similar between the two groups, except for race and inpatient status. In the olanzapine/sertraline group, 85.3% participants were white, 13.2% were African American, and 1.6% were Asian when compared with 83.1%, 9.2%, and 7.7%, respectively, in the olanzapine/placebo group ($P = 0.05$). Frequency of inpatient status at baseline was 75.2% in the olanzapine/sertraline group and 63.1% in the olanzapine/placebo group ($P = 0.05$). The mean age of the participants was 57.4 (SD = 18.0) years in the olanzapine/sertraline group and 58.5 (17.5) years in the olanzapine/placebo group. The mean age of younger adults was 41.3 (10.8) years ($n = 117$) vs. 71.7 (7.8) years in older adults ($n = 142$).

Sixty-three percent (81 out of 129) of participants in the olanzapine/sertraline group completed the 12-week study when compared to 47% (61 out of 130) of participants in the olanzapine/placebo group. Fifty-four of the 129 participants (41.9%) in the olanzapine/sertraline group responded to treatment when compared with 31 of 130 (23.9%) participants in the olanzapine/placebo group ($P = 0.002$). Treatment interactions with race, site, or inpatient status were not significant. Participants in the olanzapine/sertraline group had lower HAM-D scores ($P<0.001$) and lower CGI-S scores ($P = 0.02$) than those in the olanzapine/placebo group. Participants in the olanzapine/sertraline group also had higher rates of remission than those in the olanzapine/placebo group (66.7% vs. 49.2%; $P = 0.04$). However, there was no significant difference in the SADS delusional item score in the two groups ($P = 0.26$). Combination therapy was superior in both younger adults (OR=1.25; 95% CI, 1.05–1.50; $P = 0.02$) and older adults (OR = 1.34; 95% CI, 1.09–1.66; $P = 0.01$). A three-way interaction between age, treatment, and time was found to be insignificant (OR = 1.05; 95% CI, 0.80–1.37; $P = 0.75$).

A total of 12.4% (16/129) of participants in the olanzapine/sertraline group dropped out due to clinical worsening when compared to 10% (13/130) of participants in the olanzapine/placebo group ($P = 0.54$). A total of 3.1% (4/129) of participants in the olanzapine/sertraline group dropped out due to poor tolerability when compared to 6.9% (9/130) of participants in the olanzapine/placebo group and ($P = 0.16$).

The most common side effects were weight gain, sedation, and orthostatic dizziness (54.3%, 28.7%, and 15.5%, respectively, in the olanzapine/sertraline group; 53.4%, 30.8%, and 10.0% respectively, in the olanzapine/placebo group), with no significant difference between the two groups. Five participants (four in the olanzapine/sertraline group) had increased suicidal thinking or behavior, and one participant in the olanzapine/sertraline group completed suicide at week 4 (3.1% vs. 0.7%; Fisher exact, $P = 0.21$).

Younger subjects were significantly more likely than older subjects to meet UKU criteria for significant weight gain (65.0% vs. 45.1%, $P = 0.001$) but were less likely to experience pedal edema (4.3% vs. 13.4%, $P = 0.01$). There were no differences in incident akathisia or tardive dyskinesia by age group. Older subjects had higher extrapyramidal symptom scores during the trial; the interaction between age group and extrapyramidal symptom severity was not significant ($P = 0.21$). Rates of attrition due to poor tolerability in younger and older subjects were statistically comparable (4.3% vs. 5.6%, $P = 0.62$).

The investigators found increased cholesterol and triglyceride concentrations in both age groups ($P<0.001$) without significant interactions with age. Increased glucose concentration was observed only in the younger adults and the interaction between age group and glucose increases was not significant ($P = 0.16$). The investigators found significant weight increases in both age groups, with greater increases in participants <60 years of age (6.5 kg vs. 3.3 kg, $P = 0.001$).

Conclusions Evidence from this 12-week randomized, double-blind, and placebo-controlled trial indicates that a combination of olanzapine and sertraline is more effective than olanzapine alone in reducing symptoms of major depression with psychosis among adults ≥60 years in age and is generally well tolerated.

Strengths of the study

1. Randomized, double-blind, and placebo-controlled trial design.
2. The study assessed on the basis of Jadad score indicates that this was a high-quality study with a score of 5 out of 5 [2].

Questions Yes (1) No (0)	Was the study described as random?	Was the randomization scheme described and appropriate?	Was the study described as double-blind?	Was the method of double blinding appropriate? (Were both the patient and the assessor appropriately blinded?)	Was there a description of dropouts and withdrawals?	Total score Range of score quality 0–2 Low 3–5 High
Score	1	1	1	1	1	5

3. The study sample included a substantial number of older adults (≥60 years).
4. All participants had moderate to severe depression symptoms based on the HAM-D score.
5. The study included participants admitted to inpatient psychiatry (75.2% in the olanzapine/sertraline group and 63.1% in the olanzapine/placebo group).

Limitations of the study

1. A short duration of study period of 12 weeks.
2. The recruitment was completed through advertisements and referrals.
3. A restrictive sample which excluded participants with a diagnosis of dementia, neurological conditions, comorbid mood or psychotic disorders, unstable medical illness, and active alcohol or substance use disorder.
4. 85.3% of participants in the olanzapine/sertraline group and 83.1% in the olanzapine/placebo group were white.
5. There was a 45.2% rate of attrition.
6. There was exclusion of participants receiving ECT.

Take-home points Despite some limitations, this high-quality randomized, double-blind, and placebo-controlled trial indicates that a combination of olanzapine and sertraline is more efficacious than olanzapine alone in reducing symptoms of major depression with psychosis among adults ≥60 years in age. Older adults were not more likely to experience falls, sedation, or extrapyramidal symptoms than younger adults and had less weight gain than younger adults.

Practical applications of the take-home point Among older adults who present with major depression with psychotic features with moderate to severe symptoms, a combination of olanzapine and sertraline is an efficacious and well-tolerated treatment option.

References

1. Meyers BS, Flint AJ, Rothschild AJ, Mulsant BH, Whyte EM, Peasley-Miklus C, Papademetriou E, Leon AC, Heo M, STOP-PD Group. A double-blind randomized controlled trial of olanzapine plus sertraline vs olanzapine plus placebo for psychotic depression: the study of pharmacotherapy of psychotic depression (STOP-PD). Arch Gen Psychiatry. 2009;66(8):838–47.
2. Jadad AR, Moore RA, Carroll D, Jenkinson C, Reynolds DJ, Gavaghan DJ, McQuay HJ. Assessing the quality of reports of randomized clinical trials: is blinding necessary? Control Clin Trials. 1996;17:1–12.

Chapter 37
Speed of Remission in Elderly Patients with Depression: Electroconvulsive Therapy Versus Medication

Peter Ureste

Authors of the original article Harm-Pieter Spaans, Pascal Sienaert, Filip Bouckaert, Julia F van den Berg, Esmée Verwijk, King H Kho, Max L Stek, Rob M Kok

Journal published *The British Journal of Psychiatry*

Year of publication 2015

Type of study Randomized controlled trials

Funding sources Kok et al. were supported by a research grant from Wyeth (grant number 100186). For Spaans et al., none reported.

Objectives To compare the speed of remission using electroconvulsive therapy (ECT) versus medication in older adults [1].

Methods The authors compared two randomized controlled trials (RCTs): one comparing the efficacy of ECT techniques, while the other examined the efficacy of antidepressants [2, 3]. The ECT trial investigated the efficacy and cognitive side effects of brief pulse versus ultrabrief unilateral stimuli in 116 subjects (18 years of age and older) over 6 weeks. The medication trial studied the efficacy and side effects of nortriptyline versus venlafaxine in 81 subjects (60 years of age and older) over 12 weeks. All participants in both trials were inpatients and met Diagnostic and Statistical Manual of Mental Disorders, 4th Edition (DSM-IV) criteria for major

P. Ureste (✉)
Department of Psychiatry and Behavioral Sciences, University of California San Francisco, San Francisco, CA, USA
e-mail: Peter.Ureste@ucsf.edu

R. R. Tampi et al. (eds.), *Essential Reviews in Geriatric Psychiatry*,
https://doi.org/10.1007/978-3-030-94960-0_37

depression. The diagnosis of major depression was confirmed using the Mini-International Neuropsychiatric Interview in the ECT trial and the International Diagnosis Checklist in the medication trial.

The severity of depressive symptoms was assessed weekly in the ECT trial and in weeks 1, 3, 5, 7, 9, and 12 in the medication trial using the Montgomery-Asberg Depression Rating Scale (MADRS) and Hamilton Rating Scale for Depression (HRSD, 17-item version). The following exclusion criteria were implemented in the ECT trial:

1. Age less than 60 years
2. MADRS score <20
3. Diagnosis of bipolar depression

Of the 47 subjects included in the ECT trial, 44.7% ($N = 21$) received brief pulse ECT and 55.3% ($N = 26$) ultrabrief pulse ECT. In the medication trial, all participants ($N = 81$) were included and made up the medication arm. Of these subjects, 49.4% ($N = 40$) were treated with venlafaxine and 50.6% ($N = 41$) with nortriptyline. For all groups, assessments were available at baseline and at weeks 1, 3, and 5.

The primary outcome measure was the difference between the two groups in the time to achieve remission, defined as a MADRS score <10 within 5 weeks. Secondary outcome measures were the differences in the time to achieve remission based on an HRSD remission score <8 and the hazard ratios (HRs) of achieving remission within 5 weeks.

Possible differences in baseline variables between the ECT and medication arms were analyzed with chi-squared tests for categorical variables, two-sided Student's t-test for normally distributed continuous variables, and Mann-Whitney U-tests for nonparametric analysis of continuous variables. A Cox proportional hazards model analysis with time to remission was used to compare trajectories of the ECT and medication groups. HRs with 95% confidence intervals (CIs) of achieving remission with ECT compared with medications were calculated. Whole ECT group (brief and ultrabrief pulse) and whole medication group (venlafaxine and nortriptyline) were compared with Cox's regression model to confirm whether grouping was justified.

Results There were no statistical differences at baseline between the ECT and medication groups in age, gender, proportion of subjects with psychotic features, symptom severity, duration of current episode, and proportion of subjects with late onset first episode of depression. The ECT group had used a greater number of different antidepressants during the study period compared with the medication group (average of 2.4 vs. 0.9, $P<0.001$).

The average time to remission was shorter for the ECT group (3.07 weeks) compared to the medication group (3.95 weeks) based on MADRS scores ($P = 0.008$). On the other hand, when based on the HRSD, the average time to remission for the ECT group was 3.07 weeks compared to 3.5 weeks for the medication though this was not found to be statistically significant ($P = 0.229$). The HR for remission within 5 weeks of treatment based on the MADRS for ECT compared with medication was 3.4 (95% CL 1.9–6.2, *P*<0.001) after adjustment for age, gender, presence of psychotic depression, symptom severity, and if it was considered late onset of first depression. The HR after additional adjustment for the duration of their current depression episode and number of antidepressants to treat the current episode was 8.2 (95% CI 3.6–19.0, *P*<0.001). The results for remission defined as a score of <8 on the HRSD as a secondary outcome were 2.7 (95% CI 1.5–4.9, *P* = 0.001) and 4.5 (CL (5% 2.0–10.2, *P*<0.001), respectively.

Using additional Cox's regression analysis, ECT brief and ultrabrief pulse subgroups were compared to both medication subgroups. The HRs for achieving remission within 5 weeks using MADRS were the following: 3.9 (95% CI 1.7–8.7, *P* = 0.001) for brief pulse ECT versus nortriptyline, 5.9 (95% CI 2.1–16.6, *P* = 0.001) for brief pulse ECT versus venlafaxine, 2.3% (95% CI 1.1–5.2, *P* = 0.036) for ultrabrief pulse ECT versus nortriptyline, and 3.6 (95% CI 1.4–9.2, *P* = 0.007) for ultrabrief pulse ECT versus venlafaxine.

Conclusions Older adult inpatients with severe major depression achieved remission, as defined by a MADRS score <10, significantly faster when treated with ECT compared to antidepressants. Within 5 weeks, 63.8% (30/47) of older adults treated with ECT achieved remission according to the MADRS scores, compared with only 23.5% (19/81) treated with medication. This finding was not confirmed when analyzing HRSD scores though this could be due to missing HRSD data in the ECT group and HRSD scores reporting an extra remission in the medication group. The final remission rates of 63.8% (30/47) after 6 weeks in the ECT group and 33.3% (27/81) after 12 weeks in the medication group imply ECT being more advantageous as a treatment modality.

Strengths of the study

1. This study was the first RCT to assess speed of remission as an outcome criterion in older adults with severe major depression.
2. Both trials were randomized in design.
3. The study sample included only older adults (≥60 years).
4. All participants had moderate to severe depressive symptoms based on the MADRS.

Limitations of the study

1. A small sample size of 47 participants received ECT.
2. A short study period of 5 weeks.
3. The study results used came from two RCTs.
4. Cognition, somatic, and psychiatric comorbidities were assessed differently in each of the original trials and could therefore not be evaluated as potential confounders.
5. Assessments of participants were carried out by different groups of researchers, although both were trained on the use of depression rating scales.

6. The study assessments of the medication group were only available at baseline and in weeks 1, 3, and 5, whereas weekly assessments in the ECT trial were available.
7. To allow comparison between the groups at the four time points (baseline and weeks 1, 3, and 5), three remissions that occurred in week 4 of the ECT study were counted in week 5, which resulted in a slight underestimation of the speed of remission with ECT.

Take-home points This study comparing data of two RCTs indicates that ECT was faster in achieving remission of severe depressive symptoms compared to treatment with antidepressants.

Practical applications of the take-home point Among older adults with moderate to severe major depression, ECT had a substantially faster speed of remission compared to antidepressants. ECT deserves a more prominent position for the treatment of older adults with severe major depression.

References

1. Spaans HP, Sienaert P, Bouckaert F, van den Berg JF, Verwijk E, Kho KH, et al. Speed of remission in elderly patients with depression: electroconvulsive therapy v. medication. Br J Psychiatry. 2015;206(1):67–71.
2. Spaans HP, Verwijk E, Comijs HC, Kok RM, Sienaert P, Bouckaert F, et al. Efficacy and cognitive side effects after brief pulse and ultrabrief pulse right unilateral electroconvulsive therapy for major depression: a randomized, double-blind, controlled study. J Clin Psychiatry. 2013;74(11):e1029–36.
3. Kok RM, Nolen WA, Heeren TJ. Venlafaxine versus nortriptyline in the treatment of elderly depressed inpatients: a randomised, double-blind, controlled trial. Int J Geriatr Psychiatry. 2007;22(12):1247–54.

Chapter 38
A Systematic Review and Meta-analysis of Psychotherapy for Late-Life Depression

Jason Gandelman and Peter Ureste

Authors of the original article Alice X Huang, Kevin Delucchi , Laura B Dunn, J Craig Nelson

Journal published *American Journal of Geriatric Psychiatry*

Year of publication 2015

Type of study Systematic review and meta-analysis

Funding sources University of California, San Francisco, Epstein Endowment

Objectives To determine the efficacy of psychotherapy for the treatment of late-life depression (LLD) and to determine the effect of the type of control group on the magnitude of psychotherapy effects [1].

Methods The authors identified studies through a systematic search of English-language articles in PubMed, PsycINFO, and Cochrane Central Register of Controlled Trials. Search criteria included MeSH and keyword terms: psychotherapy, counseling, therapy, aged, aging, elder, elderly, geriatric, late life, later life, old, older, and depressed, depression, and depressive disorder. Articles were also found through examining recent reviews.

The inclusion criteria for studies chosen for this meta-analysis were as follows: acute-phase randomized, controlled trials of psychotherapy published in

J. Gandelman · P. Ureste (✉)
Department of Psychiatry and Behavioral Sciences, University of California San Francisco, San Francisco, CA, USA
e-mail: Jason.Gandelman@ucsf.edu; Peter.Ureste@ucsf.edu

R. R. Tampi et al. (eds.), *Essential Reviews in Geriatric Psychiatry*,
https://doi.org/10.1007/978-3-030-94960-0_38

peer-reviewed journals from the inception of the above online databases and study participants all had age older than 55 years. Psychotherapy intervention did not need to be of a particular methodology, but did need to meet two of three criteria: (1) the treatment was based on psychological principles, (2) the treatment was offered to the psychological community (e.g., there was a manual available), and (3) the treatment had specific components that were intended to be therapeutic. The authors included bibliotherapy studies for LLD in this meta-analysis, although this therapy is not exclusively administered face to face.

The exclusion criteria for studies chosen for this meta-analysis were as follows: psychotherapy interventions that were adjunctive to pharmacotherapy or other therapy, maintenance and prevention trials, trials with no depression criteria, trials that included patients with dementia, and trials limited to one medical disease (e.g., when participants were selected for Parkinson's disease or stroke).

Standardized mean difference scores (SMDs) were used as the primary outcome and measure of effect size, as the included studies used different outcome scales. The SMD is defined as the difference between the mean change scores of the treatment and control groups divided by the standard deviation of the difference. SMDs are thus weighted by the sample size when combined in the meta-analysis. If change scores and their standard deviations (SDs) were not reported, they were calculated by the meta-analysis authors and SD was estimated using a formula from the Cochrane Handbook [2].

SMDs with 95% confidence intervals (CIs), z score, and P values were calculated for each treatment-control contrast (some trials had multiple treatment groups). For the meta-analysis, SMDs were combined using a random-effects model for a meta-analytic summary of all treatments and then grouped by type of control condition.

Sensitivity analyses were also completed, which stratified trials in the meta-analysis based on certain dichotomous characteristics to determine if those characteristics changed the effect of psychotherapy significantly.

Exploratory analyses assessed whether certain trial characteristics were correlated with SMD including mean age of the sample, duration of the trial, number of sessions, baseline depression severity, sample size, publication year, and the study quality.

Scale totals were converted to 17-item Hamilton Rating Scale for Depression [HRSD] scores. To evaluate publication bias and determine the association of sample size with the SMD, the authors created a funnel plot and performed an Egger analysis.

To evaluate the quality of studies included in the meta-analysis, the authors used the 25-item psychotherapy quality rating scale (RCT-PQRS) developed by the American Psychiatric Association's Committee on Research on Psychiatric Treatments.

Results The authors ultimately selected a total of 27 studies for inclusion in this meta-analysis. All 27 studies were randomized, controlled trials (RCTs). In 11 of the studies, raters were explicitly blinded to treatment assignment. Trial duration ranged from 4 to 26 weeks (median = 7 weeks), with 4 to 12 psychotherapy sessions (median = 8 sessions). The types of psychotherapy included were cognitive behavioral therapy (CBT), cognitive therapy, behavioral therapy, problem-solving therapy (PST), interpersonal therapy, brief dynamic therapy, bibliotherapy, reminiscence therapy, and a "Coping with Depression" course. The types of control groups used in the selected RCTs were categorized into five types: (1) waitlist, (2) treatment as usual (TAU), (3) attention, (4) supportive therapy, and (5) placebo.

Based on the RCT-PQRS criteria (possible range from 0 at worst to 48 at best quality), the study quality of 27 selected RCTs was highly variable, ranging from "very poor" to "exceptionally good" with corresponding numeric total scores ranging from 18 to 43. Mean RCT-PQRS total score was 27.4 corresponding to "average" overall study quality.

The full combined meta-analytic SMD for all psychotherapy treatments versus all control types demonstrated psychotherapy was more effective than control: SMD = 0.73 (95% CI: 0.51–0.95, $z = 6.42$, $P<0.00001$). For context, SMD=0 would mean that the change in depression score for the treatment group was the same as the control group.

The type of control group used in RCT had a significant impact on SMD and in fact was the greatest moderator of treatment-control difference ($\chi 2 = 35.67$, df = 4, $P<0.0001$). The "attention" control group had the largest SMD = 1.36 (95% CI: 0.36–2.37, $z = 2.67$, $P<0.008$). The "placebo" control group had the smallest SMD = 0.05 and thus treatment was not significantly different from control (95% CI: −0.16–0.26, $z = 0.45$, $P = 0.66$).

Sensitivity analysis demonstrated that type of therapy and site of care did significantly moderate treatment-control differences, but stratification by trials that used HRSD, minimum age >60, or face-to-face therapy did not. Group therapy was associated with significantly different (greater) SMD than individual therapy or bibliotherapy ($\chi 2 = 6.45$, df = 2, $P<0.04$), suggestive of group therapy associated with greatest depression symptom improvement. Site of care at home was associated with significantly different (greater) SMD than site of care at clinic ($\chi 2 = 14.14$, df = 1, $P<0.0002$), suggestive of home care associated with relatively greater depression symptom improvement.

Exploratory analyses revealed that the SMD was strongly associated with the study quality, sample size, and year of publication, modestly associated with trial duration, and not significantly associated with mean age, depression severity, or the number of sessions. Interestingly, trial quality by RCT-PQRS and recency (year of publication) was inversely related to the SMD. This suggests that quality and methodological rigor appeared to improve in recent studies resulting in more conservative estimates of effects. Studies that were larger also tended to yield smaller SMD effect sizes.

Conclusions This meta-analysis confirmed that psychotherapy is an effective treatment for LLD and the magnitude of the effect varies significantly by the type of control group chosen as a comparison.

Strengths of the study

1. This meta-analysis included only RCTs, which is the highest available category of evidence.
2. Systematic reviews with meta-analyses are theoretically less susceptible to bias and the pooling of multiple studies and subjects can enhance the precision of estimated odds ratio (OR), i.e., tighter confidence intervals, and thus reduce the probability of false-negative results.
3. The study sample included only older adults (≥55 years).
4. The study conducted sensitivity and exploratory analyses to investigate the moderators of effect size.
5. The quality of meta-analyses is discussed by Higgins et al. [3] using a qualitative 43-question list that is grouped into four categories (see table below for our evaluation of this meta-analysis).

Questions **Yes** **Probably yes** **Unclear** **Probably no** **No** **Not applicable**	**(A) Data sources:** Were the review methods adequate such that biases in location and assessment of studies were minimized or able to be identified?	**(B) Analysis of individual studies by the meta-analyst:** Were the individual studies analyzed appropriately and without avoidable bias?	**(C) General meta-analysis:** Were the basic meta-analysis methods appropriate?	**(D) Reporting and interpretation:** Are the conclusions justified and the interpretations sound?
Answer	Probably yes	Probably yes	Yes	Yes

Limitations of the study

1. Meta-analysis authors conducted funnel plot and Egger's test of the combined trials, which suggested potential publication bias. In particular, the meta-analysis included several small trials with large SMDs. Analysis by control type divided studies into subgroups that were sometimes comprised of a small number of trials. All of this limits the conclusions that can be drawn from this meta-analysis.
2. This meta-analysis used an inclusive approach to trial selection; thus, a variety of psychotherapy methodologies were combined and conclusions about specific psychotherapy modalities, for example, CBT for LLD, cannot be made.
3. This meta-analysis was not intended or powered to show that specific psychotherapy modalities were more or less effective.
4. This meta-analysis included many additional exploratory analyses that were not corrected for multiple comparisons.

Take-home points Despite limitations, this high-quality meta-analysis showed that psychotherapy is an effective treatment for LLD. While it is difficult to compare psychotherapy studies to antidepressant studies, the benefit of psychotherapy appears to have a similar or superior effect size for LLD.

Practical applications of the take-home point Among older adults who present with LLD, psychotherapy is an effective treatment option.

References

1. Huang AX, Delucchi K, Dunn LB, Nelson JC. A systematic review and meta-analysis of psychotherapy for late-life depression. Am J Geriatr Psychiatry. 2015;23(3):261–73.
2. Cochrane Handbook for Systematic Reviews of Interventions. https://training.cochrane.org/handbook/current/chapter-06. Accessed 10 May 2021.
3. Higgins JP, Lane PW, Anagnostelis B, Anzures-Cabrera J, Baker NF, Cappelleri JC, Haughie S, Hollis S, Lewis SC, Moneuse P, Whitehead A. A tool to assess the quality of a meta-analysis. Res Synth Methods. 2013;4(4):351–66.

Chapter 39
A Novel Strategy for Continuation ECT in Geriatric Depression: Phase 2 of the PRIDE Study

Paul A. Parcon and Peter Ureste

Authors of the original article Charles H Kellner, Mustafa M Husain, Rebecca G Knapp, W Vaughn McCall, Georgios Petrides, Matthew V Rudorfer, Robert C Young, Shirlene Sampson, Shawn M McClintock, Martina Mueller, Joan Prudic, Robert M Greenberg, Richard D Weiner, Samuel H Bailine, Peter B Rosenquist, Ahmad Raza, Styliani Kaliora, Vassilios Latoussakis, Kristen G Tobias, Mimi C Briggs, Lauren S Liebman, Emma T Geduldig, Abeba A Teklehaimanot, Mary Dooley, Sarah H Lisanby, CORE/PRIDE Work Group

Journal published *American Journal of Psychiatry*

Year of publication 2016

Type of study Two-phased randomized placebo-controlled trial

Funding sources Supported by National Institute of Mental Health (NIMH) grants U01MH055495, U01MH081362, U01MH086127, U01MH086127, U01MH086130, U01MH08612005, U01MH084241, and U01MH086122

Objectives This study evaluated the efficacy and tolerability of continuation ECT plus medication when compared to medication alone in depressed geriatric patients

P. A. Parcon
Molecular Imaging Branch, National Institute of Mental Health, Bethesda, MA, USA
e-mail: paul.parcon@nih.gov

P. Ureste (✉)
Department of Psychiatry and Behavioral Sciences, University of California San Francisco, San Francisco, CA, USA
e-mail: Peter.Ureste@ucsf.edu

R. R. Tampi et al. (eds.), *Essential Reviews in Geriatric Psychiatry*,
https://doi.org/10.1007/978-3-030-94960-0_39

after a successful course of ECT for reduction of depressive symptom severity and relapse [1].

Methods This study is a continuation of a multi-site study of ultrabrief right unilateral electroconvulsive therapy (ECT) for depressed geriatric patients, and compared continuation of ECT with medication compared to medication alone [2]. Patients enrolled into phase 1 were ≥60 years, with unipolar depression without a diagnosis of dementia, and pre-treatment Hamilton Depression Rating Scale (HAM-D) scores ≥21. Patients in the initial study were considered to be remitters if (1) they had a score ≤10 on HAM-D on two consecutive ratings and (2) the HAM-D score did not increase >3 points on the second rating, or it remained ≤6. Exclusion criteria included diagnoses of bipolar disorder, schizophrenia, schizoaffective disorder, dementia, delirium, intellectual disability, substance abuse or dependence in the last 6 months, or neurological or medical conditions assumed to affect cognition or treatment response. Patients with contraindications to venlafaxine or lithium were also excluded.

The sample in the randomized phase (phase 2) included 120 patients who were considered remitters after an acute course of right unilateral ultrabrief pulse ECT [1]. They were randomized into two groups: a medication-only arm where patients were treated with venlafaxine plus lithium over 24 weeks and an ECT plus medication arm, which included four continuation treatments over 1 month, with additional ECT as needed, alongside continuation of venlafaxine plus lithium. Intervention in the ECT arm included a fixed ECT schedule of four treatments in 1 month. Additional ECT treatments were performed based on the Symptom-Titrated, Algorithm-Based Longitudinal ECT (STABLE) algorithm, based on HAM-D scores that were performed on a fixed schedule of twice-monthly clinic visits with telephone HAM-D screens on intervening weeks. Both arms received venlafaxine open-label with titration to 225 mg a day as tolerated, and lithium on moderate doses with lithium levels in the range of 0.4–0.6 mg. Lithium was held for 24 hours before each ECT treatment.

Primary efficacy outcome measures were the HAM-D scores, with the week 24 assessment as the primary time point. Secondary analyses included the Clinical Global Impression-Severity (CGI-S) rating scale and Mini-Mental State Examination (MMSE) scores. Efficacy was also measured with relapse status and time to relapse, with relapse categorized as two consecutive HAM-D scores ≥21, psychiatric hospitalization, or suicidality, with relapse analyses considered descriptive. Safety was evaluated using adverse events.

Results Among the 240 patients who started phase 1, 62% (148) achieved remission. Of the 148 patients, 120 patients consented for phase 2 and received at least 1 randomized treatment. These individuals were included in the intent-to-treat sample.

Efficacy data based on mean HAM-D scores for the ECT plus medication group at 24 weeks was (mean = 5.5, 95% CI = 3.7–7.3). These scores were significantly lower than that of the medication-only group (mean = 9.4, 95% CI = 7.5–11.3). The effect size was 3.9 points ($P = 0.004$), which after adjustment for site and psychosis was 4.2 points ($P = 0.002$). A steeper decline in HAM-D scores over time was noted for the ECT plus medication group ($P<0.001$) when compared to the medication-only group ($P = 0.398$).

The odds of patients in the ECT plus medication group being rated as "not at all ill" at study end on the CGI-S score were significantly higher when compared to the medication-only group [odds ratio (OR) = 5.2, 95% CI = 1.5–17.7, $P = 0.009$] using the generalized linear mixed model where the baseline CGI-S, site, and psychosis were used as covariables.

A total of 20 of the 120 patients relapsed (16.7%), with 8/61 (13.1%) in the ECT plus medication group relapsed when compared to 12/59 (20.3%) in the medication-only arm. The odds of relapse were 1.7 times higher for the medication-only group.

The median time to relapse was longer in the ECT plus medication group when compared to medication-only group (7.5 weeks vs. 6.0 weeks). A total of 72/120 (60%) of patients did not relapse or drop out at the end of the study: ECT plus medication group [39/61, 64%] and medication-only group [33/59, 56%]. At week 24 for completers and time of exit for dropouts, the mean last observed HAM-D score was 7.7 [standard deviation (SD) = 5.5] for the ECT plus medication group versus 10.5 (SD = 8.2) for the medication-only group (effect size = 2.8 points, 95% CI = −0.2–5.8, $P = 0.065$).

During weeks 5–24 (flexible phase), 21/61 (34.4%) of patients in the ECT plus medication group received at least one additional ECT treatment. Among these 21 patients, only 7 of them received 1 additional treatment beyond the 4 fixed sessions. Only three of the patients relapsed despite additional treatment. Additionally, 4 patients had HAM-D scores of 11–15 and 14 patients had HAM-D scores ≤10 at the end of the study. Receipt of rescue ECT resulted in an immediate large decrease in HAM-D scores.

There was no statistically significant difference observed on the mean MMSE scores between the two treatment arms at the primary end point at 24 weeks (effect size = −0.38 points, 95% CI = −1.0–0.2). There was no difference in the occurrence or type of adverse events between the two treatment groups. Only two adverse events were identified as being related to ECT: one patient developed reduced heart rate and one patient had a sinus pause. Suicidal ideation occurred in three patients in the ECT plus medication arm. None of these events were thought to be related to ECT or lithium. In one patient suicidal ideation was thought to be possibly related to venlafaxine. One patient in the medication-only group developed lithium toxicity and was discontinued from the study. There were no serious adverse events that were judged to be due related in any way to ECT. There were no deaths in the phase 2 of the study.

The average venlafaxine dose was 191.6 mg a day with no significant differences noted between the two treatment groups. The mean lithium blood levels were 0.5 mEq/L in the medication-only group and 0.36 mEq/L in the ECT plus medication group. The level was lower in the ECT plus medication group as the lithium doses were held 24 hours prior to ECT treatments.

Conclusions Evidence from this 24-week study of 120 geriatric depressed patients indicates that right unilateral ultrabrief pulse ECT plus medication is more effective at maintaining remission and preventing relapse of unipolar depression when compared to medication alone. This intervention is also fairly well tolerated, with no remarkable differences in the occurrence or type of adverse events and no serious adverse events that were attributable to ECT.

Strengths of the study
1. Randomized, multi-site design with appropriate randomization.
2. The study sample size was sufficiently large (120 patients) and the duration was sufficiently long (24 weeks).
3. Results were significantly efficacious with large effect size.
4. The proposed protocol for continuation ECT provides strong efficacy with as few treatments as possible, increasing access and convenience for patients and providers.
5. Provides strong evidence (along with phase 1 of the study) for use of right unilateral ultrabrief ECT, which has fewer cognitive adverse effects and is more tolerable when compared to other forms of ECT.

Limitations of the study
1. Self-reported non-generalizability, given the complexity of research study. Despite symptom severity based on HAM-D scores, many patients in clinical practice may be too ill to participate in such a study. In fact, 69% of all eligible patients did not consent to the initial phase 1 of the study.
2. Complex algorithm for additional ECT, while necessary for standardization, possibly not generalizable to clinical practice.
3. Medication-only arm performed well compared to other studies of post-acute ECT, possibly implying participants were healthier than previous studies (38% relapse rate when compared to 20% relapse rate in this study).
4. No comparison with traditional continuation ECT, in which treatments are "tapered" at increasing intervals over the 6-month period, thereby proposing a new algorithm for ECT continuation without comparing to current practice.

Take-home points This high-quality randomized control trial demonstrates that rescue ECT on a flexible basis is more efficacious in reducing symptom severity and perhaps more efficacious in preventing relapse in depressed older adults when compared to medication alone.

Practical applications of the take-home point In older adults who have achieved remission of depression from ECT, a flexible schedule of additional rescue ECT treatments is more efficacious at reducing symptom severity and preventing relapse when compared to medication alone. Rescue ECT should be considered for up to 6 months post-remission to treat depression in older adults.

Author's Disclaimer "This review was prepared or accomplished by Dr. Parcon in his personal capacity. The opinions expressed in this book chapter are the author's own and do not reflect the view of the National Institutes of Health, the Department of Health and Human Services, or the United States government."

References

1. Kellner CH, Husain MM, Knapp RG, WV MC, Petrides G, Rudorfer MV, Young RC, Sampson S, SM MC, Mueller M, Prudic J, Greenberg RM, Weiner RD, Bailine SH, Rosenquist PB, Raza A, Kaliora S, Latoussakis V, Tobias KG, Briggs MC, Liebman LS, Geduldig ET, Teklehaimanot AA, Dooley M, Lisanby SH, CORE/PRIDE Work Group. A novel strategy for continuation ECT in geriatric depression: phase 2 of the PRIDE study. Am J Psychiatry. 2016;173(11):1110–8.
2. Kellner CH, Husain MM, Knapp RG, McCall WV, Petrides G, Rudorfer MV, Young RC, Sampson S, McClintock SM, Mueller M, Prudic J, Greenberg RM, Weiner RD, Bailine SH, Rosenquist PB, Raza A, Kaliora S, Latoussakis V, Tobias KG, Briggs MC, Liebman LS, Geduldig ET, Teklehaimanot AA, Lisanby SH, CORE/PRIDE Work Group. Right unilateral ultrabrief pulse ECT in geriatric depression: phase 1 of the PRIDE study. Am J Psychiatry. 2016;173(11):1101–9.

Chapter 40
Right Unilateral Ultrabrief Pulse ECT in Geriatric Depression: Phase 1 of the PRIDE Study

Alba E. Lara and Erica C. Garcia-Pittman

Authors of the original article Charles H Kellner, Mustafa M Husain, Rebecca G Knapp, W Vaughn McCall, Georgios Petrides, Matthew V Rudorfer, Robert C Young, Shirlene Sampson, Shawn M McClintock, Martina Mueller, Joan Prudic, Robert M Greenberg, Richard D Weiner, Samuel H Bailine, Peter B Rosenquist, Ahmad Raza, Styliani Kaliora, Vassilios Latoussakis, Kristen G Tobias, Mimi C Briggs, Lauren S Liebman, Emma T Geduldig, Abeba A Teklehaimanot, Sarah H Lisanby

Journal publisher *American Journal of Psychiatry*

Year of publication 2016

Type of study First phase of a randomized, open-label prospective multicenter two-phase study

Funding sources NIMH

Objectives To evaluate the efficacy of right unilateral ultrabrief pulse ECT combined with venlafaxine for the treatment of geriatric depression, including functional outcomes and tolerability [1].

Methods This study recruited a total of 240 adults, >60 years in age from 8 sites to participate in the acute treatment phase of an open-label study consisting of 3 times

A. E. Lara · E. C. Garcia-Pittman (✉)
The University of Texas at Austin Dell Medical School, Department of Psychiatry and Behavioral Sciences, Austin, TX, USA
e-mail: ecgarcia-pittman@ascension.org

R. R. Tampi et al. (eds.), *Essential Reviews in Geriatric Psychiatry*,
https://doi.org/10.1007/978-3-030-94960-0_40

weekly ultrabrief right unilateral ECT combined with venlafaxine for the treatment of major depressive disorder. Participants were either inpatients or outpatients referred for ECT to the study sites. Those who met criteria for a unipolar major depressive episode per the Structured Clinical Interview for DSM-IV Axis I Disorders (SCID-I) or Mini International Neuropsychiatric Interview and had a score of >21 on the Hamilton Depression Rating Scale (HAM-D) were included. Exclusion criteria included diagnosis of bipolar disorder, schizoaffective disorder, dementia, intellectual disability, or substance use disorder in the past 6 months; active medical or neurological condition that would have affected cognition or treatment response; contraindications to lithium or venlafaxine; and history of failure to respond in the current episode to an adequate trial of venlafaxine plus lithium or to ECT.

Assessments for depression included the HAM-D and Clinical Global Impressions severity scale (CGI-S) at baseline and three times weekly. Global cognitive function was measured using the Mini-Mental State Examination (MMSE) at baseline and three times weekly. Suicidal ideation was assessed using the Beck Scale for Suicide Ideation. Baseline medical burden was assessed using the Cumulative Illness Rating Scale for Geriatrics. Time to reorientation was measured by the ability to correctly answer five orientation questions during treatments 1–3 at minutes 3, 5, 10, 15, and 20 after ECT treatment. Safety measures were monitored externally.

In this study, medications were discontinued within 1 week of acute phase ECT initiation. Open-label venlafaxine was started at 37.5 mg within 5 days of initiation and titrated by increments of 37.5 mg every 3 days until a target dose of 225 mg daily was achieved, then continued. ECT was standardized with three times weekly standard right unilateral placement. Sites used either a Somatics Thymatron System IV with a pulse width 0.25 ms and current 0.89 A or a MECTA spECTrum device with a pulse width 0.3 ms and current 0.8 A. Dose titration was conducted to determine seizure threshold at the initial treatment, then dosed at 6 times the seizure threshold, with an adequate motor seizure defined as >15 seconds. If the HAM-D score improved by <25% from baseline by session 6, stimulus dose was increased by 50%. If the HAM-D score improved by <25% from baseline at treatment 9, stimulus dose was again increased by 50%.

The primary efficacy outcomes were remission status and trajectory of HAM-D scores. Remission was defined as a HAM-D score of <10 on two consecutive ratings, if the HAM-D did not increase >3 points on the second rating or it remained <6. The minimum number of ECT treatments required for remission was 2, but there was no maximum. Non-remitters were defined as not meeting remission criteria with at least 12 treatments and reached a plateau with no clinical improvement. Study non-completers or dropouts were defined by not meeting remission or non-remission criteria and discontinued ECT prior to 12 treatments. Secondary efficacy outcomes included response status, defined by at least 50% decrease from baseline on HAM-D, and speed of remission as defined by the number of ECT treatments required to achieve remission.

The statistical analysis included frequency distributions to describe categorical variables and means with standard deviations for continuous variables. The investigators used a paired t-test to evaluate the difference in mean change from baseline of HAM-D scores at each ECT session to describe the trajectory of symptom severity for the total sample and within outcome categories (remitters, non-remitters, dropouts). For some statistical analyses, the investigators combined study dropouts and non-remitters as they were considered to have had similar baseline and outcome characteristics.

Results Of the 240 patients who enrolled in the study, 172 completed the study. Most patients who were ineligible for the study had a diagnosis of bipolar depression (24%) or dementia (11%). The mean age of participants was 69.9 years. Females made up 57.5% of the study population and 95% of the study population was Caucasian. The participants' baseline subtypes of major depression were categorized as melancholic (59%), psychotic (11.7%), recurrent (87.5%), and atypical (2.1%). Mean HAM-D score was in the severe range (31.2), mean MMSE was normal (27.5), and mean CGI-S was "markedly ill" (5.3). Participants had an average of 2.4 prior hospitalizations and 2.4 prior antidepressant trials. Participants with a Beck Scale for Suicide Ideation score of 0 made up 52% of the sample.

As far as primary outcomes, there were 148 patients who remitted (61.7%; 95% CI = 55.2, 67.9) and 24 who did not remit (10.0%; 95% CI = 6.5, 14.5). Secondary efficacy outcomes revealed that 169 patients (70.4%; 95% CI 64.6, 76.2) were responders. Among remitters, the mean decrease in HAM-D score was 24.7 points (95% CI 23.5, 25.9; $p<0.001$) with mean final HAM-D score of 6.2 (SD 2.5). Among all participants, the mean percentage change from baseline in HAM-D score was 19.1 (95% CI = 17.7, 20.5, $p<0.001$) and mean percent change from baseline was 60.5% (95% CI = 56.8, 64.1).

As far as trajectory of ECT treatments, there was an initial rapid decrease in depression symptom severity for the entire sample, followed by a general downtrend through ECT treatment number 14 for remitters and the total group. The mean number of ECT treatments to achieve remission was 7.3 (SD 3.1). Among remitters, 19.6% required 4 or fewer treatments, 45% remitted within 2 weeks (6 treatments), and 74.3% remitted within 3 weeks (9 treatments). However, 25% of remitters required 10+ treatments for remission.

Cognitive results included relatively stable global cognitive function during the ECT treatment course, with no significant difference between baseline and post-ECT mean MMSE scores (27.5 [SD = 2.4] and 27.6 [SD = 2.6], respectively). Reorientation was achieved at 10 minutes post-ECT at sessions 1, 2, and 3 by 60.8%, 24.8%, 46.2% of patients.

This study found several predictors of a positive outcome. Patients aged >70 significantly more likely to remit with odds 1.89 times greater (95% CI = 1.11, 3.22, $p = 0.020$, logistic regression) than 60–69 y/o group. Patients with a Beck Scale of Suicide Ideation score of 0 had odds of remission that were twice as high compared to those with score >0 (OR = 2.0, 95% CI = 1.11, 3.57; $p = 0.021$, logistic regression). Early changes in HAM-D also predicted response. Each 1-point decrease after ECT session 1 was associated with a 5% increase in odds of remission (OR = 1.05, 85% CI = 1.001, 1.09; $p = 0.045$) and each 10-point decrease after session 1 was associated with approximately 60% odds of remitting (OR = 1.57, 95% CI = 1.01, 2.43).

Regarding treatment conditions, the mean seizure threshold for the total sample was 30.5 mC (SD 14.3) and 84% of patients required only one stimulus for an adequate seizure at the first treatment. A venlafaxine dose of 225 mg/day was achieved by 52.3% of patients and the mean dose of those not achieving target dosing was 113.7 mg/day. There were 16 severe adverse events affecting 13 patients that were potentially related to ECT and venlafaxine. These included confusion, tardive seizure, atrial fibrillation, urinary retention, hyponatremia, and syncope.

Conclusions Right unilateral ultrabrief pulse ECT with venlafaxine is a fast, highly effective treatment option for severe geriatric depression w/ excellent safety and tolerability. This study is comparable with other studies of mixed-age adults with ultrabrief right unilateral ECT in remission rates (ranges of remission are reported to be from 23.4% to 73% in mixed ages). Some prior studies have shown non-inferiority of right unilateral ultrabrief ECT to regular brief pulse ECT.

When compared to other techniques, this study reported slightly lower, but expected remission results (compared to prior CORE group studies). Right unilateral ultrabrief pulse ECT is effective with rapid remission speeds averaging 7.3 weeks with no significant cognitive changes. Additionally, in this study 84% of patients achieved an adequate seizure with one ultrabrief stimulus with mean seizure threshold of 30.5 mC. This suggests that clinicians using this method can minimize the risk of adverse cognitive effects from a higher absolute stimulus charge and increase the dose if clinically indicated.

Though recent meta-analyses did not find a significant difference in acute antidepressant effect with adding antidepressant medication to ECT, these authors added venlafaxine to prepare for phase 2 and prevent relapse. This study also did not show a difference in remission results when compared with high- versus medium-dose venlafaxine, so rates of remission were likely indicative of ECT efficacy.

Strengths of the study

1. Moderately large sample size with good power.
2. The sample included only older adults (>60 years).
3. All participants had severe depressive symptoms based on the HAM-D.
4. Standardized ECT methods were used.
5. Completion rate of 71.66%.

Limitations of the study

1. Limited generalizability. Most people were Caucasian, and the sample did not include common comorbidities including dementia, serious medical illness, or neurological comorbidity.

2. Patients with bipolar depression were excluded.
3. Open-label study.
4. No control group, but we can glean data from other studies without venlafaxine.

Take-home points
1. Right unilateral ultrabrief pulse ECT is relatively fast with this dose titration method.
2. Safety/tolerability is comparable to other ECT trials.
3. Efficacy is comparable to conventional brief pulse ECT.
4. Fewer cognitive side effects compared to brief pulse ECT and to bilateral ECT.

Practical applications of the take-home point Ultrabrief pulse width stimulation has evidence for rapid response and efficacy compared with conventional brief pulse ECT, with excellent safety and tolerability. Clinicians may consider starting with this technique for the majority of patients who will not clearly require bilateral ECT in order to reduce the potential for cognitive side effects. A reasonable course of action would be to start with right unilateral ultrabrief pulse ECT and change course if not progressing as desired by week 2.

Reference

1. Kellner CH, Husain MM, Knapp RG, WV MC, Petrides G, Rudorfer MV, Young RC, Sampson S, SM MC, Mueller M, Prudic J, Greenberg RM, Weiner RD, Bailine SH, Rosenquist PB, Raza A, Kaliora S, Latoussakis V, Tobias KG, Briggs MC, Liebman LS, Geduldig ET, Teklehaimanot AA, Lisanby SH, CORE/PRIDE Work Group. Right unilateral ultrabrief pulse ECT in geriatric depression: phase 1 of the PRIDE study. Am J Psychiatry. 2016;173(11):1101–9.

Chapter 41
Improvement in Depression Is Associated with Improvement in Cognition in Late-Life Psychotic Depression

Gregg A. Robbins-Welty and Paul A. Riordan

Authors of the original article Lindsay W Victoria, Ellen M Whyte, Meryl A Butters, Barnett S Meyers, George S Alexopoulos, Benoit H Mulsant, Anthony J Rothschild, Samprit Banerjee, Alastair J Flint

Journal published *American Journal of Geriatric Psychiatry*

Year of publication 2017

Type of study Secondary analysis of a double-blind, randomized, controlled trial

Funding sources For this specific study, they note that only the National Institute of Mental Health (NIMH) provided grants. Eli Lilly provided olanzapine, and Pfizer provided sertraline (or matching placebo) for the STOP-PD clinical trial, but per authors, neither provided funding nor otherwise participated in the trial. The authors also provide a list of other grant supports they have received including from various other sources including pharmaceutical companies as disclosures on potential conflicts of interest.

Objectives To investigate the relationship between change in cognition, depression, and psychosis after treatment among older adults with major depressive disorder with psychotic features [1]

G. A. Robbins-Welty
Durham Veterans Affairs Medical Center, Department of Psychiatry, Durham, NC, USA
e-mail: Gregg.robbinswelty@duke.edu

P. A. Riordan (✉)
Durham Veterans Affairs Medical Center, Department of Psychiatry and Behavioral Sciences, Duke University School of Medicine, Durham, NC, USA
e-mail: paul.riordan@duke.edu

R. R. Tampi et al. (eds.), *Essential Reviews in Geriatric Psychiatry*,
https://doi.org/10.1007/978-3-030-94960-0_41

Methods
Patient Selection

Included study participants were a subgroup of study participants from the Study of the Pharmacotherapy of Psychotic Depression (STOP-PD) [2] who were 60 years and older with an episode of major depressive disorder with psychotic features, which was defined as at least one associated delusion and a 17-item Hamilton Depression Rating Scale (HAM-17) total score greater than 21. Exclusion criteria included patients with another mood or psychotic disorder, substance abuse or dependence in the 3 months preceding evaluation, neurologic or neuromuscular disease, unstable medical illness, DSM-IV-defined dementia, or other clinically significant cognitive impairment before index episode of depression.

Study Design

The STOP-PD trial was a double-blinded, randomized controlled treatment efficacy trial in which olanzapine plus sertraline was tested against olanzapine plus placebo for psychotic depression. This sub-analysis of STOP-PD separated participants into "young old" (aged 60–71 years) and "older old" (aged 72–86 years) age groups. Baseline data was compared to data at the end of treatment (week 12) or at termination for those who did not complete the study. Outcomes included psychiatric symptom severity using the Brief Psychiatric Rating Scale (BPRS), depression severity using HAM-17, intensity of delusions and hallucination using the Schedule for Affective Disorders and Schizophrenia (SADS), cognitive function using the Mini-Mental State Examination (MMSE), information processing speed using the Stroop Word and Color tasks, executive function using the Stroop Color-Word interference task as well as the Initiation/Perseveration subscale of the Dementia Rating Scale (DRS I/P), and medical comorbidity as assessed by the Cumulative Illness Rating Scale (CIRS). The study investigators hypothesized that depressive symptoms would improve with treatment regardless of baseline cognitive functioning and that cognitive function would improve in both age groups as depressive and psychotic symptoms improved.

Statistical Analysis

Study investigators used t-tests to compare baseline and treatment end demographic data, Pearson correlation(r) calculations to assess associations between cognitive test performance and depression severity changes, and a linear regression model including education, age, change in HAM-17 score, and days on study medication to identify predictors of global cognitive impairment.

Results One-hundred and thirty-eight of 142 participants completed the MMSE at baseline and 122 at week 12. Severity of depression, delusions, or cognitive function did not differ significantly at baseline between young old and older old groups. There was evidence for significant impairment in cognition, information processing speed, and executive function among both the young old and older old group when compared to normative data. About 20% of participants in both the young old and older old group had significant cognitive impairment with MMSE scores less than 25. On the DRS I/P (an executive function test), the groups scored at the fifth and sixth percentiles. Both groups scored more than 2 standard deviations below the

Table 41.1 Percent change in symptoms from baseline

Group	HAM-17 (% change)	Delusions (% change)	BPRS (% change)
Young old	−51.7% ($P < 0.001$)	−53.9% ($P < 0.001$)	−36.4% ($P < 0.001$)
Older old	−44.3% ($P < 0.001$)	−49.3% ($P < 0.001$)	−29.2% ($P < 0.001$)

mean on both the Stroop Word Reading test, but on the Stroop Color naming task they performed normally for their ages.

At the end of the trial, young old and older old patients both experienced statistically significant reductions in the HAM-17 (95% CI: 44.3–51.7%), in the BPRS (95% CI: 29.2–36.4%), and in delusions (95% CI: 49.3–53.9%) (Table 41.1). Baseline cognitive function did not influence clinical improvement in depression or psychotic symptoms as demonstrated by a statistically insignificant association between baseline MMSE scores and change in HAM-17 or SADS in either group (young old group: HAM-17: $r(66) = 0.18$, $P = 0.15$; SADS: $r(66) = -0.05$, $P = 0.69$; older old group: HAM-17: $r(66) = 0.07$, $P = 0.60$; SADS: $r(66) = 0.21$, $P = 0.08$).

Young old participants with psychotic depression demonstrated a greater degree of improvement in cognitive function from baseline than older old participants (mean increase in MMSE of 1.0 points versus −0.2 points [standard deviation (SD) 3.4 vs 3.0]). There was a correlation between change in MMSE and HAM-17 in the young old group ($r(58) = -0.34$, $P = 0.007$, 95% confidence interval: −0.55 to −0.10) but not in the older old group ($r(58) = -0.11$, $P = 0.40$, 95% confidence interval: −0.35 to 0.15). Despite this correlation in the young old group, there was no correlation between improvement in MMSE and reduction in delusions (SADS) in either the young old group ($r(58) = -0.2$, $P = 0.1$) or the older old group ($r(58) = -0.05$, $P = 0.7$).

In the linear regression analysis, improvement in depressive symptoms (HAM-D), younger age, and higher education all predicted improvement in cognition (MMSE) (HAM-17 score: $b = -0.33$, $t(141) = -2.76$, $P < 0.01$; younger age $b = -0.18$, $t(141) = -2.03$, $P < 0.05$; higher education $b = 0.20$, $t(139) = 2.30$, $P < 0.05$). Days on study medication, type of medication, and medical comorbidity in either age group did not predict improvement in cognitive function (days on study medication: $b = -0.16$, $t(1398) = 1.33$, $P = 0.19$; olanzapine + sertraline: mean: 0.3, SD:2.6; olanzapine + placebo: mean: 0.5, SD: 3.8; $t(118) = 0.5$, $P = 0.7$; medical comorbidity young old: $r(57) = -0.08$, $P = 0.55$; older old: $r(57) = 0.05$, $P = 0.70$).

Conclusions This study showed that there is only a mild improvement in cognition even with clinically significant improvement in depressive symptoms. The improvement in cognition is further limited by age with only young old patients (60–71 years) showing statistically significant cognitive improvement on the MMSE with improvement in depressive symptoms. Furthermore, baseline cognitive functional status did not impact improvement in depressive symptoms in either group. It is unclear why the treatment of depression does not seem to significantly improve cognition. One possibility is that commonly used antidepressants might worsen cognitive impairment in elderly patients with dementia, as was noted in the citalopram for Alzheimer's disease (CiTAD) trial [3]. Lastly and notably, improvement in psychotic features did not affect cognitive function for either group.

Strengths of the Study

1. This study represents a relatively large sample of older adults with psychotic depression with multiple well-validated outcome measures allowing for a rigorous correlational analysis.
2. Study data was collected as part of a double-blind, randomized controlled treatment trial from four different academic sites.

Limitations of the Study

1. While the primary discovery of this trial was that cognitive impairment did not improve significantly as a result of improvement in cognition or delusions in older patients, the data collected was limited in regard to neuropsychological assessment. The MMSE is a commonly used screening tool for dementia syndromes but does not adequately characterize specific patterns of cognitive function or allow for a deeper understanding of underlying neuropathology. While a statistically significant effect was found, it is unclear if a 1-point improvement on the MMSE is clinically significant.
2. All secondary and subgroup analyses of data collected from randomized controlled trials must be interpreted cautiously due to the correlational natures of such studies and because the original studies are not adequately powered to test secondary outcomes [4].
3. There is no mention of inter-rater reliability or method of data collection/test administration in this article.

Take-Home Points

1. Cognitive dysfunction in older adults with psychotic depression receiving treatment did not prevent improvement of depressive or psychotic symptoms.
2. Cognitive function improved mildly with treatment of depressive symptoms in patients aged 60–71 years, but not in older participants (aged 72–86 years) with psychotic depression. This improvement was independent of medical comorbidity or baseline cognitive impairment.

Practical Applications of the Take-Home Points

1. Cognitive dysfunction may not impede successful treatment or clinical improvement of depressive or psychotic symptoms in older adults with psychotic depression.
2. Cognitive function might be expected to improve more so in young old (60- to 71-year-old) patients than in older old (72- to 86-year-old) patients with successful treatment of depressive symptoms in patients with psychotic depression.
3. Older patients (aged 72–86 years old) with psychotic depression and cognitive impairment should be considered and monitored for possible emerging dementia syndromes.

References

1. Victoria LW, Whyte EM, Butters MA, Meyers BS, Alexopoulos GS, Mulsant BH, Rothschild AJ, Banerjee S, Flint AJ. Improvement in depression is associated with improvement in cognition in late-life psychotic depression. Am J Geriatr Psychiatry. 2017;25(6):672–9.
2. Meyers BS, Flint AJ, Rothschild AJ, Mulsant BH, Whyte EM, Peasley-Miklus C, Papademetriou E, Leon AC, Heo M, STOP-PD Group. A double-blind randomized controlled trial of olanzapine plus sertraline vs olanzapine plus placebo for psychotic depression: the study of pharmacotherapy of psychotic depression (STOP-PD). Arch Gen Psychiatry. 2009;66(8):838–47.
3. Porsteinsson AP, Drye LT, Pollock BG, Devanand DP, Frangakis C, Ismail Z, Marano C, Meinert CL, Mintzer JE, Munro CA, Pelton G, Rabins PV, Rosenberg PB, Schneider LS, Shade DM, Weintraub D, Yesavage J, Lyketsos CG, CitAD Research Group. Effect of citalopram on agitation in Alzheimer disease: the CitAD randomized clinical trial. JAMA. 2014;311(7):682–91.
4. Wallach JD, Sullivan PG, Trepanowski JF, Sainani KL, Steyerberg EW, Ioannidis JP. Evaluation of evidence of statistical support and corroboration of subgroup claims in randomized clinical trials. JAMA Intern Med. 2017;177(4):554–60.

Part VI
Electroconvulsive Therapy

Chapter 42
Continuation/Maintenance Treatment with Nortriptyline Versus Combined Nortriptyline and ECT in Late-Life Psychotic Depression: A Two-Year Randomized Study

Jennifer Tu and Paul A. Riordan

Authors of the original article Victor Navarro, Cristóbal Gastó, Xavier Torres, Guillem Masana, Rafael Penadés, Joana Guarch, Mireia Vázquez, Montserrat Serra, Nuria Pujol, Luis Pintor, Rosa Catalán

Journal published *American Journal of Geriatric Psychiatry*

Year of publication 2008

Type of study Single-blind randomized control trial

Funding sources Unknown. No financial disclosures are mentioned in the article.

Objectives To assess the 2-year tolerability and efficacy of continuation/maintenance electroconvulsive therapy + nortriptyline (ECT + NT) versus nortriptyline alone (NT) in elderly patients with psychotic depression in remission after acute ECT [1]

Methods This study recruited a total of 38 adults, ≥60 years in age, from in- and out-patients at Hospital Clinic of Barcelona, Spain, to participate in a 2-year randomized, single-blind controlled trial of continuation/maintenance ECT plus nortriptyline for psychotic depression. In order to minimize the risk of diagnostic error,

J. Tu
Duke University School of Medicine, Durham, NC, USA
e-mail: jennifer.tu@duke.edu

P. A. Riordan (✉)
Durham Veterans Affairs Medical Center, Department of Psychiatry and Behavioral Sciences, Duke University School of Medicine, Durham, NC, USA
e-mail: paul.riordan@duke.edu

R. R. Tampi et al. (eds.), *Essential Reviews in Geriatric Psychiatry*,
https://doi.org/10.1007/978-3-030-94960-0_42

the authors included only patients who fulfilled DSM-IV criteria for current severe major depressive episode with psychotic symptoms, had a pre-treatment Hamilton Depression Rating Scale (HDRS) score of ≥21 (severe symptoms), did not meet DSM-IV criteria for dementia, and had a Mini-Mental State Examination (MMSE) score >25.

Additional exclusion criteria were neurological disorders affecting the central nervous system (CNS); uncontrolled medical illness at the time of recruitment; conditions that contraindicated the use of any of the study treatments; any history of mania, hypomania, or nonaffective psychosis; and current substance dependence.

During the acute treatment phase, all patients received ECT three times weekly until patients either were remitters or had shown no further improvement over the course of three consecutive treatments. Psychoactive drugs were not allowed during this acute treatment phase, with the exception of nortriptyline and trazodone used as an anxiolytic/hypnotic.

The follow-up phase of the study included patients who achieved remission, defined by a 17-item HDRS score below 8 and complete resolution of psychotic features. Patients were randomized to either continuation/maintenance nortriptyline alone or combined ECT plus nortriptyline (ECT + NT) in a 1:1 ratio. Continuation/maintenance therapy began 1 week after completion of the acute phase. Nortriptyline treatment was titrated to serum levels of approximately 100 ng/mL for all patients. Based on the authors' clinical experience and common practice, the non-ECT group received combined treatment with risperidone in a dose of up to 2 mg/day for 6 weeks and then were tapered off it over a 4-week period. The ECT + NT group received ECT treatments weekly for the first month, every 2 weeks for the following month, and then monthly. The technical characteristics of the electrical stimulus and the anesthetic drugs used during maintenance ECT sessions were similar to those for acute ECT.

In the follow-up phase, the participants were assessed at rating visits, which occurred at weeks 0 (baseline), 2, and 4 and then monthly for 2 years or until relapse/recurrence. Evaluators (two of the authors, JG and MS) and the data analyst (author XT) were blind to treatment assignment. The primary outcome in this study was defined by time to relapse/recurrence according to the first of two consecutive visits with a diagnosis of relapse/recurrence. Relapse was defined as the re-emergence of depressive symptoms within 6 months of remission from the index episode of depression. Recurrence was defined as a new episode of depression occurring after at least 6 months without a relapse. Relapse and recurrence were diagnosed when a patient met symptomatic criteria for DSM-IV major depression and had a Hamilton score of 16 or above in two consecutive visits.

Secondary and tolerability outcomes included the MMSE, Udvalg for Kliniske Undersogelser (UKU) side effect scale, blood pressure, and electrocardiography (ECG) at baseline and endpoint visits.

Statistical analyses of efficacy and tolerability included all patients randomized to a treatment who took their assigned continuation/maintenance treatment for at least 1 week, i.e., until the first session of ECT in the case of the ECT group. Survival analysis and Kaplan-Meier product-limit estimations were used to describe the probability and incidence of relapse/recurrence in each of the two study groups. The log-rank test was used to compare both survival curves, and a hazard ratio was calculated to show clinical significance. The student's t-test and chi-square test were used to compare clinical and demographic data between the two groups.

Results Of the 38 patients in the acute treatment phase, only 1 did not achieve remission. Four others dropped out of the study for various reasons. Thirty-three of the original 38 participants were randomized into the follow-up phase. Of these 33, 17 were randomly assigned to the maintenance NT group and 16 to the maintenance ECT+NT group. No significant differences in sex, age, baseline and post-acute ECT HDRS and MMSE scores, age at onset, proportion of inpatient participants, and previous history of depression were found between subgroups at baseline. However, while not statistically significant, 64.68% of patients in the NT group had prior depression as compared to only 56.29% of participants in the NT + ECT group. The mean age was 70.65 years for the NT group and 70.38 years for the combined ECT + NT group. Of all 33 patients, 14 had initially received pharmacological treatment with no response prior to acute ECT. They were distributed between the two groups, so that there was no significant difference in antidepressant use pre-ECT.

There were four "premature exits" for each group. In the NT group, there were one death from myocardial infarction, one loss of follow-up, one adverse event (severe urinary retention), and one protocol violation (did not follow treatment). In the ECT + NT group, there were one case of breast cancer leading to withdrawal, one adverse event, and two protocol violations (did not attend scheduled visits). As a result, 25 of the 33 patients enrolled (76%) completed the follow-up phase.

In terms of efficacy among "completers," 8 of the 13 completers in the NT group had disease relapse ($n = 2$) or recurrence ($n = 6$) by 2 years. The percent of relapse for NT completers was 15.4% at 6 months, 46.2% at 12 months, and 61.5% at 2 years. The authors did not report an intent-to-treat (ITT) analysis, but if premature exits are counted, the percent of participants whose depression relapsed/recurred increases to 35.3% at 6 months, 58.8% at 12 months, and 70.6% at 24 months (Table 42.1). The mean survival time for completers was 16 months (95% confidence interval (CI): 12–20 months). By contrast, only 1 of the 12 completers in the ECT + NT group had disease relapse (during the sixth month of follow-up, with no psychotic features), and there were no recurrences. In total, only 8.3% of

Table 42.1 Relapse/recurrence rates among nortriptyline (NT) vs. ECT + NT groups, per protocol vs. calculated intention-to-treat analysis

	NT monotherapy		ECT + NT combined treatment	
	Per protocol ($n = 13$)	ITT ($n = 17$)	Per protocol ($n = 12$)	ITT ($n = 16$)
6 months	15.4%	35.3%	8.3%	31.3%
12 months	46.2%	58.8%	8.3%	31.3%
24 months	61.5%	70.6%	8.3%	31.3%

completers in the ECT + NT group experienced relapse/recurrence, which increases to 31.3% if premature exits are counted in an ITT analysis (Table 42.1). The mean survival time until relapse for ECT + NT completers was 23 months (95% CI: 21–25 months).

In terms of tolerability, the authors reported that both treatments had only mild to moderate adverse effects. Statistical tests (chi-square or t) showed that changes in UKU score, blood pressure, heart rate, PR and QTc intervals, and MMSE score were statistically insignificant over the course of follow-up.

Conclusions In contemporary practice, ECT is typically administered acutely and abruptly stopped, and relapse/recurrence rates are high after cessation [4]. Evidence from this 2-year randomized, single-blind controlled trial indicates that for elderly patients whose depression with psychosis remits after acute-phase ECT, the combination of ECT + nortriptyline is more effective than nortriptyline alone in preventing relapse/recurrence, with no observed differences in tolerability. In a similar study, Kellner et al. [3] showed that combination nortriptyline-lithium could have as much of an effect as maintenance ECT. When accounting for ITT, the percentage of relapse at 6 months among subjects on maintenance ECT in Kellner et al.'s study (37.1% by modified ITT) was similar to our calculated 31.3% percent ITT relapse/recurrence in this study.

Strengths of the Study

1. The study sample included only older adults (≥60 years).
2. The authors used strong inclusion and exclusion criteria (diagnosis based on DSM-IV criteria and HDRS scores) to ensure subjects had depression rather than organic cognitive impairment.
3. The 2-year duration of follow-up is longer than prior studies that examined maintenance ECT for elderly patients.
4. The two treatment groups were similar in demographic and clinical characteristics, with no statistically significant differences.
5. There was a 76% completion rate for the study.

Limitations of the Study

1. Because patients could not be blinded to their assigned treatment group, the study could only be single-blinded. As a result, the Jadad Score indicates that its methodological quality was intermediate, with a score of 3 out of 5 (4–5 "high," 3 "intermediate," 1–2 "low") (Table 42.2) [2].
2. The overall sample size was small ($n = 33$) and homogenous from a single facility (the Hospital Clinic of Barcelona, Spain).
3. There was no placebo control group or sham ECT group to make comparisons with. The ECT + NT group may have received indirect support through their monitoring and conversations with healthcare staff during ECT sessions, which took place weekly for the first month, every 2 weeks for the following month, and then monthly.

Table 42.2 Jadad scoring for methodological quality of study

Questions Yes (1) No (0)	Was the study described as random?	Was the randomization scheme described and appropriate?	Was the study described as double-blind?	Was the method of double blinding appropriate? (Were both the patient and the assessor appropriately blinded?)	Was there a description of dropouts and withdrawals?	Total score
Score	1	1	0 (single-blind)	0/1 (evaluators and data analyst blinded; patients could not be)	1	3/5

4. There was no intent-to-treat analysis performed that accounted for "premature exits" that are noted in the participant flowchart. We calculated ITT relapse rates in Table 42.1.
5. In their tolerability results, the authors did not report of the specific nature of adverse effects, only describing them as mild to moderate, making it difficult to ascertain the clinical relevance of these adverse effects.
6. Due to limitations of using the MMSE to measure cognition (as acknowledged by the authors), the question of whether maintenance ECT might result in cognitive impairment in the vulnerable population of the elderly remains mostly unanswered.
7. The authors correctly note that given the small nature of this study, the findings should be considered as preliminary. For clinical application, many questions about the precise duration of maintenance ECT and the benefit of concurrent pharmacological treatment require further study.

Take-home points Despite some limitations, this randomized, single-blind, and controlled trial indicates that continuation/maintenance therapy with nortriptyline combined with ECT was more efficacious than nortriptyline alone for the prevention of relapse/recurrence among older adults in remission from psychotic depression, based on observation over 2-year follow-up. Combination treatment with ECT was tolerated well, similar to nortriptyline alone.

Practical applications of the take-home point Among older adults who achieve remission from psychotic depression after acute ECT, combined continuation/maintenance ECT and pharmacologic treatment may be an efficacious and well-tolerated treatment option to prevent relapse/recurrence.

References

1. Navarro V, Gastó C, Torres X, Masana G, Penadés R, Guarch J, Vázquez M, Serra M, Pujol N, Pintor L, Catalán R. Continuation/maintenance treatment with nortriptyline versus combined nortriptyline and ECT in late-life psychotic depression: a two-year randomized study. Am J Geriatr Psychiatry. 2008;16(6):498–505.
2. Jadad AR, Moore RA, Carroll D, Jenkinson C, Reynolds DJ, Gavaghan DJ, McQuay HJ. Assessing the quality of reports of randomized clinical trials: is blinding necessary? Control Clin Trials. 1996;17:1–12.
3. Kellner CH, Knapp RG, Petrides G, Rummans TA, Husain MM, Rasmussen K, Mueller M, Bernstein HJ, O'Connor K, Smith G, Biggs M, Bailine SH, Malur C, Yim E, McClintock S, Sampson S, Fink M. Continuation electroconvulsive therapy vs pharmacotherapy for relapse prevention in major depression: a multisite study from the Consortium for Research in Electroconvulsive Therapy (CORE). Arch Gen Psychiatry. 2006;63(12):1337–44.
4. Schneider LS, Olin JT. Efficacy of acute treatment for geriatric depression. Int Psychogeriatr. 1995;7 Suppl:7–25.

Chapter 43
Safety and Utility of Acute Electroconvulsive Therapy for Agitation and Aggression in Dementia

Padmapriya Marpuri, Martin Witkin, and Rajesh R. Tampi

Authors of the Original Article Deepa Acharya, Ph.D., David G. Harper, Ph.D., Eric D. Achtyes, M.D., M.S., Stephen J. Seiner, M.D., Jack A. Mahdasian, M.D., M.A., Louis J. Nykamp, M.D., Lesley Adkison, R.N., Lori Van der Schuur White, R.N., Shawn M. McClintock, Ph.D., MSCS, Manjola Ujkaj, M.D., Ph.D., Donald A. Davidoff, Ph.D., and Brent P. Forester, M.D., M.Sc.

Journal Published International Journal of Geriatric Psychiatry.

Year of Publication 2015.

Type of Study Prospective study.

Funding Sources None reported.

P. Marpuri (✉)
Attending Geriatric Psychiatrist, Frontier Psychiatry, Billings, MT, USA

M. Witkin
PGY-4 Psychiatry Resident, Einstein Medical Center, Philadelphia, PA, USA
e-mail: witkinma@einstein.edu

R. R. Tampi
Creighton University School of Medicine, Omaha, NE, USA
e-mail: rajesh.tampi@yale.edu

R. R. Tampi et al. (eds.), *Essential Reviews in Geriatric Psychiatry*,
https://doi.org/10.1007/978-3-030-94960-0_43

Objectives In this study, the investigators examined the safety and efficacy of ECT in the treatment of behavioral disturbances among individuals with dementia. It was hypothesized that treatment with ECT would lead to a reduction in both agitation and aggressive behaviors among the participants of this study at discharge when compared to baseline [1].

Methods All the participants were recruited from the Geriatric Neuropsychiatry Unit at McLean Hospital in Belmont, MA, and the Older Adult Unit at Pine Rest Christian Mental Health Services in Grand Rapids, MI, from 2010 to 2012. Inclusion criteria for this study were as follows: 1. a diagnosis of dementia according to the DSM-IV criteria; 2. a referral for ECT by the treating psychiatrist exclusively for the treatment of agitation and/or agitation irrespective of mood symptoms; and 3. a baseline Mini-Mental State Examination (MMSE) score of ≤24 at baseline. On the Cohen-Mansfield Agitation Inventory Short Version (CMAI-short form), the minimal cutoff scores were defined as ≥4 on at least one item, a score of 3 on at least two items, or a score of 2 on at least three items. The exclusion criteria for this study were as follows: 1. a diagnosis of delirium at study entry; 2. a history of substance abuse in the past 12 months; and 3. the use of ECT treatment 90 days prior to enrollment into this study. A written informed consent was obtained from the authorized healthcare representative (AHCR) and assent from study participants. The study was approved by the institutional review board at each study site.

Agitation, aggression, and other neuropsychiatric symptoms of dementia were evaluated using the Cohen-Mansfield Agitation Inventory Short Version (CMAI-short form), Neuropsychiatric Inventory (NPI)-Nursing Home Version, Cornell Scale for Depression in Dementia (CSDD), and Clinical Global Impression (CGI) Scale. Global cognitive functioning was assessed using the MMSE and Severe Impairment Battery (SIB). The functional ability was evaluated using the Alzheimer's Disease Cooperative Study Group-Activities of Daily Living (ADCS-ADL) Scale.

Based on the determination of the treating psychiatrist and the ECT treatment team, all the participants in the study completed an inpatient acute ECT course. The assessment schedule for the participants in the study were as follows: (1) calculation of the CMAI, NPI, CSDD, and CGI scores at baseline; after the 3rd, 6th, 9th, and 12th (where applicable) ECT sessions; and within 72 h prior to discharge; (2) administration of the MMSE, SIB, and ADCS-ADL at baseline and within 72 h of discharge; (3) completion of CMAI, NPI, CSDD, and ADSC-ADL by a trained nurse and the completion of the CGI by the treating psychiatrist; and (4) completion of MMSE and SIB by a neuropsychologist or a trained nurse. For each participant in the study, the comorbid medical and psychiatric diagnoses were also recorded.

An ECT-credentialed psychiatrist completed an ECT consultation prior to treatment administration. The ECT devices that were used were the MECTA SPECTRUM 5000Q ECT (MECTA Corporation, Tualatin, Oregon) or Thymatron System IV (Somatics, LLC, Lake Bluff, IL). On the first treatment, the seizure threshold was determined using the empirical dose titration method. During the treatment course, the stimulus parameters were adjusted on an as-needed basis, depending on the seizure quality and treatment efficacy. The treating physician decided on the initial electrode placement based on their clinical assessment. Right unilateral electrode placement was chosen for most participants by the clinicians, as it is associated with less cognitive side effects. A brief pulse width (0.5–1.0 millisecond) at approximately four to six times the seizure threshold was also chosen. Bitemporal electrode placement with a brief pulse width (0.5–1 millisecond) at about 1.5–2.5 times the seizure threshold was used among individuals who had no clinical response to treatment using the right unilateral electrode placement.

The schedule for ECT treatments was three times per week, but it was done less frequently if clinically indicated. The anesthesia induction was done using methohexital, and succinylcholine was used for muscle relaxation. Etomidate could be substituted for methohexital for anesthesia induction among individuals having inadequate seizure duration or quality. Adequate seizure duration monitoring was performed using an electroencephalogram (EEG). As-needed medications could be used for the following reasons: ondansetron for nausea; ketorolac, ibuprofen, or acetaminophen for headache; esmolol or labetalol for elevated blood, pressure, or heart rate; atropine or glycopyrrolate for bradycardia; and midazolam, lorazepam, and/or propofol to prevent post-ictal agitation.

The investigators constructed linear mixed-effects models, incorporating time as a fixed effect and subject as a random effect for each of the behavioral scales. They also included all subjects who were enrolled in the study, irrespective of the treatment duration in the analysis. The investigators also tested the CMAI-short form using a multiple degree of freedom comparison of scores. In the post hoc analyses, the baseline score of CMAI was compared to the CMAI scores at the 3rd, 6th, 9th, and 12th (when applicable) ECT sessions. The investigators also evaluated the effect of ECT treatment on the secondary outcome measures including the NPI and CSDD using the same model. In addition, they completed a four-factor model analysis of the NPI using a similar methodology.

All antipsychotic medications that were used in the study were converted to chlorpromazine equivalents. This was done in order to analyze the change in dosage and number of antipsychotic medications used across the course of ECT treatments. The investigators used a linear mixed-effects model to assess the change in standing antipsychotic dosages. In addition, they constructed a separate linear mixed-effects model to examine the cumulative use of "as-needed" medications over 1–3 treatments, 4–6 treatments, and 7–9 treatments, respectively. The investigators tested their hypothesis using the Kenward-Rogers adjustment. In addition, they applied the Bonferroni corrections separately for the planned comparisons of CMAI, CSDD, and NPI. All the statistical tests were two-tailed.

Results There were a total of 23 participants in this study. A total of 14 individuals were admitted from McLean Hospital, and the remaining 9 were from Pine Rest Christian Mental Health Services. The investigators noted that when compared to baseline, there was a statistically significant decline in the CMAI-short form scores at discharge ($P = 0.006$) on the regression analyses. Additionally, the CMAI-short form scores showed a decline from baseline to 3thd, 6th, 9th, and 12th ECT treatments on the post hoc *t*-tests. However, the CMAI-short form scores remained fairly stable from the ninth session through to discharge.

Among the participants in the study, the investigators noted a reduction in NPI scores from baseline to discharge ($P < 0.001$). Additionally, the NPI scores declined from baseline to the 3rd ($P < 0.001$), 6th ($P < 0.001$), 9th ($P < 0.001$), and 12th ($P < 0.001$) ECT sessions. Furthermore, there was a decline from baseline to discharge on the NPI subdomain scores of behavioral dyscontrol ($P < 0.001$) and agitation ($P < 0.001$). It was noted that the behavioral dyscontrol subdomain scores declined from baseline to the 3rd ($P < 0.001$), 6th ($P < 0.001$), 9th ($P < 0.001$), and 12th ($P < 0.001$) ECT sessions on the post hoc *t*-tests. The agitation subdomain scores also declined from baseline to the 3rd ($P < 0.01$), 6th ($P < 0.001$), 9th ($P < 0.001$), and 12th ($P < 0.001$) ECT sessions on the post hoc *t*-tests. The investigators did not find a statistically significant decline from baseline to discharge on the mean scores of NPI subdomains of mood and psychosis.

On the mean CSDD scores, the investigators did not find any significant change from baseline to discharge ($P = 0.07$). They also noted that there was minimal change from baseline to discharge on the average CGI scores from "markedly agitated/aggressive" to "borderline agitated/aggressive."

The need for antipsychotic medications also declined from baseline to the third ECT session (average chlorpromazine equivalent dosage of 7.8–1.6). Additionally, there was decline in the need for antipsychotics between the sixth and ninth ECT sessions ($P = 0.018$). The standing antipsychotic medications did not change from baseline to discharge ($P = 0.764$).

Among the participants in the study, the ADCS-ADL scores did not change significantly from baseline to discharge ($P = 0.289$). There was a modest improvement on the average MMSE scores from 8.2 to 10.1, among the ten participants who completed the assessment at baseline and at discharge. The average SIB total score improved from 55.8 to 65 among the six participants who completed the assessment baseline and at discharge.

The ECT was discontinued in two of the participants due to poor treatment response. One participant died the day before discharge to a nursing home with palliative care. The cause of death was determined to be unrelated to the use of ECT and related to the end-stage dementia. The ECT was discontinued in two of the participants due to delirium that was unrelated to the ECT treatment. One participant who developed atrial fibrillation was transferred to a general medical hospital. This participant continued with the ECT under medical supervision.

Conclusions This naturalistic and prospective study indicates that among older adults with dementia who do not respond to psychopharmacological interventions, ECT is effective in reducing symptoms of agitation and aggression.

Strengths of the Study

1. This is the first naturalistic and prospective study to investigate the efficacy and safety of ECT in the treatment for agitation and aggression among individuals with dementia.

2. This study used validated rating scales to assess the neuropsychiatric symptoms, cognition, and function among individuals with dementia.
3. The CMAI, NPI, CSDD, and ADSC-ADL were completed by a trained nurse, the CGI was completed by the treating psychiatrist, and the MMSE and SIB were completed by a neuropsychologist or a trained nurse.
4. This study used an ECT-credentialed psychiatrist to complete an ECT consultation prior to treatment administration.

Limitations of the Study

1. There were a limited number of participants in the study.
2. This was a naturalistic study where there was no control group.
3. This study also had an open-labelled and non-randomized design.
4. The investigators were unable to consistently collect neurocognitive data for all the participants at baseline and at post-ECT time points due to severity of agitation.
5. The investigators did not have a consistent clinical algorithm to determine the number of medication trials that was required before the participants could be referred for ECT, thus impacting the clinical response to ECT.
6. The naturalistic study design prevented the control factors such as the concomitant use of psychotropic medications by the participants while they were enrolled in the study.
7. The study design prevented the comparison between the efficacy and safety of ECT and pharmacotherapy in managing agitation and aggression among individuals with dementia.
8. This study included participants with dementias of various etiologies which contributed to diagnostic heterogeneity within the study.

Take-Home Points

Among certain individuals with dementia who do not respond adequately to or do not tolerate standard behavioral interventions and/or pharmacotherapy, ECT may be a rapidly acting, effective, and safe treatment for behavioral symptoms.

Practical Applications of the Take-Home Points

ECT may be an effective and safe treatment among older adults with dementia who exhibit agitation and aggression which does not respond adequately to standard behavioral or pharmacological interventions.

Reference

1. Acharya D, Harper DG, Achtyes ED, Seiner SJ, Mahdasian JA, Nykamp LJ, Adkison L, Van der Schuur WL, McClintock SM, Ujkaj M, Davidoff DA, Forester BP. Safety and utility of acute electroconvulsive therapy for agitation and aggression in dementia. Int J Geriatr Psychiatry. 2015;30(3):265–73.

Chapter 44
Electroconvulsive Therapy and Risk of Dementia in Patients with Affective Disorders: A Cohort Study

Padmapriya Marpuri, Clay Gueits, and Rajesh R. Tampi

Authors of the Original Article Merete Osler, Maarten Pieter Rozing, Gunhild Tidemann Christensen, Per Kragh Andersen, Martin Balslev Jørgensen.

Journal Published Lancet Psychiatry.

Year of Publication 2018.

Type of Study Retrospective Cohort Study.

Funding Sources The Danish Council for Independent Research, the Danish Medical Research Council, the Velux Foundation, the Jascha Foundation, and the Doctor Sofus Carl Emil Friis and Olga Doris Friis grant.

P. Marpuri (✉)
Attending Geriatric Psychiatrist, Frontier Psychiatry, Billings, MT, USA

C. Gueits
Psychiatry Resident, Einstein Medical Center, Philadelphia, PA, USA
e-mail: gueitscl@einstein.edu

R. R. Tampi
Creighton University School of Medicine, Omaha, NE, USA
e-mail: rajesh.tampi@yale.edu

R. R. Tampi et al. (eds.), *Essential Reviews in Geriatric Psychiatry*,
https://doi.org/10.1007/978-3-030-94960-0_44

Objectives In this study, the investigators examined the association between ECT and risk of subsequent dementia among individuals with a first-time hospital diagnosis of affective disorder [1].

Methods In this cohort study, the investigators included all citizens of Denmark who were ≥10 years in age with a first-time hospital contact for an affective disorder between January 1, 2005, and December 31, 2015. They included both inpatients and outpatients with ICD-10 codes F30.0–F39.9 (affective disorders) who were identified from the Danish National Patient Registry (DNPR). This registry includes information regarding the diagnosis and the time of admission for all inpatient and outpatient hospital contacts in Denmark since 1995. The investigators also identified men with a first-time hospital contact for an affective disorder from January 1, 2005, through December 31, 2015, from the Danish Conscription Database (DCD). This study received approval from the Danish Data Protection Agency.

The investigators also obtained information regarding electrode placement and the number of ECT sessions from the DNPR. The number of ECT sessions as was dichotomized as ≤10 or >10 sessions based on the median number of ECT sessions required for remission [2].

The primary outcome was incidental dementia as ascertained by the physician diagnosis from DNPR database. The investigators also obtained diagnostic information from January 1, 2005, to October 31, 2016, for all first emergency department, inpatient or outpatient hospital contacts for individuals with ICD-10 diagnosis codes of F00.0 to F03.9 and G30.0 to G30.9 (dementia). The investigators also had access to data on previous dementia diagnoses that was registered in the DNPR or Danish Psychiatric Central Register since 1969. Additionally, they included individuals who filled at least one prescription for an acetylcholinesterase inhibitor which was identified by the Anatomical Therapeutic Chemical Classification System codes (N06D) in the Danish National Prescription Registry. A report that was based on national register data provided the investigators with the information regarding the incidence of dementia in the general Danish population.

The investigators also analyzed the effect of electrode placement and the number of ECT sessions on the risk of developing dementia. In a secondary analysis, they evaluated whether individuals with low premorbid cognitive ability had greater risk for developing dementia after receiving ECT treatment when compared to those individuals who had higher cognitive scores.

The investigators used the Cox proportional hazard regression [hazard ratio (HR) and 95% confidence interval (CI)] to analyze the association of first ECT with incidental dementia, using age as the underlying timescale and ECT as a time-dependent variable. They used the chi-square and log-rank tests to examine the difference in distributions of ECT and dementia in relation to the covariates. The participants were followed from the age when they were first registered as having an affective disorder until the age that they were first registered as having a diagnosis of dementia, they emigrated, or they died or till the end of the follow-up period, whichever came first.

The researchers used multiple regression model to adjust for confounding variables including age, sex, history of cerebrovascular accident, schizophrenia, alcohol or substance abuse, antidepressant use, lithium, and antipsychotic use. Participants were matched one to one using a propensity score estimated by using Cox regression analysis. The investigators repeated the analyses after a lag period of 2 years after study entry using the stsplit option in STATA version 14, to eliminate the bias of physicians interpreting the cognitive deficits as side effects of ECT rather than dementia.

Results A total of 168,015 individuals (mean age 47.1 years) were included in the study. Of these, a total of 5901 participants (3.5%) were treated with ECT. ECT was most commonly used among individuals 50–69 years in age (5.7%). The percentage of participants who developed dementia was 0.1% among individuals 1–49 years in age, 2.7% among individuals aged 50–69 years in age, and 12.5% among individuals 70–108 years in age. The investigators found that among the three age groups, ECT was most commonly used among participants with a diagnosis of severe episode of depression in either a single episode or recurrent episodes with comorbid schizophrenia or among those individuals who used antidepressants or antipsychotic medications at the time of entry into the study. Bilateral electrode placement was the most commonly used electrode placement among participants who received ECT at 51% followed by unilateral electrode placement at 13%.

The investigators found that 3.1% of the participants developed dementia during the median follow-up of 4.9 years, with an incidence of 59.0 cases per 10,000 person-years. Individuals ≥70 year in age who were treated with ECT had the highest incidence rate of dementia at 12.5%. Among individuals ≥70 year in age, the incidence of dementia was lowest among those participants with a diagnosis of bipolar disorder, comorbid schizophrenia, comorbid alcohol abuse, and mixed substance abuse and among individuals who used tricyclic antidepressants at the time of entry into the study. Among individuals 10–69 years in age, the incidence of dementia was lowest among those individuals with a diagnosis of bipolar disorder and higher among individuals with only basic education, comorbid schizophrenia, stroke, or comorbid abuse of alcohol with mixed substances.

The investigators found that the unadjusted incidence rate of dementia was greater among individuals treated with ECT when compared to those who did not receive ECT (70.4 per 10,000 person-years vs. 59.2 per 10,000 person-years, respectively). Among individuals ≥70 years in age, the incidence of dementia was lower among individuals who received ECT when compared to those who did not receive ECT (284.7 per 10,000 person-years vs. 420.4 per 10,000 person-years, age-adjusted hazard ratio [HR] = 0.68 $P < 0.0001$, and adjusted HR = 0.62, $P < 0.0001$). In the propensity score-matched sample, the HR for incident dementia for those who received ECT was not significantly different from those individuals who did not receive ECT (HR = 0.77, $P = 0.062$). Among individuals 10–49 years in age, the use of ECT was not associated with an increased risk of dementia (age-adjusted HR = 1.51, $P = 0.32$; adjusted HR = 1.42, $P = 0.41$; and propensity score-matched sample HR = 2.36, $P = 0.11$). Among individuals 50–69 years in age, ECT was not associated with an increased risk of dementia when matched for age and compared with individuals not receiving ECT (age-adjusted HR = 1.15, $P = 0.22$; adjusted HR = 1.28, $P = 0.072$; and propensity score-matched sample HR = 1.45, $P = 0.081$).

The investigator also found that 17.6% of the participants died (mortality rate of 35.7 per 1000 person-years). The risk for dementia was not significantly affected by ECT for the participants ≥70 years in age when the presence of the competing mortality risk was taken into account (HR = 0.98, $P = 0.24$).

It was noted that among individuals who received ECT, 47.6% of the individuals had more than ten sessions. Among individuals ≥70 years in age, receiving >10 ECTs was associated with a lower incidence of dementia per 10,000 person-years in both the original sample and the propensity score-matched sample (HR = 0.54, $P < 0.0001$, and HR = 0.59, $P = 0.0031$). Despite the presence of a competing mortality risk, individuals who had >10 sessions in the propensity score-matched sample were found to have lower risk of developing dementia (subdistribution HR = 0.84, 95% $P = 0.0014$). Among individuals who were younger, those who received ≤10 ECT sessions did not have a greater risk for developing incidental dementia in the original sample (HR = 1.51, $P = 0.15$). Although the registration data for electrode placement was incomplete, available evidence indicated that bilateral electrode placement did not appear to increase the risk for incidental dementia.

The investigators found that among the sample of men where there was data on young adult cognitive ability, the use of ECT did not increase the risk of incidental dementia (unadjusted HR = 0.92, $P = 0.58$; adjusted HR = 0.93, $P = 0.64$; and propensity score-matched sample HR = 1.05, $P = 0.72$). Among individuals with lowest premorbid cognitive ability (defined as the lowest 10% cognitive scoring), the use of ECT was associated with increased risk of incidental dementia when compared with those with higher cognitive scores (the 90% highest cognitive scoring), although this result was not significant ($P = 0.08$).

Conclusions This register-based cohort study of individuals with affective disorders indicated that the use of ECT was not associated with an increased risk of incidental dementia after the data was corrected for the potential effect of participant selection or competing mortality. Among individuals ≥70 years in age, the use of ECT was associated with a reduced risk for incidental dementia after adjustment for important covariates.

Strengths of the Study

1. The use of nationwide population-based registers in Denmark provided the investigators with access to large and relatively unselected groups of study participants.
2. The investigators were able to obtain complete follow-up information of the participants for diagnosis, migration, and death from the different registries.
3. The DNPR contained information regarding 90% of ECT treatments [2], and the registers included information regarding 2/3 of expected dementia cases in the population.

4. This study used data on individuals who had a first-time hospital admission due to an affective disorder, and as ECT occurs mainly in a hospital setting, it was assumed that the full ECT history for the participants was available.

Limitations of the Study

1. There was incomplete registration of electrode placement for ECT in the DNPR which hindered the validity of the estimates based on this data.
2. The possibility of residual confounding associated with selection of individuals for ECT could not be guaranteed despite the investigators using different approaches to account for potential confounding factors.
3. As this study used register-based data, there is a risk that the information may not have provided a complete picture of the participants demographic, social, and health status and their ability to consent for ECT and thereby the subsequent risk for developing dementia.
4. The analysis of individuals in the younger age cohort was affected by an absence of statistical power especially since dementia occurs less frequently in this age group.
5. The long-term effects of ECT may be missed as the mean follow-up of 5 years might be too short.

Take-Home Points

The findings from this study show that the use of ECT did not increase the risk of incidental dementia among older adults with an affective disorder. This data supports the continued use of ECT among this population for the treatment of severe episodes of depression.

Practical Applications of the Take-Home Points

When older individuals present with severe depressive episodes, ECT can be used to treat these episodes without increasing the risk for incidental dementia among these individuals.

References

1. Osler M, Rozing MP, Christensen GT, Andersen PK, Jørgensen MB. Electroconvulsive therapy and risk of dementia in patients with affective disorders: a cohort study. Lancet Psychiatry. 2018;5(4):348–56.
2. Hundrup E, Osler M, Jørgensen MB. Time trends and variations in electroconvulsive treatment in Denmark 2008 to 2014: a nationwide register-based study. J ECT. 2017;33(4):243–8.

Chapter 45
Electroconvulsive Therapy and Risk of Dementia: A Nationwide Cohort Study in Taiwan

Clay Gueits, Padmapriya Marpuri, and Rajesh R. Tampi

Authors of the Original Article Ching-Wen Chu, Wu-Chien Chien, Chi-Hsiang Chung, Pei-Chun Chao, Hsin-An Chang, Yu-Chen Kao, Yu-Ching Chou, and Nian-Sheng Tzeng.

Journal Published Frontiers in Psychiatry.

Year of Publication 2018.

Type of Study Retrospective, matched-cohort design.

Funding Sources Tri-Service General Hospital Research Foundation (TSGH-C105-130, TSGH-C106-002, TSGH-C106-106, and TSGH-C107-004) and the Medical Affairs Bureau, Ministry of Defence of Taiwan (MAB-107-084).

C. Gueits
Psychiatry Resident, Einstein Medical Center, Philadelphia, PA, USA
e-mail: gueitscl@einstein.edu

P. Marpuri (✉)
Attending Geriatric Psychiatrist, Frontier Psychiatry, Billings, MT, USA

R. R. Tampi
Creighton University School of Medicine, Omaha, NE, USA
e-mail: rajesh.tampi@yale.edu

R. R. Tampi et al. (eds.), *Essential Reviews in Geriatric Psychiatry*,
https://doi.org/10.1007/978-3-030-94960-0_45

Objectives In this study, the investigators evaluated whether the use of ECT among individuals with schizophrenia, bipolar disorder, and major depressive disorder is associated with an increased risk for dementia by using the data from the National Health Insurance Research Database (NHIRD) in Taiwan [1].

Methods The NHIRD is a comprehensive database containing encrypted information about inpatient and ambulatory care, prescription drug treatment, as well as sex and date of birth of the enrolled population. The diagnoses in the NHIRD are coded according to the International Classification of Disease, Ninth Revision, Clinical Modification (ICD-9-CM). All the diagnoses of dementia were made by board-certified psychiatrists or neurologists, and the diagnoses of schizophrenia, bipolar disorder, and major depressive disorder were made by board-certified psychiatrists.

This study was a retrospective, matched-cohort study where individuals with schizophrenia, bipolar disorder, or major depressive disorder who had undergone ECT treatment in a 12-month period from January 1 to December 31, 2000, were selected from the NHIRD.

Inclusion criteria was a ICD-9-CM diagnosis of schizophrenia, bipolar disorder, or major depressive disorder as well as having made at least three outpatient visits during this 1-year study period for dementia, in addition to having received ECT.

Exclusion criteria for this study were a diagnosis of schizophrenia, bipolar disorder, or major depressive disorder prior to the year 2000 and the receipt of ECT prior to 2000. Individuals with cancer, other organic brain syndromes, Parkinsonism, stroke, and brain surgery and those age ≤20 years were excluded from the study.

The investigators included a total of 3796 participants: 994 individuals who received ECT (mean age 39.65 ± 12.76) and 2982 control subjects who did not receive ECT (mean age 40.40 ± 13.30) who were matched for sex and age from the NHIR.

The investigators used sex, age, geographical area of residence, urbanization level of residence, and insurance premiums as covariates. They used the Charlson comorbidity index to adjust for comorbidities. For adverse effects, the investigators recorded post-ECT prolonged seizures, in-hospital delirium, acute myocardial infarction (AMI), acute stroke, coronary artery disease (CAD), dysrhythmia, cardiac shock, and deaths during the hospital stay when ECT was used.

The data on all the study participants was collected January 1 to December 31, 2000, until the onset of dementia, withdrawal from the National Health Institute (NHI) program, or the end of the year in 2010. The primary outcome measure was the development of dementia. The diagnosis of dementia in this study included Alzheimer's type, vascular type, or other dementias as defined by the DSM-IV-TR criteria and recorded using the ICD-9-CM codes.

Results The investigators did not find any difference between the two study groups in terms of sex, age, psychiatric disorders, and insurance premiums. One difference was that the individuals in the ECT cohort lived more urban areas and in the northern and central areas of Taiwan ($P < 0.001$). Additionally, there were more women in the bipolar and major depressive disorder groups when compared to the schizophrenia group.

The investigators found that on the Kaplan-Meier analysis, the cumulative incidence of dementia (of all types) was no different between the ECT and control groups, respectively (4.53% vs 5.0%, $P = 0.308$). At the end of the follow-up period, there were only slight differences between the ECT and control groups, respectively, for prolonged seizures (0.7% vs 0.03%, $P < 0.001$) and delirium/confusion (0.2% vs 1.17%, $P = 0.004$). The overall re-admission rate was more than 80% with the rate of re-admission for ECT being about 20% among the three diagnostic groups.

Fine and Gray's survival analysis showed that the participants in the ECT cohort, following adjustments for age, sex, income, urbanization level, geographic region, and comorbidities, were not more likely to develop dementia [adjusted hazard ratio (aHR) = 0.992, $P = 0.882$] when compared to individuals who did not receive ECT.

Men were more likely to develop dementia when compared to women, aHR = 2.063, $P < 0.001$. Individuals who were >65 years of age were more likely to develop dementia when compared to individuals 20–64 years in age, aHR = 2.268, $P < 0.001$. Individuals who had prolonged seizures, in-hospital delirium, and acute stroke were all at higher risk for developing dementia; aHR = 2.063, 2.268, 5.260, 5.623, and 2.086, respectively, all $P < 0.001$. There was no increase in risk for dementia among the subgroups of individuals with schizophrenia (aHR = 0.518, $P = 0.152$), bipolar disorder (aHR = 1.616, $P = 0.228$), and major depressive disorder (aHR = 0.865, $P = 0.208$). The risks of dementia after ECT within the first 0–1 year, 3–6 years, and ≥6 years were as follows: aHR = 0.991, $P = 0.213$; aHR = 1.821, $P = 0.198$; and aHR = 0.685, $P = 0.114$, respectively.

Conclusions The evidence from this study indicates that the use of ECT was not associated with an increased risk for developing dementia among individuals with schizophrenia, bipolar disorder, and major depressive disorder. Among individuals who received ECT, men, individuals ≥65 years in age, and those who developed prolonged seizures, in-hospital delirium, and acute stroke had greater risk for developing dementia.

Strengths of the Study

1. The diagnoses were based on ICD-9 codes which have demonstrated accuracy and validity within the NHIRD for several other diagnoses.
2. The cumulative incidence rates for dementia in the ECT cohort (4.53%) and in the control group (5.0%) are similar to the outcomes noted in a previous nationwide survey done in Taiwan [2].
3. The selected population can be considered as representative for this type of cohort study.
4. The study had a 10-year follow-up period.

Limitations of the Study

1. Given the insidious onset of dementia, a follow-up period of 10 years could be considered inadequate for studying the risk for developing dementia.
2. The data in this study is retrospective and is dependent on the ICD-9-CM codes instead of a direct patient assessment.

3. The database does not provide detailed information regarding the severity of disease.
4. The investigators only studied individuals with three specific psychiatric diagnoses, so the effect of other psychiatric diagnoses on the risk of developing dementia following ECT cannot be ruled out.
5. Protopathic bias although mitigated by sensitivity analysis may have occurred, as only newly developed dementia diagnosis was included in the follow-up period.

Take-Home Points

The use of ECT does not appear to be associated with an increased risk for dementia among individuals with a diagnosis of schizophrenia, bipolar disorder, and major depressive disorder. The risk for developing dementia was greater among men, individuals ≥65 years in age, and those individuals who developed prolonged seizures, in-hospital delirium, and acute stroke from the ECT, so it is important to monitor these individuals closely following ECT.

Practical Applications of the Take-Home Points

Among individuals with schizophrenia, bipolar disorder, and major depressive disorder, the use of ECT does not appear to be associated with an increased risk for dementia. Status post ECT, there should be careful monitoring of men, individuals ≥65 years in age, and individuals who develop prolonged seizures, in-hospital delirium, and acute stroke from the ECT, as these individuals appear to be at greater risk for developing dementia.

References

1. Chu CW, Chien WC, Chung CH, Chao PC, Chang HA, Kao YC, Chou YC, Tzeng NS. Electroconvulsive therapy and risk of dementia-a nationwide cohort study in Taiwan. Front Psych. 2018;9:397.
2. Sun Y, Lee HJ, Yang SC, Chen TF, Lin KN, Lin CC, Wang PN, Tang LY, Chiu MJ. A nationwide survey of mild cognitive impairment and dementia, including very mild dementia, in Taiwan. PLoS One. 2014;9(6):e100303.

Part VII
Grief

Chapter 46
Treatment of Complicated Grief in Elderly Persons: A Randomized Clinical Trial

Jennie B. Davidow and Juan Carlos Urizar

Authors of the Original Article M Katherine Shear, Yuanjia Wang, Natalia Skritskaya, Naihua Duan, Christine Mauro, Angela Ghesquiere.

Journal Published JAMA Psychiatry.

Year of Publication 2014.

Type of Study Randomized Control Trial, double blind.

Funding Sources Grant R01MH070741 from the National Institute of Mental Health.

Objectives The investigators wanted to assess whether there will be greater improvements in complicated grief (CG) and depressive symptoms with complicated grief treatment (CGT) when compared to grief-focused interpersonal psychotherapy (IPT) [1].

Methods The participants for this study were recruited through community outreach. To be included, participants had to be age 50 or older in age, with a score of 30 on the Inventory of Complicated Grief (ICG) and confirmed by a study author to have complicated grief on a clinical interview establishing prolonged acute grief

J. B. Davidow
Mass General Brigham Geriatric Psychiatry Fellowship, Harvard Medical School Clinical Fellow, Boston, MA, USA
e-mail: jdavidow@partners.org

J. C. Urizar (✉)
Department of Psychiatry Brigham and Women's Hospital, Mass General Brigham Geriatric Psychiatry Fellowship and Harvard Medical School Instructor, Boston, MA, USA
e-mail: jurizar@bwh.harvard.edu

R. R. Tampi et al. (eds.), *Essential Reviews in Geriatric Psychiatry*,
https://doi.org/10.1007/978-3-030-94960-0_46

symptoms with complicating dysfunctional thoughts, feelings, or behaviors. Participants with a current substance use disorder, psychosis, bipolar I disorder, active suicidality, Mini-Mental State Examination (MMSE) score below 24, or a pending lawsuit or disability claim relating to the death or who were already in psychotherapy were excluded. The concurrent use of antidepressant and anxiolytic was permitted in this study [1].

Complicated grief therapy (CGT) has roots in interpersonal therapy (IPT) and cognitive behavior therapy (CBT) as well as motivational interviewing. CGT utilizes attachment theory, targeting loss-related processes as well as symptoms of painful intrusive memories and behavioral avoidance using techniques derived from prolonged exposure therapy as well [2]. A previous randomized clinical trial showed better response to CGT than IPT for complicated grief symptoms among middle-aged adults [3].

In this study, different therapists with similar levels of experience (who were doctoral-level students, social workers, and psychologists) who were trained and certified administered either CGT or IPT. CGT was delivered based on an unpublished manual by the study authors and was informed by the dual-process model which places emphasis on components of grief relating to the loss and focused on the restoration of routine activities. Treatment was divided into phases, with phase 1 involving reviewing the participants' experience, introducing a grief-monitoring diary, and beginning work on aspirational goals, and included a conjoint session with a significant other. Phase 2 included exposure-based procedures, termed imaginal and situational revisiting work, with memories and pictures to focus on personal goals. Phase 3 was a review of the first two phases, and a phase 4 added an imaginal conversation with the deceased and completion and consolidation of treatment aims and termination [1].

IPT, which has previously shown efficacy in the treatment of major depressive disorder related to bereavement [4], was delivered according to a published manual. In phase 1, mood symptoms were reviewed and identified, the model was explained, and the therapists used a grief focus accompanied by secondary focus on role transition or interpersonal disputes if needed. In the next phase, the therapist discussed how bereavement and interpersonal events can affect emotions, discussed the patient's relationship with the deceased in a realistic way, and worked to help patients develop satisfying relationships and activities in the present. In the termination phase, the therapist reviewed gains, made plans for the future, and discussed termination [1].

Each participant received 16 sessions over 20 weeks. Data was collected at baseline and weeks 8, 16, and 20 and then monthly, with participants also self-reporting data at week 12. Data was collected on the Structured Clinical Interview for DSM-IV axis I disorders with supplemental model for complicated grief, the Columbia Suicide Severity Rating Scale, and a complicated grief-focused Clinical Global Improvement scale (CGI-I). Patients self-reported their symptoms on the Inventory of Complicated Grief (ICG), the Work and Social Adjustment Scale, the Grief-Related Avoidance Questionnaire, and the Beck Depression Inventory (BDI) [1].

Independent evaluators were mental health professionals who were blinded to treatment assignment and trained to achieve acceptable reliability on rating instruments. Rating scales were completed beginning at week 8, with nine instances of unblinding. Assessments were audiotaped and randomly selected sample was co-rated, and questions about ratings were discussed in weekly meetings [1].

Results A total of 151 participants were randomized to CGT ($n = 74$) or IPT ($n = 77$) treatment. Among those who began treatment, there were an 82% completion rate for CGT and an 81% completion rate for IPT. The sample had an average age of 66.1 years, and 81.5% of the sample was female, and the two groups had similar baseline characteristics except for the rate of post-traumatic stress disorder (PTSD) being higher in the complicated grief treatment group (21.6% vs. 9.1% in the IPT group, $P = 0.03$).

Differences in scores were analyzed at 20 weeks based on the intention-to-treat (ITT) principle, including all randomized participants. The rate of response was statistically and significantly greater for those who received CGT when compared to IPT. A total of 52 individuals (70.5%) responded to CGT when compared with 24 (32%) of the IPT group. When adjusted for current PTSD, relative risk (RR) was 2.08. The number needed to treat (NNT) with CGT was found to be 2.60 [1].

On secondary outcome measures, as measured by the CGI severity subscale score, 64.1% of participants in the IPT group were still ill at week 20 when compared to 35.2% of the CGT group ($P = 0.001$). There was also a greater reduction on the ICG scores in the CGT group when compared to the IPT group (21.10 point reduction for CGT when compared to 15.00 reduction in IPT, $T(633) = 2.58$; $P = 0.01$). There was more improvement per week noted on the Work and Social Adjustment Scale (0.63 points per week compared with 0.39 points per week, $P = 0.004$) and on the Grief-Related Avoidance Questionnaire (0.56 points per week with CGT and 0.33 points per week with IPT, $P < 0.05$) and the BDI (0.60 points per week with CGT and 0.41 points per week with IPT ($P = 0.03$)) [1].

At 6-month follow-up, data was obtained for 112 of the participants, with results revealing that 100% of CGT responders (38/38) had maintained their response, while 19 out of 22 IPT responders (86.4%) maintained a response [1].

Conclusions Evidence from this blinded, randomized study indicated that CGT is statistically and clinically superior to IPT in ameliorating cognitive grief symptoms and was statistically superior in rate of improvement in depression. The therapy was well tolerated, with no discontinuation due to adverse effects reported and a similar dropout rate in both groups [1].

Strengths of the Study

1. This was a randomized controlled trial where the evaluators were blinded.
2. There were steps taken to ensure interrater reliability on the instruments that were used.

3. The study had a large sample size, samples overall comparable in demographic measures.
4. The instruments used were gold standards for measurement of each outcome variable.
5. Jadad score [5] indicates that this was a high-quality study with a score of 5 out of 5.

Questions Yes (1) No (0)	Was the study described as random?	Was the randomization scheme described and appropriate?	Was the study described as double-blind?	Was the method of double blinding appropriate? (Were both the patient and the assessor appropriately blinded?)	Was there a description of dropouts and withdrawals?	Total score Range of score quality0–2 low3–5 high
Score	1	1	1	1	1	5

Limitations of the Study

1. The sample was predominantly female, white, and highly educated, so the results may not generalize to other groups.
2. Percentage of patients with a diagnosis of PTSD was significantly different at baseline between patients who received CGT and those who received IPT. This may have affected the results, especially given that CGT incorporates elements of therapies targeted toward PTSD symptoms such as prolonged exposure and conceptualizes complicated grief as a stress disorder similar to PTSD, which IPT does not.

Take-Home Points

Despite some limitations, this high-quality randomized trial indicates that CGT, a model of therapy conceptualizing complicated grief as a stress disorder different from major depressive disorder (MDD), outperformed IPT on measures of complicated grief symptoms and depression, delivered over 20 weeks, with results being sustained at 6 months.

Practical Applications of the Take-Home Points

For older adults who present with symptoms of complicated grief, CGT may be more helpful when compared to other types of treatment including IPT. Additionally, it is helpful to conceptualize complicated grief as different from grief-related MDD and recognize that it may respond to different types of treatment.

References

1. Shear MK, Wang Y, Skritskaya N, Duan N, Mauro C, Ghesquiere A. Treatment of complicated grief in elderly persons: a randomized clinical trial. JAMA Psychiatry. 2014;71(11):1287–95.
2. Wetherell JL. Complicated grief therapy as a new treatment approach. Dialogues Clin Neurosci. 2012;14(2):159–66.
3. Shear K, Frank E, Houck PR, Reynolds CF 3rd. Treatment of complicated grief: a randomized controlled trial. JAMA. 2005;293(21):2601–8.
4. Miller MD, Frank E, Cornes C, Imber SD, Anderson B, Ehrenpreis L, Malloy J, Silberman R, Wolfson L, Zaltman J, Reynolds CF 3rd. Applying interpersonal psychotherapy to bereavement-related depression following loss of a spouse in late life. J Psychother Pract Res. 1994;3(2):149–62.
5. Jadad AR, Moore RA, Carroll D, Jenkinson C, Reynolds DJ, Gavaghan DJ, McQuay HJ. Assessing the quality of reports of randomized clinical trials: is blinding necessary? Control Clin Trials. 1996;17(1):1–12.

Part VIII
Pain Disorders

Chapter 47
Association Between Psychological Interventions and Chronic Pain Outcomes in Older Adults: A Systematic Review and Meta-Analysis

Michael G. Li and Erica C. Garcia-Pittman

Authors of the Original Article Bahar Niknejad, Ruth Bolier, Charles R. Henderson Jr., Diana Delgado, Elissa Kozlov, Corinna E. Löckenhoff, M. Carrington Reid.

Journal Published JAMA Internal Medicine.

Year of Publication 2018.

Type of Study Systematic review and meta-analysis.

Funding Sources National Institute on Aging; Pfizer Pharmaceuticals; Howard and Phyllis Schwartz Philanthropic Fund.

Objectives To determine the efficacy of psychological interventions in older adults with chronic pain and whether treatment effects vary by participant, intervention, and study characteristics [1].

Methods In accordance with the Preferred Reporting Items for Systematic Reviews and Meta-Analyses (PRISMA), this study searched online databases for clinical trials that evaluated one or more psychological interventions for the treatment of chronic pain in older adults. The search was conducted with subject headings and keywords including *chronic pain*, *noncancer pain*, *arthritis*, *cognitive therapy*, *mindfulness*, and *elderly*.

M. G. Li · E. C. Garcia-Pittman (✉)
The University of Texas at Austin Dell Medical School, Department of Psychiatry and Behavioral Sciences, Austin, TX, USA
e-mail: michael.li@phhs.org; ecgarcia-pittman@ascension.org

R. R. Tampi et al. (eds.), *Essential Reviews in Geriatric Psychiatry*,
https://doi.org/10.1007/978-3-030-94960-0_47

Studies were included if they used a randomized clinical trial design, evaluated cognitive behavioral techniques in both combination or monotherapy strategies, enrolled participants with chronic pain defined as pain lasting longer than 3 months by the time of enrollment, focused on adults aged 60 or older, and reported preintervention and postintervention quantitative data for each assessment. Studies were excluded if they were not published in a peer-reviewed journal, were written in a non-English language, or had patients with pain due to cancer or chronic headaches.

Two researchers independently screened the titles and abstracts of the search results and conducted a full-text inspection of potentially eligible articles. Disagreements were resolved by consensus from the entire research team.

The researchers included data from the intervention and control groups in order to normalize the data for comparison from all the eligible studies. In studies that had multiple control groups, the researchers pooled data from the active control groups. In studies with multiple intervention modalities, the researchers analyzed only the interventions that addressed chronic pain and excluded comorbid conditions like insomnia. One study had two intervention groups, including a group-based intervention and an individual-based intervention. The researchers reported the posttreatment outcomes data as pooled data from the two intervention groups. The quality of the eligible studies was determined by the quality rating scale developed by Yates et al. [2].

This study extracted data on outcomes that previous research has shown to be positively affected by psychological therapies. A total of eight outcomes (pain intensity, pain-related interference, depressive symptoms, anxiety, catastrophizing beliefs, self-efficacy in pain management, physical health, and self-reported physical function) were extracted and organized into three domains including pain, psychological, and functional. For each outcome, the mean and standard deviation were extracted for intervention and control groups at the pretreatment and posttreatment phase. The researchers defined posttreatment period as any assessment that took place less than 12 weeks after completing the treatment. Mid-term outcomes were defined as assessments taking place between 12 and 24 weeks after treatment. Long-term outcomes were defined as those taking place longer than 24 weeks after treatment.

Meta-analyses were carried out in statistical mixed models. The effect of the intervention on study outcomes was examined by the *treatment* × *time* interaction and separated into three time periods: baseline to first follow-up, baseline to mid-term follow-up, and baseline to long-term follow-up. The primary outcome of interest was the baseline to first follow-up because all studies reported outcomes at this time point. Results were reported as the differences of standardized mean differences (d_D) due to the numerous measurement instruments and scale ranges used by the studies for each outcome. The researchers used mixed models in which studies are assumed to be random rather than fixed, as they accounted for the variability of effect sizes across all studies. They computed the Cochran Q statistic and Higgins-Thompson H^2 and I^2 values to examine the heterogeneity across studies.

Results Initial database searches identified 2391 articles. Researchers selected 238 studies based on title and abstract for full-text review to determine eligibility. Ultimately, a total of 22 studies with 2608 participants were included in the final sample. The treatment interventions in the studies were psychological modalities based on the principles of mindfulness, physical exercise, and cognitive behavioral therapy. A summary of the participants characteristics is outlined below (Table 47.1).

A summary of the study characteristics is outlined in the following table (Table 47.2).

According to the Yates quality rating scale scores which range from 0 to 35, with higher scores indicating better quality, the quality of the studies had a mean (range) score of 24.5 (13–33). Researchers determined that studies with a score of 22.7 or greater had excellent methodologic quality. Twelve studies (55%) met criteria for minimizing possibility of measurement bias, and ten studies (45%) were judged to be at low risk for allocation bias. The Cochran Q and I^2 scores for the key variable of pain intensity, 25.9% and 27.6%, respectively, indicated a modest degree of heterogeneity.

The treatment interventions in all of the studies were psychological modalities based on the principles of mindfulness, cognitive behavioral therapy, and physical exercise. The results of eight treatment outcomes, reported as d_D, with respective P values, are as follows: pain intensity ($d_D = -0.181$, $P = 0.006$), pain interference ($d_D = -0.133$, $P = 0.12$), depressive symptoms ($d_D = -0.128$, $P = 0.14$), anxiety ($d_D = -0.205$, $P = 0.09$), catastrophizing beliefs ($d_D = -0.184$, $P = 0.046$), self-efficacy for managing pain ($d_D = 0.193$, $P = 0.02$), physical function ($d_D = 0.006$, $P = 0.96$), and physical health ($d_D = 0.160$, $P = 0.24$). The treatment result for pain intensity persisted up to 24 weeks after treatment completion ($d_D = -0.251$, $P = 0.002$). There was no evidence that treatment results persisted beyond 24 weeks, but this was also limited by the small number of studies that assessed long-term follow-up. The effect sizes of each study that assessed pain intensity were modest due to smaller sample size, but overall their summation indicated a statistically significant difference in favor of the treatment groups over the control groups.

Table 47.1 Participant characteristics

Total number of participants	2608
Number (%) of women	1799 (69.0%)
Mean [SD] pain duration	16.1 [13.9] years
Mean [SD] age	71.9 [7.1] years

Table 47.2 Study characteristics

Total number of studies	22
Mean [range] length of intervention period	9.4 [4–35] weeks
Mean [range] number of treatments	8.4 [6–14]
Number (%) of studies with group-based approach	15 (68.1%)
Number (%) of studies with in-person treatment	19 (86.4%)

Researchers determined whether treatment effects differed by the level of potentially modifying variables to the primary model of *treatment* × *time*. These variables fell under three broad areas: participant characteristics, study characteristics, and intervention characteristics. Across all of the outcomes and possible modifying variables, only the mode of therapy (group vs. individual therapy) showed a consistent pattern of results in favor of group-based interventions.

There were three studies that assessed the harms and adverse outcomes of therapy treatment. Two studies identified a mild increase in pain with an exercise and behavioral skills protocol, and one study found no adverse events with a meditation mindfulness-based protocol.

Conclusions Psychological interventions in the treatment of chronic pain in older adults have a measurable benefit with improving pain intensity, catastrophizing beliefs, and self-efficacy in pain management. Moderator analyses demonstrated that the mode of therapy (i.e., group versus individual) was the most consistent pattern of results in favor of group-based approaches. Out of all the treatment outcomes, only pain intensity reduction was observed to persist up to 6 months after completion of treatment.

Strengths of the Study

1. The study included participants only aged 60 years or older.
2. The participants had chronic pain much greater than a 3-month period.
3. The study included studies that had an excellent methodological quality as determined by the quality rating scale from Yates et al. [2].
4. The study analyzed variables that could potentially modify treatment outcomes (i.e., mode of therapy, study quality, level of therapist training).

Limitations of the Study

1. The study did not include publications that reported treatment-related reduction in pain medication use.
2. The study only used English language publications.
3. There was a lack of long-term studies beyond a 6-month period after treatment completion.
4. Lack of heterogeneity across intervention characteristics (e.g., treatment length, number of treatments) made it difficult to conclude if there was a correlation between treatment dose and outcome.
5. Only three publications included in this study examined adverse outcomes related to treatment.

Take-Home Points

Psychological interventions delivered in-person within a group environment can provide measurable improvements in treating chronic pain in older adults, primarily within pain intensity, catastrophizing thoughts, and self-efficacy in managing pain. While there is a lack of long-term data, benefits in reducing pain intensity can last up to 6 months after completing treatment.

Practical Applications of Take-Home Points

Older adults with chronic pain should be encouraged to attend group-based psychological treatments of pain as they may provide safe interventions with improvements that could last up to 6 months.

References

1. Niknejad B, Bolier R, Henderson CR Jr, Delgado D, Kozlov E, Löckenhoff CE, Reid MC. Association between psychological interventions and chronic pain outcomes in older adults: a systematic review and meta-analysis. JAMA Intern Med. 2018;178(6):830–9.
2. Yates SL, Morley S, Eccleston C, de C Williams AC. A scale for rating the quality of psychological trials for pain. Pain. 2005;117(3):314–25.

Part IX
Psychotic Disorders

Chapter 48
A Randomized Controlled Trial of Cognitive Behavioral Social Skills Training for Middle-Aged and Older Outpatients with Chronic Schizophrenia

Avee Champaneria and Paul A. Riordan

Authors of the Original Article Eric Granholm, John R McQuaid, Fauzia Simjee McClure, Lisa A Auslander, Dimitri Perivoliotis, Paola Pedrelli, Thomas Patterson, Dilip V Jeste.

Journal Published American Journal of Psychiatry.

Year of Publication 2005.

Type of Study Randomized Controlled Trial.

Funding Sources NIH.

Objectives To assess whether CBT + social skills training provided as group therapy would improve social functioning in middle-aged and older adults (>40 years old) with chronic schizophrenia [1].

Methods The sample population was recruited from patients between the ages of 42 and 74, with DSM-IV diagnoses of schizophrenia or schizoaffective disorder, in San Diego County from 1999 to 2003. Investigators excluded persons with disabling medical problems that could interfere with testing, absence of medical records to confirm diagnosis, and the diagnosis of a substance use disorder other

A. Champaneria
Fellow in Geriatric Psychiatry, Duke University School of Medicine, Durham, NC, USA
e-mail: avee.champaneria@duke.edu

P. A. Riordan (✉)
Durham Veterans Affairs Medical Center, Department of Psychiatry and Behavioral Sciences, Duke University School of Medicine, Durham, NC, USA
e-mail: paul.riordan@duke.edu

R. R. Tampi et al. (eds.), *Essential Reviews in Geriatric Psychiatry*,
https://doi.org/10.1007/978-3-030-94960-0_48

Table 48.1 Patients' psychotropic medications at baseline

Psychotropic medications at baseline	Number of patients
Atypical antipsychotics	46
Typical antipsychotics	17
Typical + atypical antipsychotics	7
No antipsychotic	6
Antidepressants	36
Mood stabilizers	22

than nicotine or caffeine within the past 6 months. Patients' baseline psychotropic medications are listed in Table 48.1.

To decrease non-adherence to therapy due to transportation issues, CBT + social skills was delivered both at the research center ($N = 52$) and at various board-and-care facilities in the community ($N = 24$). Randomization was stratified by location to one of the two treatment conditions: (1) treatment as usual or (2) treatment as usual plus cognitive behavioral social skills training (CBT + social skills). Only the project coordinator and the therapists knew group membership with all assessors blinded. Investigators tested the blind by having the assessors guess group membership at each assessment by using a 7-point Likert scale.

Investigators measured outcomes at baseline, 3 months, and 6 months (at the end of treatment). Investigators adapted the Independent Living Skills Survey (ILSS) and the University of California at San Diego (UCSD) Performance-Based Skills Assessment to assess social functioning as the primary outcome. They excluded five domains in the ILSS (food preparation/storage, care of personal possessions, job seeking, job maintenance, and money management) because the majority of participants in the study lived in board-and-care settings. Investigators also used standardized role-playing situations in the UCSD Performance-Based Skills Assessment, to assess five domains of functioning—household chores, communication, finance, transportation, and planning recreational activities.

Investigators assessed secondary outcomes with the Positive and Negative Syndrome Scale and the Hamilton Depression Rating Scale [2]. They measured process variables using the Beck Cognitive Insight Scale and the Comprehensive Module Test. Finally, they tracked baseline psychotropic medications (antipsychotic, antidepressant, mood stabilizers) and psychotropic medication changes.

Both groups continued to receive treatment as usual with their psychiatric medications managed by their psychiatrists.

In the CBT + social skills group, patients also received weekly 2-h group psychotherapy sessions (with half-hour lunch break) over a 24-week period. A treatment manual was developed combining cognitive behavioral therapy and social skills training [3], with modifications to address the unique needs of older patients. Participants completed three 4-week modules twice. The domains are detailed in Table 48.2.

Each group was led by two therapists, with requirements of at least a master's level of training and 2 years of clinical experience or having a doctorate in clinical

Table 48.2 Module domains

Module	Focus
Thought-Challenging	Identify the relationship among thoughts, feelings, and behaviors; identify and challenge age-relevant beliefs cognitive distortions
Asking for Support	Improve communication skills and social interactions through age-relevant role-playing
Solving Problems	Target problems related to illness and disability

psychology. The Cognitive Therapy Rating Scale for Psychosis was used to rate therapist competence from 30 randomly selected videotaped sessions. The investigators used intent-to-treat analysis to examine all outcome variables with missing data imputed by within-group means of the missing values. For their primary analysis, investigators used an analysis of covariance (ANCOVA) to test differences between the groups.

Results A total of 72% of the eligible patients consented to the study, with 39 patients randomized to treatment as usual only and 37 to treatment as usual with CBT + social skills. The two groups did not differ significantly at baseline. Notably, most patients were high school-educated, Caucasian non-veteran males, who lived in assisted housing. Participants had a mean illness duration of about 30 years. Treatment Adherence Retention of participants at the end of treatment was 86%. Four participants assigned to the combined treatment group did not become engaged in treatment. All participants who engaged in receiving combined treatment completed all three modules at least once (12 sessions). The mean number of sessions attended was 22 (95% confidence interval (CI) = 21–23), and the mean percentage of homework assignments completed was 75% (95% CI = 66–84%, range = 0–100%). The treatment group effect was statistically significant at improving frequency of social activities, cognitive insight, and mastery of cognitive behavioral social skills training. No other significant associations were found. Table 48.3 details the effect sizes for all outcomes per the ANCOVA model.

Psychiatric hospitalizations during enrollment in the study were uncommon with two participants in treatment as usual hospitalized for suicidal ideation and two from the combined treatment group hospitalized, one for suicidal ideation and one for agitation/paranoia after medication changes. The differences between treatment groups were similar at mid-treatment and at the end of treatment for all outcome variables. The efficacy of the intervention was not significantly affected by site of delivery.

The treatment group effect at the end of treatment was not significant for the dose of antipsychotic medication or the dose of anticholinergic medication.

Conclusions This is the first published non-pilot randomized controlled trial investigating whether adding a cognitive behavioral and skills-based group psychotherapy intervention to treatment as usual improved social functional outcomes in middle-aged and older patients with schizophrenia or schizoaffective disorder. The

Table 48.3 The effect sizes for all outcomes per the ANCOVA model

Outcome	Eta squared (effect size)	P value
Independent Living Skill Survey (ILSS)	0.08	0.02[a]
UCSD Performance-Based Skills Assessment	0.05	0.052
PANSS positive symptoms	0.03	0.13
PANSS negative symptoms	0.01	0.52
Beck Cognitive Insight Scale	0.12	0.002[a]
Comprehensive Module Test	0.33	<0.001[a]
Hamilton Depression Rating Scale	0.01	0.37

[a]Authors set statistical significance at $P < 0.05$ in this study

patients who received treatment as usual plus cognitive behavioral social skills training performed social functioning activities significantly more frequently than patients in treatment as usual. The cognitive behavioral social skills training specifically focused on challenging illness-related thoughts and beliefs (e.g., paranoia) and thoughts that interfere with the execution of daily activities, increasing the likelihood that the patients would engage in social activities. The treatment groups failed to differ significantly in their general skill at performing specific everyday functioning activities which may be due to the fact that the cognitive behavioral social skills training does not specifically train all the skills measured by this test. There was not any significant benefit from repeating the modules, indicating that 12-week-long therapy is likely sufficient for teaching the three domains offered in this CBT + social skills group therapy protocol.

Strengths of the Study

1. Patients were randomly assigned to the two treatment groups with groups having similar baseline characteristics. All assessors were blind.
2. Intervention was manualized, and treatment fidelity was monitored.
3. Participants had excellent attendance and had a low dropout rate likely due to the investigators providing transportation to therapy and/or conducting sessions at board-and-care facilities in the community.
4. Improvement in cognitive insight may be a possible mechanism of symptom change in cognitive behavioral therapy [4]. Patients in the combined treatment group showed significantly greater cognitive insight after treatment in comparison to the patients in the treatment as usual group.

Limitations of the Study

1. The study has a relatively small sample size.
2. Generalizability is limited as most participants were Caucasian males without comorbid substance use disorder.
3. Limited generalizability to application of treatment intervention by clinicians in the community who are not the experts who developed the interventions.
4. It is unknown for how long after the study the acquired skills were retained.

5. There was no therapy control group to determine if effects were due to additional contact with a clinician or due to the CBT + social skills intervention.
6. The effects size of the treatment on one of primary outcomes was small (0.08 for frequency of social activities), but statistically significant. The effect size on the other measure of social functioning (UCSD Performance-Based Skills Assessment) was even smaller (0.05) and not statistically significant.

Take-Home Points

This study adds to the growing base of evidence for cognitive behavioral therapy for schizophrenia. It shows that the addition of cognitive behavioral social skills training to treatment as usual with psychotropics leads to a mild improvement in social functioning in middle-aged and older adults with chronic schizophrenia or schizoaffective disorder; however, the generalizability of this to other population subgroups is limited.

Practical Applications of the Take-Home Point

Social impairment in chronic schizophrenia in older adults is only mild to moderately addressed by psychotropics [5]; thus, psychotherapeutic interventions should be considered to improve social functioning in this population. Age-specific barriers (such as transportation) to treatment should be identified and addressed to improve overall adherence to interventions for older adults.

References

1. Granholm E, McQuaid JR, McClure FS, Auslander LA, Perivoliotis D, Pedrelli P, Patterson T, Jeste DV. A randomized, controlled trial of cognitive behavioral social skills training for middle-aged and older outpatients with chronic schizophrenia. Am J Psychiatry. 2005;162(3):520–9.
2. Hamilton M. Development of a rating scale for primary depressive illness. Br J Soc Clin Psychol. 1967;6(4):278–96.
3. McQuaid JR, Granholm E, McClure FS, Roepke S, Pedrelli P, Patterson TL, Jeste DV. Development of an integrated cognitive-behavioral and social skills training intervention for older patients with schizophrenia. J Psychother Pract Res. 2000;9(3):149–56.
4. Beck AT, Baruch E, Balter JM, Steer RA, Warman DM. A new instrument for measuring insight: the Beck Cognitive Insight Scale. Schizophr Res. 2004;68(2–3):319–29.
5. Huhn M, Nikolakopoulou A, Schneider-Thoma J, Krause M, Samara M, Peter N, Arndt T, Bäckers L, Rothe P, Cipriani A, Davis J, Salanti G, Leucht S. Comparative efficacy and tolerability of 32 oral antipsychotics for the acute treatment of adults with multi-episode schizophrenia: a systematic review and network meta-analysis. Lancet. 2019;394(10202):939–51.

Chapter 49
Safety and Tolerability of Oral Paliperidone Extended-Release Tablets in Elderly Patients with Schizophrenia: A Double-Blind, Placebo-Controlled Study with Six-Month Open-Label Extension

Elizabeth Qin and Peter Ureste

Authors of the Original Article Andreas Tzimos, Viktor Samokhvalov, Michelle Kramer, Lisa Ford, Cristiana Gassmann-Mayer, Pilar Lim, Mariëlle Eerdekens.

Journal Published American Journal of Geriatric Psychiatry.

Year of Publication 2008.

Type of Study Randomized double-blind placebo-controlled trial.

Funding Sources Johnson & Johnson Pharmaceutical Research and Development, LLC.

Objectives To determine the safety and tolerability of paliperidone extended-release tablets in older adults with schizophrenia from a double-blind, randomized, placebo-controlled trial, which was extended to a 6-month open-label extension period [1].

Methods This study employed two phases: first, a 6-week, double-blind, randomized phase, and second, an optional 24-week open-label extension phase. The study was conducted across multiple centers internationally. One hundred thirty-one individuals, ≥65 years in age, were screened, and those individuals who met the Diagnostic and Statistical Manual of Mental Disorders, fourth edition (DSM-IV), criteria for schizophrenia for at least 1 year and experienced an acute episode

E. Qin · P. Ureste (✉)
Department of Psychiatry and Behavioral Sciences, University of California San Francisco, San Francisco, CA, USA
e-mail: Elizabeth.Qin@ucsf.edu; Peter.Ureste@ucsf.edu

R. R. Tampi et al. (eds.), *Essential Reviews in Geriatric Psychiatry*,
https://doi.org/10.1007/978-3-030-94960-0_49

(Positive and Negative Syndrome Scale [PANSS] total score of 70–120) were enrolled in the double-blind phase.

Exclusion criteria for this study were as follows: a DSM-IV diagnosis other than schizophrenia or of substance dependence; significant risk of suicidal or aggressive behavior or other unstable disease; medical conditions that could alter the pharmacology of the study medication; known allergic reactions to multiple medications (barbiturates, carbamazepine, lamotrigine, phenytoin, paliperidone, or risperidone); previous lack of response to risperidone; recent use of depot antipsychotic, experimental treatment, or electroconvulsive therapy; or involuntary admission to a psychiatric hospital.

Prior to the study, participants were expected to discontinue all antipsychotics and benzodiazepines at least 3 days before baseline assessment. Oral benzodiazepines were allowed for the treatment of agitation, anxiety, or sleep, among individuals who were taking a stable dose for 3 months before baseline assessment. Additional medications that were allowed were as follows: oral benztropine or biperiden for the treatment of extrapyramidal symptom (EPS), β-adrenergic blockers for treatment-emergent akathisia, beta-adrenergic blockers for hypertension among individuals stabilized before screening, and antidepressants [except monoamine oxidase inhibitors MAOIs)] if an individual was taking a stable for at least 3 months before screening.

In the 6-week double-blind phase, participants were randomized 2:1 to receive either flexibly dosed paliperidone ER (3–12 mg) or placebo. Participants taking paliperidone ER started at 6 mg/day, with dose adjustments by 3 mg increments. Doses were permitted to be increased at weekly intervals or decreased at any time for concerns for safety and tolerability. Participants were hospitalized for at least 14 days for close monitoring.

An open-label extension phase was subsequently conducted, with eligible participants receiving paliperidone extended-release (ER), with similar dose-adjustment protocols as in the double-blind phase. Eligible participants were those who completed the double-blind phase or discontinued due to lack of efficacy [defined as an increase in the Positive and Negative Syndrome Scale (PANSS) score by at least 20%].

The primary outcome measures in this study were PANSS total and factor scores, Clinical Global Impressions Scale-Severity score (CGI-S), Personal and Social Performance Scale, and the Schizophrenia Quality of Life Scale. The study also evaluated safety by assessing for adverse events, laboratory tests (including prolactin, insulin, and C-peptide), vital signs and physical exam, electrocardiograms, and movement disorder rating scales [Simpson Angus Scale, Barnes Akathisia Rating Scale, and Abnormal Involuntary Movement Scale (AIMS)].

The investigators assessed safety and tolerability by descriptive statistics, without formal statistical analyses. For efficacy analyses, the investigators compared the change from baseline of PANSS, Personal and Social Performance Scale, and Schizophrenia Quality of Life Scale using estimated least squares mean changes and two-sided 95% confidence intervals. They also compared PANSS total score over time through the double-blind and open-label extension phases for the paliperidone vs placebo groups.

Results From a total of 131 individuals who were screened to participate in the study, a total of 114 patients enrolled in the double-blind phase. Three participants had an adverse event, and 14 participants were excluded for a reason designated "other." A total of 88 participants continued on to the open-label phase.

Of the 114 participants in the double-blind phase, 73% were female and 99% were white. The mean age was 70 years. The demographics for the paliperidone ER and placebo groups were similar. The distribution of demographics was also similar between the participants in the double-blind phase and those who continued on to the open-label phase. All participants had moderate to severe schizophrenia (99%), with 85% having paranoid schizophrenia. A total of 77% of participants had used typical antipsychotics before screening, with the most common medication being haloperidol (49%). Common preexisting medical conditions including cardiovascular disorders, hypertension, and diabetes. About 80% of participants completed the 6-week double-blind phase, with the most common reason for discontinuation being lack of efficacy (16% in the placebo group, 4% in the paliperidone ER group). Adverse effects that led to discontinuation occurred at similar rates in the two groups. In the open-label phase, the most common adverse event leading to discontinuation was a "confusional" state which occurred in two patients in the paliperidone ER/paliperidone ER group.

The median doses of paliperidone ER were 8.4 mg/day in the double-blind phase and 7.4–8.5 mg/day in the open-label extension phase.

Regarding safety and tolerability, adverse events that did not lead to discontinuation also occurred at similar rates in the two groups. There was an age-related increase in somnolence noted during the double-blind phase (7% in ages 64–69 years, 11% in ages 70–75 years, 14% in ages >75 years). Three participants in the paliperidone ER groups experienced orthostatic hypotension. There was a higher incidence of tachycardia (heart rate ≥100 beats/min) in participants in the paliperidone ER group, which was more notable in ages 70–75 years when compared to ages 64–69 years. Two participants had a prolonged QTc interval ≥500 msec in the double-blind phase and one participant in the open-label extension; it was noted that all three of these participants had a prior history of QTc prolongation. About half of participants treated with paliperidone ER had elevated prolactin levels above the normal range, with no adverse events thought to be related to prolactin during the study. There were no substantial changes in liver or renal function, hematology tests, body weight, or body mass index from baseline between the two groups. There was a low incidence of extrapyramidal symptoms, with 2–3% participants experiencing hypertonia, tremor, and akathisia. Three deaths occurred: one by cardiac arrest and one by intracranial hemorrhage in the double-blind phase and one by nontreatment-emergent bronchopneumonia in the extension phase. All three of these patients were in the placebo group.

Regarding efficacy, the investigators note that the study was not powered for efficacy; however, they did find that treatment with paliperidone ER improved

PANSS total scores. In the double-blind phase, the paliperidone ER group showed improved PANSS scores from baseline when compared to the placebo group. The analysis of covariance last-observation-carried-for-ward analysis showed a separation between treatment groups becoming noticeable from day 15 onward. In addition, when compared to placebo, the paliperidone ER-treated group showed greater improvements on the PANSS factors of positive symptoms, negative symptoms, and anxiety/depression. Between the two treatment groups, there was no statistically significant difference in the median change in CGI-S scores. The two groups did not differ significantly on Personal and Social Performance Scale or Schizophrenia Quality of Life Scale.

Individuals previously treated with paliperidone ER who continued in the extension phase maintained the improvements they had gained in the PANSS subscales, CGI-S, Personal and Social Performance Scale, and Schizophrenia Quality of Life Scale.

Conclusions Evidence from this 6-week randomized, double-blind, and placebo-controlled trial, with optional continuation to an open-label extension phase, indicates that paliperidone ER is overall well tolerated by older adults. While the study was not powered for efficacy, results suggest that paliperidone ER would be similarly beneficial in treating schizophrenia in older adults as in a younger population when compared to placebo.

Strengths of the Study

1. Randomized, double-blind, and placebo-controlled trial design, with optional continuation into an open-label extension phase.
2. The quality of study assessed on the basis of Jadad Score indicates that this was high-quality study with a score of 5 out of 5 [2].

Questions Yes (1) No (0)	Was the study described as random?	Was the randomization scheme described and appropriate?	Was the study described as double-blind?	Was the method of double blinding appropriate? (Were both the patient and the assessor appropriately blinded?)	Was there a description of dropouts and withdrawals?	Total score Range of score quality0–2 low3–5 high
Score	1	1	1	1	1	5

3. The study sample included only older adults (≥65 years).
4. A total of 99% of participants had moderate to severe schizophrenia.
5. There was a 79% completion rate for the double-blind phase of the study.

Limitations of the Study

1. A small sample size of 114 participants.
2. A short duration of double-blind study period of 6 weeks.
3. The study was supported by Johnson & Johnson Pharmaceutical Research and Development.
4. A total of 73% of the participants were female.
5. A total of 99% of the participants were white.
6. The study was not powered for an evaluation of efficacy.

Take-Home Points

Despite some limitations, this high-quality randomized, double-blind, and placebo-controlled trial, with optional continuation to an open-label extension phase, indicates that paliperidone ER has clinical (non-significant) benefit when compared to placebo for the treatment of schizophrenia among older adults over 6 weeks, with continued benefit over 6 months. Paliperidone ER was generally well tolerated when compared to placebo with the most commonly reported side effects being somnolence, tachycardia, and elevated prolactin level.

Practical Applications of the Take-Home Point

Among older adults who present with schizophrenia with moderate to severe symptoms, paliperidone ER is a beneficial and well-tolerated treatment option.

References

1. Tzimos A, Samokhvalov V, Kramer M, Ford L, Gassmann-Mayer C, Lim P, Eerdekens M. Safety and tolerability of oral paliperidone extended-release tablets in elderly patients with schizophrenia: a double-blind, placebo-controlled study with six-month open-label extension. Am J Geriatr Psychiatry. 2008;16(1):31–43.
2. Jadad AR, Moore RA, Carroll D, Jenkinson C, Reynolds DJ, Gavaghan DJ, McQuay HJ. Assessing the quality of reports of randomized clinical trials: is blinding necessary? Control Clin Trials. 1996;17(1):1–12.

Chapter 50
Antipsychotic Treatment for Elderly People with Late-Onset Schizophrenia

Christa DeFries and Peter Ureste

Authors of the Original Article Adib Essali, Ghassan Ali.

Journal Published Cochrane Database of Systemic Reviews.

Year of Publication 2012.

Type of Study Systematic review.

Funding Sources The Cochrane Library.

Objectives To find and review studies assessing the effects of antipsychotic drugs for older adults with late-onset schizophrenia [1].

Methods The authors searched the Cochrane Schizophrenia Group Trials Register, which is compiled from regular searches of CINAHL, Embase, MEDLINE, and PsycINFO. They updated a similar search that was done in 2002.

Selection criteria were for randomized controlled trials comparing typical or atypical antipsychotic drugs to placebo, to no intervention, or to another antipsychotic drug. Any dose, mode, pattern, or duration of administration was acceptable. Population was older people, at least 80% older than 65 years old. They had to have a recent diagnosis of schizophrenia or schizophrenia-like illness (including

C. DeFries
Department of Psychiatry, Baylor Scott & White Health, Temple, TX, USA
e-mail: christa.defries@bswhealth.org

P. Ureste (✉)
Department of Psychiatry and Behavioral Sciences, University of California San Francisco, San Francisco, CA, USA
e-mail: Peter.Ureste@ucsf.edu

R. R. Tampi et al. (eds.), *Essential Reviews in Geriatric Psychiatry*,
https://doi.org/10.1007/978-3-030-94960-0_50

delusional disorder, schizoaffective disorder, schizophreniform psychosis, or paraphrenia) – diagnosed within the previous 5 years.

The review wanted to look at outcome measures of mortality, global clinical response, quality of life, adverse events, cost, and service utilization, e.g., hospital admission/number of days in hospital.

Results Of 88 citations, only 1 trial was found that met the selection criteria. Among these, 35 were excluded because the intervention was not a neuroleptic medication; another 34 were excluded because they did not involve older adults or included people whose psychiatric disorder was not late-onset. Seven studies did focus on late-onset schizophrenia, but four were excluded based on incomplete randomization, and the authors did not have enough information to evaluate two studies.

The single study included 44 participants diagnosed with schizophrenia according to Chinese Classification of Mental Disorders, third version (CCDM-3), who were randomized to receive risperidone or olanzapine for 8 weeks' duration. It was not blinded. Efficacy in the study was measured by the Brief Psychiatric Rating Scale (BPRS), but data was unusable as it did not include standard deviations. Outcome data about changes in body mass index, fasting blood glucose, serum cholesterol, and serum triglycerides also did not include standard deviations.

Conclusions This review reveals that very little evidence exists for the effects of antipsychotic drugs used among older adults with late-onset schizophrenia.

Strengths of the Study

1. A thorough search of available databases.
2. In the only included study, all participants completed the 8-week trial, resulting in a 100% completion rate.

Limitations of the Study

1. Very little data is available on this topic.
2. The only included study reported outcomes for all participants, but presented continuous data without standard deviations, which prevented the authors from using data related to changes in body mass index, fasting blood glucose, serum cholesterol, and serum triglycerides.

Take-Home Points

After a thorough search in 2012, no significant data are available about antipsychotic drug treatment for older adults with late-onset schizophrenia. There is a need for further research in this area.

Practical Applications of the Take-Home Point

Until further studies are available, clinicians will have to continue to rely on clinical judgment when using antipsychotic drugs in older adults with late-onset schizophrenia. There is no trial-based evidence available for guidance.

Reference

1. Essali A, Ali G. Antipsychotic drug treatment for elderly people with late-onset schizophrenia. Cochrane Database Syst Rev. 2012;2012(2):CD004162.

Chapter 51
Schizophrenia and Risk of Dementia: A Meta-Analysis Study

Andrew Wong, Vahid Pasovic, Adan Khan, and Esther Akinyemi

Authors of the Original Article Laisheng Cai and Jingwei Huang.

Journal Publisher Neuropsychiatric Disease and Treatment.

Year of Publication 2018.

Type of Study Quantitative meta-analysis.

Funding Sources None stated.

Objectives To assess the relationship between schizophrenia and the risk of subsequent dementia using a quantitative meta-analysis [1].

Methods The authors used the Preferred Reporting Items for Systematic Reviews and Meta-Analyses (PRISMA) guidelines for this meta-analysis. The two researchers identified relevant articles from PubMed, Embase, and Web of Science published till December 23, 2017, using specific keywords. Additionally, they used Medical Subject Heading (MeSH) in PubMed and Emtree terms in Embase to identify relevant studies. The authors restricted their search to article published in the English language only. They also searched the reference lists of included studies for additional papers. Each author independently conducted the literature search, reviewed titles and abstracts, and made final decisions on eligibility on studies after a full-text review. Additionally, they extracted data independently from the identified studies.

A. Wong · V. Pasovic · A. Khan · E. Akinyemi (✉)
Henry Ford Health System, Detroit, MI, USA
e-mail: vpasovi1@hfhs.org; eakinye2@hfhs.org

R. R. Tampi et al. (eds.), *Essential Reviews in Geriatric Psychiatry*,
https://doi.org/10.1007/978-3-030-94960-0_51

The inclusion criteria were as follows: (1) studies that have a community-based or population-based design (either prospective or retrospective); (2) the data from original article was not previously published in reviews, posters, or abstracts; (3) the main diagnosis was schizophrenia; (4) a minimum of 12-month period of follow-up was present; and (5) the study provided quantitative estimates of multivariate-adjusted relative risks (RR) and 95% confidence intervals (CI) for dementia in relation to schizophrenia. The authors considered hazard ratios (HRs) and odds ratios (ORs) as being equivalent to RR. The exclusion criteria were as follows: (1) cross-sectional study design; (2) editorials, reviews, meetings proceedings, commentaries, case reports or series, meta-analyses, manuscripts that were unrelated to the research topic, and animal or cell-line studies; (3) studies having less than a 12-month follow-up period; and (4) studies with data that was insufficient to estimate adjusted RRs and 95% CI. The authors used EndNote to remove duplicate data. Additionally, the authors for studies were contacted if multiple studies were conducted at the same research center in order to remove any overlapping samples. Disagreements between the two authors on the information collected were resolved by a colleague.

The data that was extracted independently by the two authors from the individual studies included the following: the first author name, the year of publication, the design of the study, the country of origin of the study, the location, the number of participants, the number of dementia cases, the gender of sample participants, the mean age, the follow-up time, the assessment of schizophrenia and dementia, the adjusted covariates, and the quality of the study. The quality of the included studies was assessed using the Newcastle-Ottawa Scale (NOS). Studies that are graded as a 7–8 out of 9 are classified as being of good quality.

The outcomes were pooled using the random-effects model. Multivariate-adjusted RRs and 95% CIs were used in the analysis. $P < 0.05$ was considered to be statistically significant.

Results A total of six papers were included in the meta-analysis. All six studies were assessed as being of good quality based on the NOS. All six studies were rated as being satisfactory for methodological quality based on the NOS. This included a total of 5,063,316 participants and 206,694 cases of dementia. Four of the studies were conducted in European countries, one was from an Asian country, and one was from Oceania. The duration of follow-up ranged from 3 to 20 years, with three studies each having a follow-up of < and >10 years, respectively. There were four prospective studies and two retrospective studies. Only two out of the six studies reported the RR of men and women. Participants were divided into <65 and ≥65 years for age group analysis.

Individuals with schizophrenia were found to have a greater risk of developing dementia when compared to individuals without schizophrenia (RR = 2.29, 95% CI 1.35–3.88) based on the meta-analysis of the six studies. However, significant heterogeneity among the studies was noted ($P = 0.000$; $I^2 = 98.9\%$).

Subgroup analyses indicated that the estimated RR was different when comparing studies from Europe (RR = 1.66, 95% CI 1.03–2.66) to studies from non-European countries (RR = 4.70, 95% CI 4.37–5.06). The incidence of dementia was greater among individuals ≥65 years (RR = 3.56, 95% CI 3.22–3.93) when compared to individuals <65 years (RR = 3.53, 95% CI 1.04–12.03). Prospective studies found a greater incidence of dementia (RR = 2.52, 95% CI 1.47–4.34) when compared to retrospective studies (RR = 2.03, 95% CI 0.41–10.16). The pooled estimate of multivariate RRs for the incidence of dementia was slightly different among women (RR = 3.36, 95% CI 1.24–9.13) when compared to men (RR = 3.09, 95% CI 1.85–5.13). The association was found to be greater in studies that had a follow-up period of >10 years (RR = 2.08, 95% CI 1.57–2.76) when compared to studies with a follow-up period of <10 years (RR = 2.19, 95% CI 0.65–7.40). In addition, studies that had a quality rating of 8 on the NOS found a greater association for dementia (RR = 2.02, 95% CI 1.70–2.79) when compared to studies that had a rating of 9 on the NOS (RR = 2.73, 95% CI 0.75–9.92). The sensitivity analysis demonstrated that no single study had significantly influenced the statistically significant differences that were noted in the incidence of dementia among the participants of this meta-analysis.

Conclusion This meta-analysis indicates that individuals with schizophrenia may have a higher risk for developing dementia when compared to individuals without schizophrenia. Additionally, the relative risk for developing dementia may be greater among women when compared to men.

Strengths of the Study

1. The authors followed the PRISMA guidelines for the reporting of this meta-analysis.
2. The authors searched three large databases to identify possible studies for inclusion in the meta-analysis.
3. The inclusion and exclusion criteria were sufficiently broad to be as inclusive as possible with the studies.
4. The authors used the NOS to rate the quality of the included studies.
5. Subgroup and sensitivity analyses were also conducted by the authors.

Limitations of the Study

1. Literature search did not include the terms "major neurocognitive disorder" which is the official classification of dementia under DSM-5.
2. The study did not differentiate between treated and untreated individuals with schizophrenia or the modalities of treatment.
3. The study did not comment on comorbid conditions and other risk factors (poor healthcare, lifestyle, diet, poor day to day functioning) which could contribute to higher risk of dementia.
4. There was no distinction based on the different dementia subtypes.
5. There was limited demographic range (race, ethnicity) of the participants as four of the six studies were conducted in Europe.
6. Early mortality rates seen among individuals with schizophrenia may have contributed to the more conservative results noted in this meta-analysis.

Take-Home Points
This high-quality meta-analysis indicates that individuals with schizophrenia may be at greater risk for developing dementia.

Practical Applications of the Take-Home Points
Patients with schizophrenia especially those who are aging should be regularly screened for changes in cognitive functioning. Additionally, the appropriate assessment and treatment of comorbid medical conditions (vascular disease, diabetes etc.) which can increase the risk for dementia is of utmost importance, especially among individuals with chronic mental illness.

Reference

1. Cai L, Huang J. Schizophrenia and risk of dementia: a meta-analysis study. Neuropsychiatr Dis Treat. 2018;14:2047–55.

Chapter 52
Antipsychotic Treatment of Very Late-Onset Schizophrenia-Like Psychosis (ATLAS): A Randomized, Controlled, Double-Blind Trial

William B. Smith and Peter Ureste

Authors of the Original Article Robert Howard, Elizabeth Cort, Rosie Bradley, Emma Harper, Linda Kelly, Peter Bentham, Craig Ritchie, Suzanne Reeves, Waleed Fawz, Gill Livingston, Andrew Sommerlad, Sabu Oomman, Ejaz Nazir, Ramin Nilforooshan, Robert Barber, Chris Fox, Ajay Verma Macharouthu, Pranathi Ramachandra, Vivek Pattan, John Sykes, Val Curran, Cornelius Katona, Tom Dening, Martin Knapp, Richard Gray, ATLAS Trialists Group.

Journal Published Lancet Psychiatry.

Year of Publication 2018.

Type of Study Randomized placebo-controlled trial.

Funding Sources The trial was funded by the UK National Institute for Health Research's Health Technology Assessment Programme (reference 09/55/06). Two coauthors were supported by the University College Hospital NIHR Biomedical Research Centre and Medical Research Council.

Objectives This study acknowledges that there were no randomized controlled trials (RCTs) regarding the use of antipsychotic treatment for people with very late-onset schizophrenia-like psychosis (VLOSLP) at the time of publication of this study in 2018. Given this lack of RCT data, this trial focuses on the efficacy and safety of low-dose amisulpride in treating people with VLOSLP who had significant psychotic symptom burden. This study had three aims which are as follows: (1)

W. B. Smith · P. Ureste (✉)
Department of Psychiatry and Behavioral Sciences, University of California San Francisco, San Francisco, CA, USA
e-mail: william.smith2@ucsf.edu; Peter.Ureste@ucsf.edu

R. R. Tampi et al. (eds.), *Essential Reviews in Geriatric Psychiatry*,
https://doi.org/10.1007/978-3-030-94960-0_52

Determine whether 12 weeks of VLOSLP with low-dose amisulpride improves psychiatric symptom scores compared with placebo. (2) Determine whether prolonged treatment of VLOSLP for an additional 12 weeks with amisulpride 100 mg daily has additional benefit when compared with placebo. (3) Assess the side effects and serious adverse events, compliance, and effects on quality of life associated with low-dose amisulpride compared with placebo [1].

Methods This is a three-arm, double-blind, randomized controlled trial with two stages. Participants of the study were recruited from community and inpatient specialist old age psychiatric services with the National Health Service (NHS) in England and Scotland.

Inclusion criteria were as follows: onset of VLOSLP at age 60 or older with meeting criteria as defined by the International Consensus Group Criteria [2], Brief Psychiatric Rating Scale (BPRS) score of 30 or higher, and capacity to give consent to participate in trial. Exclusion criteria were as follows: cognitive impairment defined as Mini-Mental State Examination (MMSE) score of less than 25, diagnosis of an affective disorder, serious physical illness, prescribed amisulpride in 28 days prior to enrollment (other antipsychotic treatment within 28 days prior to enrollment was permissible as long as they met BPRS criteria and there were no contraindications to discontinuation of prior antipsychotic), contraindications to amisulpride, and participation in another clinical trial with an investigational medicinal product in 28 days prior to enrollment.

Participants (n = 101) were randomized into three treatment groups as follows: group (A) amisulpride 100 mg daily for 24 weeks (or 36 if enrolled prior to change in protocol); group (B) amisulpride 100 mg daily for 12 weeks followed by placebo for 12 weeks (or 24 weeks if enrolled prior to change in protocol); and group (C) placebo for 12 weeks followed by amisulpride 100 mg daily for 12 weeks (or 24 weeks if enrolled prior to change in protocol). Randomization was controlled for age, sex, living circumstances, time since onset of symptoms, prior antipsychotic use, and BPRS score severity. Participants were followed by their own clinicians, clinical study officers, and ATLAS trial research nurses who are all masked to group assignments (except statisticians). Participants were provided medications in 28-day blister packs and assessed for outcomes at 4, 12, 24, and 36 weeks (if enrolled prior to protocol change) on a modified intent to treat analysis (as long as they received at least one dose of trial medication).

Primary outcomes were as follows: (1) change in BPRS score from 0 to 12 weeks and between 12 weeks and final assessment (24 or 36 weeks depending on when patient enrolled) and (2) number of patients who withdrew from study due to perceived absence of efficacy. Secondary outcomes were as follows: extrapyramidal symptoms assessed by Simpson Angus Scale, compliance with number who discontinued medication and percentage of medication taken per review of blister packs, quality of life measures per World Health Organization (WHO) Quality of Life Scale and EuroQoL-5D scale, resource usage, and pharmacokinetics in those who consented to optional blood draws.

Results Of the 101 patients that were randomized in the study, 9 patients withdrew from the study prior to starting treatment resulting in 29 and 32 patients in groups A and B, respectively, receiving amisulpride 100 mg daily in stage 1 and 31 patients in group C receiving placebo. Participants had a mean age of 80.2 years, there were predominantly more females than males, and most individuals lived alone. Majority of participants also had symptoms for >6 months and ~50% of participants had prior antipsychotic treatment. The average BPRS score at baseline was 41.3. Notably BPRS scores decreased significantly for both treatment and placebo groups in stage 1 at 4 weeks and 12 weeks with the amisulpride group demonstrating a significantly greater decrease at 4 weeks and 12 weeks with 6.7 point and 7.7 difference, respectively (11.9 point decrease in amisulpride group when compared to 4.2 point decrease in the placebo group at 12 weeks).

In stage 2, at 24 weeks from trial initiation (or 12 weeks of stage 2 treatment), patients in group B who transitioned from amisulpride to placebo treatment had an BPRS increase of 5.2 points, while group A who continued amisulpride treatment had an additional BPRS decrease of 1.1 points. There was a significantly greater improvement in BPRS scores with amisulpride for patients who had taken antipsychotics previously, those with >6 months of symptoms, and those with more severe symptoms at baseline. A total of 67% of participants in amisulpride groups A and B when compared to 58% of participants in placebo group C completed stage 1 of the study; and fewer patients in the amisulpride groups discontinued treatment due to perceived lack of efficacy when compared to placebo ($P = 0.010$) which persisted in stage 2 when comparing those allocated to continue amisulpride versus those who switched to placebo ($P = 0.031$).

The investigators did not find any significant difference between the amisulpride and placebo groups in any of the secondary outcome measures either in stage 1 or stage 2 of the study. They did not identify any significant improvements from baseline on either the EuroQol-5D utility score or the four WHO Quality of Life Scale domains between the two groups.

With regard to adverse effects, the investigators did not find any significant differences in change in Simpson Angus Scale scores between the amisulpride versus placebo groups. Serious adverse effects were more in the amisulpride groups when compared to placebo group but were not statistically significant [stage 1 (10 vs. 1, $P = 0.05$) and stage 2 (9 vs. 6, $P = 0.19$)]. Five patients died during the study, but the deaths were not related to treatment.

Conclusions This study demonstrates that for patients with VLOSLP, the use of amisulpride 100 mg daily is an effective treatment when compared to placebo with a significant change in symptom burden per the standardized BPRS. This builds on prior results of an open label single-arm study with using amisulpride in this population showing significant efficacy [3]. The authors argue that when using a measure of 25% reduction in BPRS score as a worthwhile benefit, the number needed to treat with amisulpride 100 mg daily in this population is three patients. It is notable that the dose of amisulpride used in this study is significantly lower than the standard dose of amisulpride (400–800 mg) used in early-onset schizophrenia which is to be expected given evidence that suggests older adults tend to have higher levels of striatal dopamine receptor occupancy at a given dose compared to younger patients [4]. In regards to secondary outcome measure of impact of treatment on quality of life measures, there were no significant differences between treatment and placebo groups despite significant improvement in BPRS score with amisulpride treatment. The authors argue that this is likely due to poor insight into illness characteristic of this population and thus inability to recognize the impact of symptom burden on their subjective quality of life [5]. Overall, this study shows significant improvement in symptom burden and minimal risks with low-dose amisulpride in patients with VLOSLP when compared to placebo providing clear treatment recommendations for this largely understudied patient population.

Strengths of the Study

1. This is the only randomized controlled trial for the use of an antipsychotic medications in patients with VLOSLP, a population that is difficult to study and for which there remains a relatively dearth of robust evidenced-based treatment recommendations.
2. This study enrolled patients from the community which increases the generalizability of these positive results to the general patient population with VLOSLP.
3. The study provides strong evidence for the benefits of low-dose amisulpride in reducing symptom burden in patients with VLOSLP, a population where antipsychotics are often used at lower rates than their early-onset schizophrenia counterparts [6].

Limitations of the Study

1. Small sample size with only 100 patients randomized into the first stage of the study and only 41 patients entering the second stage of the study. However, it was sufficiently powered to determine a statistically significant difference in reduction of symptoms with amisulpride when compared to placebo.
2. The authors argue that the VLOSLP population commonly have poor insight into their condition and thus makes it challenging to obtain consent from the patient to enroll in this study. Therefore, it is likely that this study represents participants with less severe symptoms of VLOSLP, as those who have more severe symptoms are unlikely to voluntarily enroll in a clinical trial studying the efficacy of antipsychotic treatment.
3. Relatively short duration at 24–36 weeks, which may be premature to determine risk of adverse effects including metabolic syndromes and development of extrapyramidal symptoms, particularly tardive dyskinesia.

Take-Home Points

There is limited evidence currently available for the treatment of VLOSLP, specifically guidance on antipsychotic selection and dosing. The ATLAS study is the first and only double-blind randomized controlled trial for the treatment of this patient population. This study demonstrates that treatment with low-dose amisulpride (100 mg daily) is effective in significantly reducing symptoms related to VLOSLP when compared to placebo. There were no significant differences in adherence and adverse reactions including extrapyramidal symptoms (EPS) between amisulpride and placebo groups. This study is limited by a small sample size of 100 participants; however, the data remain statistically significant for the aforementioned findings.

Practical Applications of the Take-Home Point

Low-dose amisulpride (100 mg daily) is effective in treating symptoms of VLOSLP with minimal adverse drug reactions. This is the only RCT evidenced-based treatment available to date supporting any form of treatment for patients with VLOSLP. This study encourages the use of amisulpride in patients with VLOSLP and may motivate future studies for the use of psychopharmacological treatments in this patient population.

References

1. Howard R, Cort E, Bradley R, Harper E, Kelly L, Bentham P, Ritchie C, Reeves S, Fawzi W, Livingston G, Sommerlad A, Oomman S, Nazir E, Nilforooshan R, Barber R, Fox C, Macharouthu AV, Ramachandra P, Pattan V, Sykes J, Curran V, Katona C, Dening T, Knapp M, Gray R, ATLAS Trialists Group. Antipsychotic treatment of very late-onset schizophrenia-like psychosis (ATLAS): a randomised, controlled, double-blind trial. Lancet. Psychiatry. 2018;5(7):553–63.
2. Howard R, Rabins PV, Seeman MV, Jeste DV. Late-onset schizophrenia and very-late-onset schizophrenia-like psychosis: an international consensus. The International Late-Onset Schizophrenia Group. Am J Psychiatry. 2000;157(2):172–8.
3. Psarros C, Theleritis CG, Paparrigopoulos TJ, Politis AM, Papadimitriou GN. Amisulpride for the treatment of very-late-onset schizophrenia-like psychosis. Int J Geriatr Psychiatry. 2009;24(5):518–22.
4. Reeves S, McLachlan E, Bertrand J, D'Antonio F, Brownings S, Nair A, Greaves S, Smith A, Taylor D, Dunn J, Marsden P, Kessler R, Howard R. Therapeutic window of dopamine D2/3 receptor occupancy to treat psychosis in Alzheimer's disease. Brain. 2017;140(4):1117–27.
5. Almeida O, Levy R, Howard R, David A. Insight and paranoid disorders in late life (late paraphrenia). Int J Geriatr Psychiatry. 1996;11:653–8.
6. Sin Fai Lam CC, Reeves SJ, Stewart R, Howard R. Service and treatment engagement of people with very late-onset schizophrenia-like psychosis. BJPsych Bull. 2016;40(4):185–6.

Part X
Neurocognitive Disorders

Chapter 53
Efficacy and Safety of Cholinesterase Inhibitors in Alzheimer's Disease: A Meta-analysis

Chadrick E. Lane and Michelle L. Conroy

Authors of the Original Article Krista L. Lanctôt, Nathan Herrmann, Kenneth K. Yau, Lyla R. Khan, Barbara A. Liu, Maysoon M. LouLou, Thomas R. Einarson.

Journal Published Canadian Medical Association Journal.

Year of Publication 2003.

Type of Study Meta-analysis.

Funding Sources None reported.

Objectives To quantify the efficacy and safety of ChEIs in the treatment of AD [1].

Methods The authors searched MEDLINE, EMBASE, and Cochrane databases, ranging from 1980 to 2002, using cholinesterase inhibitor and Alzheimer as keywords, along with randomized controlled trials, English, and human being applied as limits. Additional searches for individual ChEIs were performed. They also searched references and bibliographies of recent review articles and published reports of clinical trials for additional studies. The study population was comprised of those clinically diagnosed with AD using either criteria set forth by the *Diagnostic*

C. E. Lane (✉)
Peter O'Donnell Jr. Brain Institute, Department of Psychiatry, UT Southwestern Medical Center, Dallas, TX, USA
e-mail: Chadrick.lane@utsouthwestern.edu

M. L. Conroy
Yale University School of Medicine, New Haven, CT, USA

VA Connecticut Healthcare System, West Haven, CT, USA
e-mail: Michelle.l.conroy@yale.edu

R. R. Tampi et al. (eds.), *Essential Reviews in Geriatric Psychiatry*,
https://doi.org/10.1007/978-3-030-94960-0_53

and Statistical Manual of Mental Disorders, fourth edition (DSM-IV), or the National Institute of Neurological and Communicative Disorders and Stroke and the Alzheimer's Disease and Related Disorders Association (NINCDS-ADRDA). Only those publications that were original research and utilizing randomized, double-blind, placebo-controlled, and parallel-group trial designs were included in the analysis. Only original research with therapeutic treatment periods of at least 12 weeks were included. The raters were blinded to potentially biasing details of each study, including authors' names, author institute, and publication date. Identified studies were then rated using the Jadad scale in an effort to characterize the quality of the trial.

The raters divided subjects into categories assessing treatment response versus no response, adverse events, discontinuation of treatment for any reason, and terminating participation due to adverse effects. The study authors used a random-effects meta-analytic model for the statistical analysis. The outcomes of interest included global response, using either the Clinical Global Impression of Change [CGIC] or Clinician Interview-Based Impression of change plus caregiver input [CIBIC+] scales, cognitive response, defined as those with at least a four-point improvement on the Alzheimer's Disease Assessment Scale-cognitive portion (ADAS-cog), as well as adverse effect reports and dropouts. All proportions were calculated using an intention-to-treat approach. The number needed to treat (NNT) and to harm (NNH) were reported. Lastly, the authors conducted sub-analyses on the impact of ethnicity, dose, specific drug, treatment duration, and the CGIC degree of change.

Results After initially identifying 40 articles, 24 were excluded for varying reasons. The resultant 16 studies were considered high enough quality for inclusion (Jadad score greater than 3, with a median score of 5), with 5159 subjects receiving active treatment and 2795 receiving placebo.

Of the 16 studies, 9 provided data for calculating differences in global response, and 5 studies for differences in cognitive response. After pooling data, the proportion of global responders receiving ChEIs exceeding that for placebo was 9% (95% confidence interval (CI), 6–12%). For cognitive response, the excess in favor for ChEIs over placebo reached 10% (95% CI, 4–17%). This latter number increased to 14% (95% CI, 8–18%) when a single study using high- and low-dose rivastigmine was excluded, resulting in the cognitive response studies no longer being heterogeneous.

In regard to safety, 14 studies provided relevant data. Those receiving ChEIs experienced higher rates of adverse effects, dropout due to any cause, and dropout due to adverse effects specifically, with the mean difference in proportion being 8% (95% CI, 5–12%), 8% (95% CI, 5–11%), and 7% (95% CI, 3–10%), respectively. It is important to note that there was statically significant heterogeneity among these 14 studies. The most common adverse effects were gastrointestinal in nature, and there were no treatment-related deaths.

The NNT for cognitive response was 10 (95% CI, 8–15%), which, again, translated to at least a four-point improvement on the ADAS-cog subscale. Relating to global response, the NNT was 7 (95% CI, 6–9%) for stabilization or better, 12 (95% CI, 9–16%) for minimal improvement or better, and 42 (95% CI, 26–114%) for marked improvement.

This meta-analysis incorporated sub-analyses by drug, by dose, by treatment duration, and by the strictness of CGIC definition. The highlights of the drug sub-analysis were as follows: (1) Excess pooled mean proportions for global response were 13% (95% CI, 8–17%) with donepezil, 5% (95% CI, 1–8%) with galantamine, and 12% (95% CI, 5–19%) in the single rivastigmine study; (2) excess pooled mean proportions for dropout were 3% (95% CI, 1–6%) with donepezil, 14% (95% CI, 8–21%) with galantamine, and 9% (95% CI, 5–12%) with rivastigmine; and (3) analysis by dose revealed excess pooled mean proportions for global response of 8% (95% CI, 5–12%) with lower doses and 11% (95% CI, 7–15%) with higher doses, both statistically significant when compared to placebo.

In regard to treatment duration, the excess pooled mean proportion of global responders was 11% (95% CI, 5–16%) with shorter-term treatment (duration of 12–14 weeks) and 9% (95% CI, 5–12%) with longer-term treatment (duration of 24–52 weeks). With increasingly strict definitions for the CGIC measured degree of improvement, the excess pooled mean proportion reached 15% (95% CI, 11–18%) for stability or better, 9% (95% CI, 6–12%) for any improvement, and 2% (95% CI, 1–4%) for more than minimal improvement.

Of note, one study included in this meta-analysis, published by Homma et al., revealed a large effect of low-dose donepezil in a primarily Japanese population [2]. This finding may suggest treatment response differences relating to population genetics.

Conclusions ChEIs can result in statistically significant global and cognitive improvement when compared to placebo in the treatment of AD, and they appear to be fairly well tolerated.

Strengths of the Study

1. This is a meta-analysis of studies utilizing randomized, double-blind, placebo-controlled, parallel-group trial.
2. All of the included studies were rated as having a Jadad quality score of greater than 3 with a median score of 5 [3].
3. The authors calculated proportions using intention-to-treat populations.
4. The primary analysis emphasized clinical global response, highlighting this as a potentially more meaningful outcome.

Limitations of the Study

1. Given negative studies are rarely published, any meta-analysis can be impacted by publication bias.
2. Only 9 of 16 studies contained data for the global response proportions; 5 of 16 studies were useful for calculating the cognitive response proportions.
3. Findings in both the primary analyses and subgroup analyses contained degrees of heterogeneity among the component studies.

4. While this study did consider long-term treatment, the upper limit of this window was 52 weeks. ChEIs may continue to differentiate from placebo with treatment even beyond 52 weeks.
5. This meta-analysis does not use studies with possibly more meaningful outcome measures, e.g., time to institutionalization and assessment of functional abilities.
6. Subjects were diagnosed with AD based on clinical criteria established by either the DSM-IV or the NINCDS-ADRDA. It is now known that the sensitivity and specificity of this diagnostic method is far from perfect; biomarker supported Alzheimer's disease, e.g., molecular imaging and/or CSF analyses, would allow for a more diagnostically homogenous study sample.

Take-Home Points

Despite some limitations, this high-quality meta-analysis indicates ChEIs are fairly well tolerated and, in the treatment of those with the clinical syndrome of AD, afford modest but statistically significant global and cognitive benefits. The NNT for benefit is relatively small and comparable to the NNTs for medications used in other neuropsychiatric diseases, e.g., schizophrenia and depression.

Practical Applications of the Take-Home Point

ChEIs provide modest benefits for patients living with AD and, while usually well tolerated, are associated with modest increases in adverse effects. Any decision to use this class of medications should be a shared process between clinician, patient, and, if applicable, a surrogate decision-maker.

References

1. Lanctôt KL, Herrmann N, Yau KK, Khan LR, Liu BA, LouLou MM, Einarson TR. Efficacy and safety of cholinesterase inhibitors in Alzheimer's disease: a meta-analysis. CMAJ. 2003;169(6):557–64.
2. Homma A, Takeda M, Imai Y, Udaka F, Hasegawa K, Kameyama M, Nishimura T. Clinical efficacy and safety of donepezil on cognitive and global function in patients with Alzheimer's disease. A 24-week, multicenter, double-blind, placebo-controlled study in Japan. E2020 Study Group. Dement Geriatr Cogn Disord. 2000;11(6):299–313.
3. Jadad AR, Moore RA, Carroll D, Jenkinson C, Reynolds DJ, Gavaghan DJ, McQuay HJ. Assessing the quality of reports of randomized clinical trials: is blinding necessary? Control Clin Trials. 1996;17(1):1–12.

Chapter 54
Depression and Risk for Alzheimer's Disease: Systematic Review, Meta-analysis, and Metaregression Analysis

Emily B. Phelps and Sandra Swantek

Authors of the Original Article Raymond L Ownby, Elizabeth Crocco, Amarilis Acevedo, Vineeth John, David Loewenstein.

Journal Published Archives of General Psychiatry.

Year of Publication 2006.

Type of Study Systematic review, meta-analysis and metaregression analysis.

Funding Sources Grant K23 AG 19745 from the National Institute on Aging.

Objectives The study's primary aim was to systematically review and complete a meta-analysis on the connectedness of a history of depression and subsequent Alzheimer's disease (AD). A secondary aim was to assess the interval between depression and AD diagnosis on observed risk for AD. The latter aim addresses the understanding of depression as either a risk factor for AD or a prodrome of it [1].

Methods Three reviewers conducted bibliographic searches of MEDLINE, PsychLit, EMBASE, and BIOSIS, emphasizing risks of depression and AD. Of the 153 identified studies, 20 met the inclusion criteria, including categorical diagnoses of depression and AD, the inclusion of a control group, and the exclusion of other types of dementia. Essential factors in study selection included data that permitted

E. B. Phelps
Mount Sinai Hospital, New York, NY, USA
e-mail: Emily.Phelps@mountsinai.edu

S. Swantek (✉)
Rush Medical College, Chicago, IL, USA
e-mail: Sandra_Swantek@Rush.edu

R. R. Tampi et al. (eds.), *Essential Reviews in Geriatric Psychiatry*,
https://doi.org/10.1007/978-3-030-94960-0_54

calculation of an odds ratio and an explicit description of diagnostic criteria. The authors assessed the quality of observational studies using the Newcastle-Ottawa Scale (such as completeness of follow-up, selection criteria, and comparability of patient groups). A funnel plot comparing studies' standard errors to effect sizes was used to assess sample publication bias. The authors conducted a separate random effects metaregression analysis for the interval between the diagnoses of depression and AD. These 20 studies comprised a sample of 102,172 people across 8 countries, with considerable heterogeneity among studies.

Results The odds ratios (OR) were stratified by study type for AD diagnosis in persons with a history of depression. The OR for case-control studies was 2.03 ($P < 0.001$) and for cohort studies, 1.9 ($P < 0.001$). Including all study types, the overall OR was 2.02 ($P < 0.001$). For cohort studies, prospective designs demonstrated an OR of 1.78 ($P = 0.008$); the decreased significance may be due to the inclusion of persons with a history of depression in one study's control group. By contrast, retrospective studies yielded an OR of 2.11 ($P < 0.001$).

When considering the clarity of diagnostic criteria, the OR was most robust for studies using explicit diagnostic criteria for both depression and AD (OR = 2.3, $P < 0.001$) compared to those for just depression (OR = 2.23, $P < 0.001$) or just AD (OR = 1.91, $P < 0.001$).

The examination of quality metrics demonstrated the greatest odds ratio strength. The OR for case-control studies after Newcastle-Ottawa Scale correction for quality was 4.14 ($P = 0.3$). The OR for cohort-control after Newcastle-Ottawa Scale correction for quality was 3.85 ($P = 0.001$).

Publication bias appeared to be present but did not significantly alter odds ratio calculations across study design (OR = 1.96, $P < 0.001$) for case-control and (OR = 1.90, $P < 0.001$) for cohort-control studies.

For the 13 studies providing interval data, metaregression of the log OR on the interval in years showed a linear, positive correlation between interval time and subsequent risk of developing AD (coefficient = 0.003, $P = 0.05$). This finding persisted after the correction of retrospective or prospective design.

Conclusions Across study types, a history of depression positively correlated with later development of AD, and the strength of this association increased with the interval time between depression and AD. As such, depression may be a distinct and modifiable risk factor for AD instead of merely a prodrome of AD.

Strengths of the Study

1. This review is the most comprehensive systematic analysis for its publication date while accounting for varied psychiatric history.
2. This review demonstrates the most robust effect size when controlling for study quality metrics per Newcastle-Ottawa criteria. Odds ratios (OR) remain significant across study design (case-control versus cohort and prospective versus retrospective).

3. Effects are most substantial among case-control, retrospective studies with strict diagnostic criteria for both depression and AD.
4. The authors examined publication bias and found that despite the potential of publication bias to exclude small studies, additional analyses suggest that small studies' omission did not significantly affect the pooled odds ratios.
5. Though analyses demonstrated heterogeneity across studies, all but one of the studies found an increased risk for developing AD in persons with a history of depression. Authors postulate that previous studies' negative findings may be attributed to a lack of significance when a nonsignificant increase in AD risk exists.
6. These studies are graded using the Newcastle-Ottawa scale for case-control studies and cohort-control studies below. These scores suggest that a majority of studies had a representative sample and adequately defined controls. For cohort studies, metrics indicated that most studies had representative samples, adequate case definitions, and appropriate controls (Tables 54.1 and 54.2).

Limitations

1. While including varying severities and occurrences of depressive episodes, the studies rely on distinct categorical diagnoses of depression and AD. In calculating odds ratios, the authors did not consider continuous variables such as the number of symptoms, duration of episodes, or cognitive function measures. Of the four cases describing diagnostic criteria for case definition and controls, the authors used DSM-IV and the NINCDS-ADRDA criteria to diagnose AD.
2. Based on the Newcastle-Ottawa scores above, case-control studies were most lacking in the assessment of AD and depression (medical records versus structured interviews) as well as controls. None of the studies describe a nonrespondent rate.

Table 54.1 Newcastle-Ottawa Scale for case-control studies ($N = 9$)

Domain	Description	Score (1 or 0)
Selection		
Is the case definition adequate?	Yes, with independent validation	4/9
Representativeness of the cases	Representative series of cases	7/9
Selection of controls	Structured interview	4/9
Definition of controls	No history of disease	7/9
Comparability		
Studies control for (most important factor; an additional factor)	Age, sex	7/9; 7/9
Exposure		
Assessment of exposure	Medical records	3/9
Same method of ascertainment for cases and controls	Yes, although sites for cases and controls varied in some studies	6/9
Nonresponse rate		0/9

Wells et al. [2]

Table 54.2 Newcastle-Ottawa Scale for cohort studies ($N = 11$)

Domain	Description	Score (1 or 0)
Selection		
Representativeness of the exposed cohort	No description of the derivations of the cohort	9/11
Selection of the nonexposed cohort	No description of the derivation of the nonexposed cohort	10/11
Ascertainment of exposure	Structured interview	7/11
Demonstration that the outcome of interest was not present at start of study	Yes	11/11
Comparability		
Studies control for (most important factor; an additional factor)	Age, sex	8/11; 8/11
Outcome		
Assessment of outcome	Record linkage	6/11
Was follow-up long enough for outcomes to occur?	Yes	8/11
Subjects lost to follow-up unlikely to introduce bias; small number lost; > % (select an adequate %) follow-up	60%	10/11

Wells et al. [2]

However, this metrics' applicability is unclear (subject attrition due to death, loss of follow-up). For cohort studies, data were lacking primarily in the assessment of AD as an outcome.

3. Missing demographic data limit the review's external validity and insight into the target population for interventions to mitigate depression as a risk factor for AD. Population-based studies with more robust controls may suggest underlying risk factors such as race, socioeconomic status, or geographic location.

Take-Home Points

Depression is a distinct and significant risk factor for AD, but depression is not excluded as a prodrome of AD.

Practical Application of the Take Home Points

Given the possible pathophysiology connecting depression and AD, depression may be considered a modifiable risk factor for AD. In the interest of prevention, clinicians must monitor for a history of depression in older adults when assessing risk factors for AD, even if this history is remote.

References

1. Ownby RL, Crocco E, Acevedo A, John V, Loewenstein D. Depression and risk for Alzheimer disease: systematic review, meta-analysis, and metaregression analysis. Arch Gen Psychiatry. 2006;63(5):530–8.
2. Wells GA, Shea B, O'Connell D, Peterson J, Welch V, Losos M, Tugwell P. The Newcastle-Ottawa Scale (NOS) for assessing the quality of nonrandomised studies in meta-analyses 2000. https://web.archive.org/web/20210716121605id_/http://www3.med.unipmn.it/dispense_ebm/2009-2010/Corso%20Perfezionamento%20EBM_Faggiano/NOS_oxford.pdf. Accessed on 17 Feb 2022.

Chapter 55
Effectiveness of Atypical Antipsychotic Drugs in Patients with Alzheimer's Disease

Emily B. Phelps and Sandra Swantek

Authors of the Original Article Lon S Schneider, Pierre N Tariot, Karen S Dagerman, Sonia M Davis, John K Hsiao, M Saleem Ismail, Barry D Lebowitz, Constantine G Lyketsos, J Michael Ryan, T Scott Stroup, David L Sultzer, Daniel Weintraub, Jeffrey A Lieberman, CATIE-AD Study Group.

Journal Published *New England Journal of Medicine.*

Year of Publication 2006.

Type of Study Randomized controlled trial.

Funding Sources Grant (NO1 MH9001) from the NIMH. AstraZeneca Pharmaceuticals, Forest Pharmaceuticals, Janssen Pharmaceuticals, and Eli Lilly provided medications for the studies.

Objectives This study assesses the effectiveness of atypical antipsychotic drugs in outpatients with Alzheimer's disease [1].

Methods In phase I of this study, individuals were randomly assigned under double-blind conditions to receive olanzapine, quetiapine, risperidone, or placebo in a 2:2:2:3 ratio. The doses of medications were adjusted as clinically indicated by study physicians. If the physicians judged that the individual's response was

E. B. Phelps
Mount Sinai Hospital, New York, NY, USA
e-mail: Emily.Phelps@mountsinai.edu

S. Swantek (✉)
Rush Medical College, Chicago, IL, USA
e-mail: Sandra_Swantek@Rush.edu

R. R. Tampi et al. (eds.), *Essential Reviews in Geriatric Psychiatry*,
https://doi.org/10.1007/978-3-030-94960-0_55

not adequate at any time after the first 2 weeks, then the treatment could be discontinued. Individuals with an adequate response continued treatment for up to 36 weeks.

To be eligible for the study, the participants had to meet the criteria for dementia of the Alzheimer's type according to the Diagnostic and Statistical Manual of Mental Disorders, fourth edition, or probable Alzheimer's disease on the basis of the history, physical examination, and results of structural brain imaging. They also should have a score on the Mini-Mental State Examination (MMSE) between 5 and 26. In addition, individuals had to be ambulatory and living at home or in an assisted living facility. Furthermore, eligible individuals should also have delusions, hallucinations, aggression, or agitation that developed after the onset of dementia severe enough to disrupt their functioning, and in the opinion of the study physicians, there was justification to treatment with antipsychotic drugs.

Exclusion criteria included a diagnosis of a primary psychotic disorder (e.g., schizophrenia), delirium, other dementia such as vascular dementia or Lewy body dementia or psychosis, agitation, or aggression that could be better accounted for by another medical condition, medication, or substance abuse. In addition, participants could be excluded if they required psychiatric admission, were suicidal, were going to receive treatment with a cholinesterase inhibitor or antidepressant medication, had previously been treated with two of the three atypical antipsychotic drugs under study, or had contraindications to any of the study drugs.

The design of the trial encouraged prescribing based on clinical practice while maintaining the randomized and double-blind treatment assignment. The starting doses of medications and the dose adjustments were based on the study physician's clinical judgment and the participant's responses. Medications were dispensed at each visit in the form of identically appearing small and large capsules containing lower and higher doses of olanzapine (2.5 mg or 5.0 mg), quetiapine (25 mg or 50 mg), risperidone (0.5 mg or 1.0 mg), or placebo.

The primary outcome measure was the time until discontinuation of treatment for any reason. The main secondary outcome measure was the attainment of minimal or greater improvement on the Clinical Global Impression of Change (CGIC) scale at week 12 while the participants continued to receive the phase I drug. The other secondary outcomes were the time to the discontinuation of treatment in phase I because of lack of efficacy and the time to the discontinuation of treatment because of adverse events, intolerability, or death. The safety of the drugs was assessed reviewing the information about the occurrence of adverse events. In addition, the participant's weight and levels of prolactin, glucose, cholesterol, and triglyceride levels were measured at weeks 12, 24, and 36.

Results From a total of 521 individuals who were screened, 421 underwent randomization and received at least 1 dose of medication. The last prescribed mean doses of medications in phase I were 5.5 mg of olanzapine per day, 56.5 mg of quetiapine per day, and 1.0 mg of risperidone per day. During the 36-week follow-up period, 82% of participants discontinued their initially assigned medication.

There were no significant differences in the time to treatment discontinuation for any reason: olanzapine (median, 8.1 weeks), risperidone (median, 7.4 weeks), quetiapine (median, 5.3 weeks), and placebo (median, 8.0 weeks) ($P = 0.52$).

The median time for discontinuing treatment due to lack of efficacy favored risperidone (26.7 weeks) and olanzapine (22.1 weeks) over quetiapine (9.1 weeks) and placebo (9.0 weeks). The hazard ratio (HR) for the discontinuation of treatment because of lack of efficacy was 0.51 ($P < 0.001$) for olanzapine when compared with placebo and 0.61 ($P = 0.01$) for risperidone when compared to placebo. For the discontinuation of treatment, olanzapine and risperidone were found to be equivalent to each other (HR = 0.84). Olanzapine was significantly superior to quetiapine (HR = 0.63, $P = 0.02$).

The time to discontinuation of treatment owing to intolerance of the study drug, adverse effects, or death favored placebo when compared to the three drugs. The discontinuation rates among individuals receiving drugs were as follows: olanzapine (24%), quetiapine (16%), and risperidone (18%) when compared to placebo (5%). All individuals who received an atypical antipsychotic drug were significantly more likely to discontinue treatment when compared to those who received placebo: olanzapine (HR = 4.32), quetiapine, (HR = 3.58), and risperidone (HR = 3.62).

At 12 weeks, a CGIC score indicating at least minimal improvement with continued use of the phase I study medication was 32% for the olanzapine group, 26% for the quetiapine group, 29% for the risperidone group, and 21% in the placebo group, with these rates being not significantly different between the groups ($P = 0.22$).

The proportion of participants who had at least one serious adverse event and the proportion of individuals who had any adverse event were no different among the groups. Greater rates of parkinsonism or extrapyramidal signs were noted in the olanzapine and risperidone groups (12% in each) when compared to the quetiapine group (2%) or the placebo group (1%). Sedation occurred more commonly with the three drugs (15–24%) when compared to placebo (5%). Confusion or changes in mental status occurred more commonly with the olanzapine (18%) and risperidone groups (11%) when compared to the placebo group (5%). The body weight and body mass index (BMI) of participants increased with the three antipsychotic drugs (by 0.4–1.0 lb) per month and 0.2 BMI unit, whereas it decreased in the placebo group (by −0.9 lb) per month and −0.2 BMI unit. Prolactin levels at week 12 were markedly elevated in the risperidone group only.

Conclusions Adverse effects offset advantages in the efficacy of atypical antipsychotic drugs for the treatment of psychosis, aggression, or agitation in patients with Alzheimer's disease.

Strengths of the Study

1. This study adheres to a placebo-controlled, double-blind, randomized controlled trial methodology with a large number of subjects across numerous sites.
2. The Jadad scale [2] used to assess the quality of a randomized controlled trial indicates that this was a well-conducted study.

Jadad scale for reporting randomized controlled trials			
Metric	Maximum score	Description	Score
Randomization	2	One point if randomization is mentioned One point if the randomization is appropriate	2
Blinding	2	One point if blinding is mentioned One additional point if the method of blinding is appropriate	2
An account of all patients	1	The fate of all patients in the trial is known. Missing data is explained	1

Jadad et al. [2]

3. The study design addresses the longitudinal outcomes of antipsychotic use in Alzheimer's disease patients [3].
4. Study physicians quickly discontinued drugs demonstrating little clinical benefit; about half of patients were discontinued or switched to another therapy within 8 weeks.
5. The study team used the time to discontinuation as a proxy for drug suitability to match the nuance of weighing efficacy versus adverse outcomes. Interestingly, time to discontinuation due to adverse effects did not match the rate of adverse effects, suggesting individual factors in clinical decision-making.

Limitations

1. While time to ending a drug trial reflects therapeutic choices, the opportunity to progress into phase II and an alternative study drug may have prompted early discontinuation in some cases.
2. Study participants frequently stopped their assigned drug (82%). This figure likely overestimates real-world clinical practice, where clinical decision-making includes medical history, polypharmacy, adverse effects, and access to care.
3. As assessed by the Clinical Global Impression of Change (CGIC), the clinical improvement is scarcely discussed while tolerating "minimal improvement" as a binary clinical marker to justify the therapeutic response. The multitude of scores (MMSE, frequency of episodes) used to justify inclusion criteria could have been applied to clinical outcomes and continuously stratified. However, the CGIC does offer a simple measure with ease of utility across each of 42 sites.
4. Similarly, lacking definitions of clinical improvement also reflect inherent gaps in internal validity. The inclusion criteria of agitation, aggression, and psychosis comprise distinct pathophysiology, with little discussion of diagnostic specifications. While outcomes were stratified based on MMSE, a lower MMSE score may confound a presentation of agitation and the inclusion criteria of episode frequency (daily or intermittently).
5. Study groups did not differ significantly in demographic or clinical variables, but racial diversity was lacking (79–81% white). Representation across race is exceedingly critical, given known barriers to care. Study participants' level of care may confound this discrepancy, primarily nursing home and assisted living facilities, while family caregiving only accounts for 5.2 h per day. Study settings

may underestimate the time to discontinuation due to inadequate access to care outside study settings.

6. The authors acknowledge a discrepancy in administered doses of quetiapine. The average quetiapine dose administered (57.0 mg) was a quarter to a half of the standard therapeutic dose, perhaps underestimating the rate of adverse effects and overestimating the weeks to reach efficacy.

Take-Home Points

1. Using time to discontinuation as a proxy for therapeutic benefit suggests that the three atypical antipsychotics in this study are equivalent in efficacy and tolerability.
2. The clinical utility of second-generation antipsychotics depends on the successful management of adverse effects and optimization of tolerability.

Practical Application of the Take-Home Points

When selecting second-generation antipsychotic agents for the treatment of psychosis, aggression, or agitation in patients with Alzheimer's disease, consider the medical history, medication list, and vulnerability to adverse outcomes.

References

1. Schneider LS, Tariot PN, Dagerman KS, Davis SM, Hsiao JK, Ismail MS, Lebowitz BD, Lyketsos CG, Ryan JM, Stroup TS, Sultzer DL, Weintraub D, Lieberman JA. CATIE-AD Study Group. Effectiveness of atypical antipsychotic drugs in patients with Alzheimer's disease. N Engl J Med. 2006;355(15):1525–38.
2. Jadad AR, Moore RA, Carroll D, Jenkinson C, Reynolds DJM, Gavaghan DJ, McQuay HJ. Assessing the quality of reports of randomized clinical trials: is blinding necessary? Control Clin Trials. 1996;17(1):1–12. ISSN 0197-2456. https://doi.org/10.1016/0197-2456(95)00134-4.
3. Schneider LS, Olin JT, Doody RS, Clark CM, Morris JC, Reisberg B, Ferris SH, Schmitt FA, Grundman M, Thomas RG. Validity and reliability of the Alzheimer's Disease Cooperative Study-Clinical global impression of change (ADCS-CGIC). In: Becker RE, Giacobini E, Barton JM, Brown M, editors. Alzheimer disease. Advances in Alzheimer disease therapy. Boston: Birkhäuser; 1997. p. 425–9.

Chapter 56
Predictors of Progression from Mild Cognitive Impairment to Alzheimer's Disease

Sarah Kim and Tracey Holsinger

Authors of the Original Article K Palmer, A K Berger, R Monastero, B Winblad, L Bäckman, L Fratiglioni.

Journal Published *Neurology.*

Year of Publication 2007.

Type of Study Prospective cohort study.

Funding Sources The Swedish Council for Working Life and Social Research (FAS), the Swedish Alzheimer Association (Alzheimerfonden), the Max Planck International Research Network on Aging (MaxnetAging), Gamla Tjanarinnor, the Loo and Hans Osterman Foundation, the Gun and Bertil Stohnes Foundation, and the Eurogendis Marie-Curie Programme (scholarship to R Monastero).

Objective to determine the occurrence of neuropsychiatric symptomatology and the relationship to future development of Alzheimer's disease in persons with and without mild cognitive impairment [1].

Methods Participants of this study were taken from the Kungsholmen Project, a longitudinal study initiated in 1987 which assessed the occurrence, risk factors, and

S. Kim
Duke University Department of Psychiatry and Behavioral Sciences, Durham, NC, USA
e-mail: kyung.kim@duke.edu

T. Holsinger (✉)
Duke University Department of Psychiatry and Behavioral Sciences, Durham, NC, USA

Durham VA Medical Center, Durham, NC, USA
e-mail: Tracey.holsinger@duke.edu

R. R. Tampi et al. (eds.), *Essential Reviews in Geriatric Psychiatry*,
https://doi.org/10.1007/978-3-030-94960-0_56

evolution of dementia in individuals aged 75 years and above living in the Kungsholmen area of Stockholm, Sweden. A sample of 668 individuals who had gone through a battery of clinical assessment including a psychiatric and neurologic examination as well as neuropsychological testing were considered for this analysis.

Of the sample, 225 individuals were excluded because they met the diagnostic criteria of dementia according to Diagnostic and Statistical Manual of Mental Disorders (DSM) III-R. Another 40 individuals were excluded for scoring less than 20 on the Mini-Mental State Examination (MMSE), unknown educational level, or age over 95 years. Of the remaining, 296 individuals underwent neuropsychological testing. Sixty-four did not fulfill the criteria for amnestic or multi-domain MCI, but also did not display a normal level of cognitive functioning. Finally, a total of 232 participants (47 individuals with MCI, either amnestic or multi-domain, and 185 individuals with normal cognitive functioning) were included in this study.

For the assessment of neuropsychiatric symptoms on the 232 participants, the investigators used the Comprehensive Psychopathological Rating Scale (CPRS) [2]. This is an inventory of 40 self-reported items and 27 observed items largely surveying anxiety, depression, and paranoia symptoms on a scale from 0 to 3. The investigators in this study incorporated elements from CPRS pertinent to three categories: mood, motivation, and anxiety. They also rated each symptom on a six-point scale, with the score of 2–6 indicating a severe symptomology. Mood symptoms included dysphoria, suicidal ideation/thoughts of death, feelings of guilt, and appetite disturbances. Motivation symptoms included a lack of interest, concentration difficulties, psychomotor disturbances, and loss of energy. Anxiety symptoms included indecision, persistent worrying, anxiety, and social withdrawal.

The participants underwent neuropsychological testing assessing three specific domains: episodic memory (various word recall tasks), language fluency (category fluency for grocery items), and visuospatial functioning (block design, clock reading, and clock setting). The MCI cohort of 47 participants were divided into MCI-amnestic (impairment in episodic memory but normal functioning on language and visuospatial tasks) and MCI-multi-domain (impairment in two or more areas of the episodic memory, language, and visuospatial domains).

Subjects were reassessed 3.4 years (SD 0.6) after baseline. Nineteen subjects dropped out, and 33 subjects had died. The remaining subjects underwent a clinical examination where the dementia diagnosis was made according to DSM III-R using a three-step procedure [3]. A preliminary diagnosis was made by the examining physician and then independently reviewed by a specialist. In case of disagreement between the examining physician and the specialist, a third specialist made the final diagnosis.

Results The mean age of the study population was 84 years (SD = 5.1), 84.9% ($n = 197$) were females, and 39.2% ($n = 91$) had high education (≥8 years). Logistic regression models and chi-squared tests were used to assess differences in the neuropsychiatric symptoms between subjects with MCI and subjects without cognitive impairment, adjusting for age, sex, and education. Of the study population, 185 subjects had normal cognitive function, 17 subjects had MCI-amnestic, and 30 subjects had MCI-multi-domain at baseline.

At baseline, mood symptoms were present in 18.4% (*n* = 34) of normal subjects and 36.2% (*n* = 17) of subjects with MCI all types (35.3% in MCI-amnestic, 36.7% in MCI-multi-domains). The odds ratio (OR) of mood symptoms in MCI all types was 2.5 (95% CI, 1.2–5.0), MCI-amnestic OR was 2.3 (95% CI, 0.8–6.8), and MCI-multi-domains OR was 2.5 (95% CI, 1.1–5.7). Anxiety symptoms were present in 24.9% (*n* = 46) of normal subjects and 46.8% (*n* = 22) of subjects with MCI all types (41.2% in MCI-amnestic, 50.0% in MCI-multi-domains). The OR of anxiety symptoms in MCI all types was 2.5 (95% CI, 1.3–5.2), MCI-amnestic OR was 2.1 (95% CI, 0.7–6.0), and MCI-multi-domains OR was 2.9 (95% CI, 1.3–6.7). Motivation symptoms were present in 13.0% (*n* = 24) of normal subjects and 36.2% (*n* = 17) of subjects with MCI all types (35.3% in MCI-amnestic, 36.7% in MCI-multi-domains). The OR of motivation symptoms in MCI all types was 3.8 (95% CI, 1.8–8.0), MCI-amnestic OR was 3.9 (95% CI, 1.3–11.9), and MCI-multi-domains OR was 3.8 (95% CI, 1.6–9.0).

At 3-year follow-up, 77.1% (*n* = 131) of cognitively normal subjects were alive without dementia; 12.9% (*n* = 22) were dead without dementia; 5.9% (*n* = 10) had been diagnosed with Alzheimer's disease (AD) and 4.1% (*n* = 7) with other dementias. For the subjects with baseline MCI, 18.6% (*n* = 8) were alive without dementia; 18.6% (*n* = 8) were dead without dementia. A total of 56.2% (*n* = 24) had been diagnosed with AD and 7.0% (*n* = 3) with other dementias. The relative risk (RR) for each neuropsychiatric symptom was assessed for progression to AD in subjects with MCI and in subjects with no cognitive impairment at baseline. There was no statistically significant increased risk for mood symptoms increasing progression from MCI to AD (RR = 0.9 [95% CI, 0.6–1.5]). Anxiety symptoms almost doubled the risk of progression to AD in subjects with MCI (RR = 1.8 [95% CI, 1.2–2.7]). Motivation symptoms did not show statistically significant increased risk of progression to AD in MCI subjects (RR = 1.1 [95% CI, 0.7–1.8]). For cognitively normal subjects, there was increased risk of developing AD when mood symptoms were present at baseline (RR = 1.9 [95% CI, 1.0–3.6]). Motivation symptoms at baseline also increased risk (RR = 1.9 [95% CI, 0.5–7.4]), but baseline anxiety symptoms did not (RR = 1.1 [95% CI, 0.5–2.3]).

Conclusions Neuropsychiatric symptoms such as mood (depression), anxiety, and motivation symptoms were more common in participants with MCI (66.0%) when compared to the population without cognitive impairment (38.9%). Among the symptoms examined, anxiety showed highest prevalence (46.8%) in participants with MCI, followed by mood (36.2%) and motivation (36.2%) symptoms. At 3-year follow-up, baseline anxiety symptoms were associated with an increased risk of progression to AD in MCI subjects (RR = 1.8), but not a significantly increased risk of developing AD in subjects who were cognitively normal at baseline (RR = 1.1). Mood and motivation symptoms did not show a statistically significant increase in risk of progression to AD in MCI subjects (RR = 0.9, RR = 1.1, respectively) but showed an increased risk of developing AD in subjects with normal cognition at baseline (RR = 1.9 for both).

Strengths of the Study

1. Longitudinal population-based cohort study.
2. This study not only assessed the effect of neuropsychiatric symptoms on progression or development of AD but also evaluated the prevalence of such symptoms in MCI population.
3. There was separation and comparison of general "mood" symptoms into depression, anxiety, and motivation.
4. The length of follow-up period (3 years).
5. The diagnosis of dementia through a three-step procedure.

Limitations of the Study

1. Small sample size in the final MCI groups.
2. Large female to male ratio (84.9% female) which can be a confounding factor for prevalence of disorders such as depression and anxiety.
3. Unclear assessment in making cognitive diagnoses of patients who had died.

Take-Home Points

Neuropsychiatric symptoms are more common in individuals with MCI. Neuropsychiatric symptoms not only increase the risk of progression of MCI to AD but also increase the risk of incidence of AD in individuals without cognitive impairment at baseline. Among the various neuropsychiatric symptoms, anxiety increases the risk of progression to AD in participants who have a MCI by twofold, and depression increases the risk of development of AD by twofold in subjects who were cognitively normal at baseline.

Practical Applications of the Take-Home Points

These findings suggest that anxiety symptoms may reflect the neuropathological changes responsible for the progression from MCI to AD. It could also be that anxiety is a subjective reaction to the neurodegenerative process in progress. Whether it be reflective of actual changes or a subjective reaction, anxiety is common in cognitive impairment, and behavioral agitation is also common in later stages of dementia. Many studies have looked at the impact of depression on dementia, but fewer have examined the effect of anxiety. This study proposes that the role of anxiety in dementia may be greater than previously known.

References

1. Palmer K, Berger AK, Monastero R, Winblad B, Bäckman L, Fratiglioni L. Predictors of progression from mild cognitive impairment to Alzheimer disease. Neurology. 2007;68(19):1596–602.
2. Asberg M, Montgomery SA, Perris C, Schalling D, Sedvall G. A comprehensive psychopathological rating scale. Acta Psychiatr Scand Suppl. 1978;271:5–27.

3. Fratiglioni L, Grut M, Forsell Y, Viitanen M, Winblad B. Clinical diagnosis of Alzheimer's disease and other dementias in a population survey. Agreement and causes of disagreement in applying diagnostic and statistical manual of mental disorders, revised third edition, criteria. Arch Neurol. 1992;49(9):927–32.

Chapter 57
Efficacy and Safety of Cognitive Enhancers for Patients with Mild Cognitive Impairment: A Systematic Review and Meta-analysis

Emily B. Phelps and Sandra Swantek

Authors of the Original Article Andrea C Tricco, Charlene Soobiah, Shirra Berliner, Joanne M Ho, Carmen H Ng, Huda M Ashoor, Maggie H Chen, Brenda Hemmelgarn, Sharon E Straus.

Journal Published *Canadian Medical Association Journal.*

Year of Publication 2013.

Type of Study Systematic review, meta-analysis.

Funding Sources Drug Safety and Effectiveness Network/Canadian Institutes of Health Research (DSEN/CIHR; grant no. 257990).

Objectives To examine the efficacy and safety of cognitive enhancers among individuals with mild cognitive impairment (MCI) via a systematic review and meta-analysis [1].

Methods The investigators conducted the systematic review based on the Preferred Reporting Items for Systematic reviews and Meta-Analysis for Protocols. In addition, they published the final systematic review protocol in an open-access journal and registered the study with PROSPERO, the international prospective register of systematic reviews with the registration no. CRD42012002234.

E. B. Phelps
Mount Sinai Hospital, New York, NY, USA
e-mail: Emily.Phelps@mountsinai.edu

S. Swantek (✉)
Rush Medical College, Chicago, IL, USA
e-mail: Sandra_Swantek@Rush.edu

R. R. Tampi et al. (eds.), *Essential Reviews in Geriatric Psychiatry*,
https://doi.org/10.1007/978-3-030-94960-0_57

Only studies that involved individuals with a diagnosis of MCI who were treated with donepezil, rivastigmine, galantamine, and memantine were compared with other cognitive enhancers; placebo and supportive care were included in this review. Additionally, only randomized clinical trials (RCTs), quasi-RCTs, non-RCTs, quasi-experimental (e.g., interrupted time series, controlled before-and-after study), and observational epidemiology (cohort study) which reported on cognition, function, behavior, global status, and mortality or harms were included in this review. There were no restrictions based on languages of dissemination, years of publication, and types of articles, i.e., published and unpublished, for inclusion in the study.

The investigators searched MEDLINE, Embase, the Cochrane Methodology Register, the Cochrane Central Register of Controlled Trials, the Cumulative Index of Nursing and Allied Health Literature, and AgeLine databases for eligible studies. They also searched trial registry websites, the websites of organizations that produce guidelines and abstracts from conference proceedings. Furthermore, the investigators contacted the manufacturers of these drugs. They also compiled a list of included studies and relevant reviews and then contacted researchers and healthcare providers who were experts and well published in this area of research. An experienced librarian conducted the literature searches on November 23, 2011. Two authors collected the title and abstract information from each citation independently using a preestablished eligibility criterion. All conflicts were resolved by discussion or with the involvement of a third reviewer. This process was also followed when screening for potentially relevant full-text articles. In cases where additional information was needed, the authors of the study were contacted to determine the eligibility of the study.

Results The investigators included a total of ten articles that fulfilled the eligibility criteria in the final review. There were seven primary publications and three companion reports that included data from a total of eight RCTs. All the RCTs were conducted between 1999 and 2007 in North America, Europe, New Zealand, Australia, South America, Israel, and Turkey. Three studies were multicenter trials. Four RCTs evaluated donepezil, one study evaluated rivastigmine, two studies evaluated galantamine, and one study examined memantine. All the RCTs compared the cognitive enhancers to placebo.

The Clinical Dementia Rating (CDR) was the commonly used rating scale to diagnose mild cognitive impairment, and the Mini-Mental State Examination (MMSE) was also used across the studies to identify cognitive deficits or to exclude dementia. The Cochrane risk-of-bias tool indicated that three studies were appraised as having a low risk of bias, one study was deemed to have a high risk of bias, and the remaining five studies were appraised as having an unclear risk of bias [2].

In the donepezil studies, there were no difference in cognition as measured by the MMSE among individuals who received donepezil versus those who received placebo (three RCTs, mean difference [MD] = 0.14).

There was no significant difference in cognition between donepezil or galantamine and placebo that was measured using the Alzheimer's Disease Assessment Scale-cognition component (five RCTs, standardized MD = −0.07). In addition, the investigators found no significant differences with this form of cognitive assessment for drugs with different modes of action (i.e., donepezil vs. galantamine). For cognition, the meta-regression analysis favored cognitive enhancers over placebo for studies with 12–84 weeks of follow-up when compared to studies with 85–96 weeks of follow-up.

There was no significant difference between individuals who received galantamine versus those who received placebo on functional status as measured by the Alzheimer's Disease Cooperative Study activities of daily living inventory (two RCTs, MD = 0.30).

In one RCT that evaluated behavioral symptoms using the Neuropsychiatric Inventory (NPI), there was no significant difference between individuals who received donepezil versus those who received placebo (MD = 0.8).

There was no difference in overall mortality rates between individuals who received a cognitive enhancer versus those individuals who received placebo (three RCTs, relative risk [RR] = 1.84, 95% confidence interval (CI), 0.41–8.20). There was no significant difference in mortality between agents with different modes of action (donepezil and rivastigmine versus galantamine). In the only RCT that reported on treatment-related mortality, there was no significant difference between donepezil and placebo (RR = 2.97).

Individuals receiving cognitive enhancers (donepezil, rivastigmine, or galantamine) had greater frequency of nausea and diarrhea when compared to individuals receiving placebo (nausea: four RCTs, RR = 3.04; diarrhea: four RCTs, RR = 2.33). Vomiting was more common among individuals receiving donepezil or rivastigmine when compared to placebo (three RCTs, RR = 4.40). Headaches were more common among individuals receiving rivastigmine or galantamine when compared to placebo (two RCTs, RR = 1.27). The frequency of serious adverse events was no different between individuals receiving cognitive enhancers versus placebo (four RCTs, RR = 0.97). There were no significant differences between agents with different modes of action across all of the harm outcomes on meta-regression and subgroup analyses. In one study, individuals receiving donepezil had more nausea (RR = 2.21), diarrhea (RR = 4.87), and headaches (RR = 2.23) when compared to placebo. In another study, greater proportion of individuals receiving galantamine experienced bradycardia (RR = 1.52) but lesser number of falls (RR = 0.71) when compared to individuals receiving placebo.

Conclusions Cognitive enhancers did not improve cognition or function among individuals with MCI. Their use was associated with a greater risk of developing of gastrointestinal side effects and headaches. The current data does not support the use of cognitive enhancers among individuals with MCI.

Strengths of the Study

1. This study provides a comprehensive review of available literature on the use of cognitive enhancers among individuals with MCI.
2. The quality of meta-analysis [3] was good based on the following criteria:

   (i) Study question clearly stated: Yes
   (ii) Comprehensive literature search: Yes
   (iii) Complete data abstraction: Yes
   (iv) Appropriate appraisal of results: Yes
   (v) Evaluation for publication bias: Yes
   (vi) Applicability of results: Yes
   (vii) Funding sources/conflicts of results noted: Unclear

Limitations of the Study

1. Despite the extensive search of literature, only eight RCTs were included in the final analysis.
2. The demographic information regarding the participants in these studies is lacking, making it difficult to generalize these results across gender, race, and socio-economic status.
3. The absence of information regarding comorbidities in the participants makes it difficult to generalize the results across all older adult population.
4. This review's main limitation is the omission of bias assessment using the Cochrane tool [2]. The Cochrane risk of bias tool assesses the reporting of results in systematic reviews and meta-analyses. The tool comprises theoretical and empirical considerations to appraise bias with particular attention to internal validity [2]. The tool suggests review teams build frameworks with parameters in mind, such as blinding, randomization, and completion of outcomes reporting [2]. Of equal importance is a discussion of the judgments made for each parameter. Of note, of the 56 Cochrane assessments completed by the study team (8 articles under 7 parameters), 25 of them were rated "unclear." The authors do not discuss explanations for these ratings, although the Cochrane risk of bias tool recommends including these judgments. It is likely that studies merely left out details of the methodology and earned an "unclear" rating on this premise.

Take-Home Points

1. Overall, cognitive enhancers do not improve cognition or function among individuals with MCI.
2. The use of cognitive enhancers was associated with greater rates of gastrointestinal side effects and headaches among individuals with MCI when compared to placebo.
3. The use of cognitive enhancers among individuals with MCI is not associated with increased risk for death when compared to placebo.

Practical Application of the Take-Home Points

Individuals with MCI are unlikely to benefit from the use of cognitive enhancers for both cognition and function. The use of these drugs is often associated with gastrointestinal side effects and headaches. Among individuals with MCI, it would be better to use non-pharmacological treatments like cognitive activities, diet, exercise, and the control of vascular risk factor to prevent further cognitive decline.

References

1. Tricco AC, Soobiah C, Berliner S, Ho JM, Ng CH, Ashoor HM, Chen MH, Hemmelgarn B, Straus SE. Efficacy and safety of cognitive enhancers for patients with mild cognitive impairment: a systematic review and meta-analysis. CMAJ. 2013;185(16):1393–401.
2. Higgins JP, Altman DG, Gøtzsche PC, Jüni P, Moher D, Oxman AD, Savovic J, Schulz KF, Weeks L, Sterne JA, Cochrane Bias Methods Group; Cochrane Statistical Methods Group. The Cochrane Collaboration's tool for assessing risk of bias in randomised trials. BMJ. 2011;343:d5928.
3. Russo MW. How to review a meta-analysis. Gastroenterol Hepatol (N Y). 2007;3(8):637–42.

Chapter 58
Personality and Risk of Alzheimer's Disease: New Data and Meta-analysis

Katherine Levine

Authors of the Original Article Antonio Terracciano, Angelina R Sutin, Yang An, Richard J. O'Brien, Luigi Ferrucci, Alan B. Zonderman, Susan M. Resnick.

Journal Published *Alzheimer's & Dementia.*

Year of Publication 2014.

Type of Study Longitudinal study and meta-analysis.

Funding Sources Intramural Research Program of the National Institute of Health, National Institute on Aging.

Objectives To determine if specific facets of personality are associated with an increased risk of developing Alzheimer's disease (AD) as seen in a long-run longitudinal study as well as by performing meta-analysis of longitudinal studies [1].

Methods This article was effectively two different studies; the first study was a long-running longitudinal study, and second study was a pooled meta-analysis [1].

The first study used participants from the Baltimore Longitudinal Study of Aging (BLSA), a prospective cohort study of physical and psychological aging. Participants ($n = 1671$) have no physical or cognitive impairments when they enter the study and are followed to see if they develop diseases or disabilities as they age [2]. Over the course of the study, participants have serial follow-ups with physical and psychological examinations. The frequency of follow-up varies with age, with increasing frequency at older ages. Participants 60–79 years old are tested every 2 years;

K. Levine (✉)
Medical College of Wisconsin, Milwaukee, WI, USA

R. R. Tampi et al. (eds.), *Essential Reviews in Geriatric Psychiatry*, https://doi.org/10.1007/978-3-030-94960-0_58

participants 80 years and older are tested approximately yearly. Subjects included in the analyses were cognitively normal at the time of the baseline personality assessment and had at least one follow-up evaluation. About 7% (n = 119) of participants in this study were lost to follow-up [1].

At enrollment, each participant was evaluated for history of cerebrovascular disease, focal neurological abnormalities, and cognitive or behavioral impairment. Follow-up evaluations included neuropsychological testing (including the Blessed Information Memory Concentration score and the Clinical Dementia Rating (CDR) scale or the Dementia Questionnaire), neurological examination, medication review, and informant/subject structured interview. Every subject with an abnormal neuropsychological test was reviewed at a diagnostic consensus conference where all diagnostic and clinical data was available for review. Diagnosis of dementia was based on DSM-III-R criteria and diagnosis of AD was based on the National Institute of Neurological and Communication Disorders and Stroke-Alzheimer's Disease and Related Disorders Association (NINCDS-ADRDA) criteria [1].

Participants completed the self-report version of the Revised NEO Personality Inventory (NEO-PI-R). The NEO-PI-R is a 240-item questionnaire that assesses 30 facets, 6 for each of the 5 major dimensions of personality – neuroticism (the tendency to experience negative emotions, such as anxiety, anger, and sadness), extraversion (an inclination toward being sociable, assertive, enthusiastic, and energetic), openness (the tendency to be imaginative, unconventional, curious, emotionally and artistically sensitive), agreeableness (an interpersonal dimension defined by altruism, trust, modesty, and cooperativeness), and conscientiousness (the tendency to be organized, strong-willed, persistent, reliable, and a follower of rules and ethical principles). Raw scores were standardized using combined-sex norms as reported in the NEO-PI-R manual. In the BLSA sample, the NEO-PI-R factor structure shows high congruence with the normative structure (Tucker's phis = 0.97–0.99), the internal consistencies for the five dimensions ranged from 0.87 to 0.92, and the test-retest correlations for the five dimensions ranged from 0.78 to 0.85 over an average interval of 10 years [1].

To test whether personality traits conferred risk of AD, proportional hazards regression models were used, controlling for age of personality assessment, sex, ethnicity (white vs. others), and education (years of schooling). The analyses were conducted separately for each of the five personality domains and each of the facets. Personality scores were standardized so that one unit corresponded to a one SD difference. In addition to the continuous scores, domain scores were recoded to provide a statistical and graphical comparison of the top and bottom quartiles of the distribution. A model that included all five factors simultaneously was tested. The time end point was the year of onset of AD-type clinical dementia. Participants who did not develop AD were censored at the time of their last clinical evaluation. Because of differences in the pathophysiologic processes among dementia subtypes, 44 participants were excluded who developed non-AD dementia (e.g., vascular, Lewy body, Parkinson disease). However, the results were similar if these 44 participants censored at time of onset of non-AD dementia were included [1].

The population attributable risk (PAR) based on the hazards ratio (HR) of incident AD associated with the top or bottom quartile of the distribution on a personality trait vs. the rest of the sample (adjusted for the demographic covariates) was estimated using the formula PAR = PRF × ((HR−1)/HR), where PRF is the prevalence of the risk factor (i.e., 25%). The PAR estimates are calculated for comparisons with established risk factors. PAR estimates, however, are generally based on clinically recognized cut points (e.g., the blood pressure value that defines hypertension), whereas this study used statistical thresholds for the personality traits. In addition, in calculating the PAR, this study is not necessarily assuming a direct causal link between the risk factor and the outcome [1].

As the APOE ε4 allele is a known risk factor for AD, secondary analyses with APOE genotype (presence vs. absence of ε4 allele) as a covariate or moderator of the association between personality and incident AD were performed for the subset of 1472 participants with available APOE genotype. The analyses were also repeated excluding individuals younger than 50 years at initial examination or those who developed AD within 2 years after the initial personality assessment. Finally, the question of whether sex moderated the association between personality traits and incident AD was evaluated. These analyses were conducted using SPSS statistical software [1].

The meta-analysis aspect of the study searched PubMed and Scopus databases up to February 2012 and screened the reference lists for relevant articles. The focus was on prospective cohort studies with five-factor model personality traits assessed at baseline in cognitively healthy participants who were evaluated at follow-up for incident AD. When there were multiple publications from the same sample, they considered one effect for each trait from each sample. To reduce variability across studies, generally the risk estimates from the main model were chosen with age, sex, education, and ethnicity as covariates. The logHR and standard error were scaled in each study to correspond to the effect associated with one SD difference on the trait [1].

The authors performed random-effects model meta-analysis. A random-effects meta-analysis model assumes that the observed estimates of treatment effect can vary across studies because of *real* differences in the treatment effect in each study as well as sampling variability (chance). Thus, even if the studies had an extremely large sample size, the observed study effects would still vary because of the *real* differences in treatment effects. Such *heterogeneity* in treatment effects is caused by differences in study populations (such as age of patients), interventions received (such as dose of drug), follow-up length, and other factors [3]. Heterogeneity was evaluated using the Q statistic, and publication bias was evaluated statistically with the Kendall's tau and Egger test. This was conducted using the Comprehensive Meta-Analysis software package [1].

Results In the BLSA, participants were monitored for a mean of 12 years (mean = 12, SD = 6, range = 1–22). Onset of clinical AD diagnosis occurred in 90 individuals within an average of 8 years (SD = 8, range = 1–18) from baseline personality assessment. The incident dementia group was older and more likely to be white. This was partially because many minorities were recruited later in the study. Sex and education were not found to be significantly associated with the onset of AD [1].

Certain personality traits were found to be significantly associated with the development of AD. For each SD increase in neuroticism, the risk of incident AD increased by more than 30% (HR, 1.37; 95% CI, 1.09–1.73). The authors calculated that more that 10% of AD cases in the population could be attributed to high neuroticism (top quartile vs. others; HR, 2.02; PAR, 13%). A similar effect was observed for conscientiousness (HR, 0.69; 95% CI, 0.55–0.87); the risk of incident AD was three times higher in the lowest vs. the highest quartile. Like neuroticism, the proportion of AD cases that could be contributed to low conscientiousness was about 10% (bottom quartile vs. others; HR, 1.74, 11%) [1].

Separate analyses were performed. One set looked to see if there was more of an association or interaction between the personality factors beyond the apparent correlation of high neuroticism and low conscientiousness. No further associations or interactions were found. Another set of analyses looked at the APOE e4 allele as an additional covariate that increased the risk of AD and was associated with scoring in the top quartile of neuroticism (HR, 3.82; 95% CI, 1.85–7.89) or the bottom quartile of conscientiousness (HR, 3.40; 95% CI, 1.39–8.28). The authors tested for additional interactions between the five factors and APOE e4 variant. High openness was protective against AD for the APOE e4 carriers (interaction term: HR, 0.58; 95% CI, 0.34–0.98). For those who were noncarriers, high agreeableness was protective against AD (interaction term: HR, 1.87; 95% CI, 1.10–3.16) [1].

At the personality facet level, the anxiety, angry hostility, and depression aspects of neuroticism increased the risk of incident AD by more than 30%; there was a trend for vulnerability ($P = 0.05$). Among the facets of conscientiousness, self-discipline had the strongest association, followed by competence, order, and dutifulness; risk of incident AD was reduced by more than 30% for each SD higher score on any of these facets. One facet of openness, openness to new ideas, was associated significantly with a 25% reduced risk of AD for each SD increase in score [1].

The meta-analysis included data from four other trials in addition to the BLSA data. Longitudinal studies looking at neuroticism and incident AD were the most common, with 5054 participant samples, but there was less available data for the remaining four personality factors, with only 3342 participants. Personality facets were unable to be analyzed due to insufficient data. The NEO-PI-R instrument was utilized in all studies. Neuroticism was found to have a highly significant effect – every SD increase in this trait increased the risk of AD by 30% (HR, 1.33; 95% CI, 1.21–1.45). This association was highly consistent across studies, and there was no statistical evidence of publication bias (Kendall's z-tau = 1.22; $P = 0.22$; and Egger's regression intercept test: $t = 1.87$; df = 3; $P = 0.16$). Low scores on conscientiousness were associated with a higher risk of incident AD (HR, 0.77; 95 CI, 0.69–0.86; $P = 2 \times 10^{-6}$). There was no evidence of heterogeneity ($P = 0.55$) or publication bias ($P > 0.05$). Openness (HR, 0.86; 95% CI, 0.77–0.96; $P = 0.008$; heterogeneity,

$P = 0.91$; publication bias, $P > 0.05$) and agreeableness (HR, 0.88; 95% CI, 0.79–0.98; $P = 0.019$, heterogeneity, $P = 0.51$; publication bias, $P > 0.05$) were also associated with a lower risk of AD, but there was no significant association for extraversion (HR, 0.96; 95% CI, 0.86–1.07; $P = 0.53$) [1].

Conclusions Neuroticism is directly and conscientiousness is inversely associated with risk of developing Alzheimer's disease. The highest quartile of neuroticism and the lowest quartile of conscientiousness each accounts for more than 10% of the cases of AD. For people who are carriers of the APOE e4 risk allele, being in the top quartile of openness is significantly protective against developing AD. For those who are noncarriers, agreeableness is significantly protective against developing AD [1].

Strengths of the Study

1. Longitudinal cohort studies are highly valid in determining long-term trends and changes over time. The Baltimore Longitudinal Study of Aging (BLSA) is the longest running study on aging in the world [2].
2. Only 7% (119) of the 1671 patients were lost to follow-up, a relatively low level of attrition given the size and duration of the study [1].
3. A robust and detailed personality assessment was used [1].
4. The meta-analyses indicated a high degree of consistency across studies which served to strengthen the overall results [1].
5. The article combined two different types of studies (a longitudinal study and a meta-analysis) and found similar results with both [1].

Limitations of the Study

1. The observational nature of the BLSA and the studies included in the meta-analysis [1].
2. The BLSA sample is not representative of the US population. For instance, the BLSA did not even include women until 1978 [2].
3. All the meta-analysis studies examined neuroticism, but not all of the meta-analysis studies examined the other four personality traits [1].
4. We do not know how stable personality is across a lifetime, which limits how much we can infer from the results. If we knew that personality is 100% stable, this data would seem to support intervening as early as possible. But, if personality can change significantly across a lifetime, perhaps the high neuroticism and low conscientiousness that we are seeing as associated with dementia is actually a type of dementia prodrome [1].

Take-Home Points

Combining the BLSA's decades of cognitive testing and personality inventories with meta-analyses shows us that high neuroticism and low conscientiousness are significant risk factors for Alzheimer's dementia [1].

Practical Applications of the Take-Home Point

Increasing our awareness of the connection between high neuroticism, low conscientiousness, and AD allows clinicians to identify individuals at greater risk of

AD. This association indicates that there may be value in more intensively monitoring or treating this population [1].

References

1. Terracciano A, Sutin AR, An Y, O'Brien RJ, Ferrucci L, Zonderman AB, Resnick SM. Personality and risk of Alzheimer's disease: new data and meta-analysis. Alzheimers Dement. 2014;10(2):179–86.
2. BLSA history | National institute on aging (nih.gov). Accessed 1 Mar 2021.
3. Riley RD, Higgins JPT, Deeks JJ. Interpretation of random effects meta-analyses. BMJ. 2011;342:d549.

Chapter 59
Modifiable Predictors of Dementia in Mild Cognitive Impairment: A Systematic Review and Meta-analysis

Emily B. Phelps and Sandra Swantek

Authors of the Original Article Claudia Cooper, Andrew Sommerlad, Constantine G Lyketsos, Gill Livingston.

Journal Published *American Journal of Psychiatry.*

Year of Publication 2015.

Type of Study Systematic review, meta-analysis.

Funding Sources No external funding source. Dr. Lyketsos was supported by National Institute on Aging grant P50 AG-005146 to the Johns Hopkins Alzheimer's Disease Research Center.

Objectives In this systematic review and meta-analysis, the investigators synthesized evidence from longitudinal observational studies regarding the modifiable risk factors that predict the conversion of individuals with mild cognitive impairment (MCI) to dementia [1].

Methods The investigators define MCI as cognitive impairment that was identified from objective neuropsychological tests, in the absence of functional impairment or dementia. They defined modifiable risk factors as factors potentially changeable through lifestyle or existing medical treatment. The investigator authors conducted

E. B. Phelps
Mount Sinai Hospital, New York, NY, USA
e-mail: Emily.Phelps@mountsinai.edu

S. Swantek (✉)
Rush Medical College, Chicago, IL, USA
e-mail: Sandra_Swantek@Rush.edu

R. R. Tampi et al. (eds.), *Essential Reviews in Geriatric Psychiatry*,
https://doi.org/10.1007/978-3-030-94960-0_59

literature searches via PubMed and Web of Knowledge for longitudinal studies connecting modifiable risk factors for the incidence of dementia among individuals with MCI using specific search terms. There were no limits applied for language or date of publication. Additionally, the authors searched the references of included articles.

One author extracted the study characteristics and findings, whereas two of the authors independently assessed the studies for bias using a criterion that was devised from published checklists (10). Studies were considered of high quality if the study subjects were a defined representative sample of participants assembled at a common point in their disease or recruited to be representative of the general older population, with a response rate of at least 60% of eligible potential participants [1]; the participants were followed-up for at least a year, with at least 70% participation; and the diagnostic criteria for MCI and dementia were objective or applied in a "masked" fashion. All disagreements were resolved by consensus. The authors graded the evidence in support of the conclusions into three grades: grade 1 evidence, consistent evidence from higher-quality studies; grade 2 evidence [1], from a single higher-quality study or was consistent with evidence from other studies; and inconsistent evidence, notably inconsistent with other studies. When the data from at least three studies could be combined, the authors conducted a meta-analysis on the findings. The study analysts calculated unadjusted pooled odds ratios for dichotomous outcomes and standardized effect sizes from means and standard deviations for continuous outcomes.

Results The systematic review yielded 62 eligible studies reported in 76 articles. The final review discusses 17 epidemiological studies and 45 clinical studies. The meta-analyses included 30 of the 62 studies, with other results being reported qualitatively.

A. Risk Factors for Cerebrovascular Disease

1. Diabetes: There is grade 2 evidence that diabetes increases the risk of Alzheimer's dementia among individuals with amnestic MCI. Diabetes also increases the risk of any-cause dementia in individuals with any-type or non-amnestic MCI (pooled odds ratio (OR) = 1.65; 95% CI, 1.12–2.43). Prediabetes predicts conversion from any-type MCI to all-cause dementia [1]. Available data from both epidemiological and clinical studies of amnestic MCI and any-type MCI appeared consistent.
2. Hypertension: Data from epidemiological and clinical studies indicates that there is grade 2 evidence that hypertension does not predict the conversion from any-type MCI to all-cause dementia (pooled OR = 1.05; 95% CI, 0.60–1.85). However, the evidence regarding conversion from amnestic MCI to Alzheimer's dementia is inconsistent.
3. Hypercholesterolemia: There is grade 2 evidence that hypercholesterolemia is not associated with risk of conversion from any-type MCI to all-cause dementia (pooled OR = 0.92; 95% CI, 0.50–1.68). However, the evidence for

the risk of Alzheimer's dementia among individuals with amnestic MCI is inconsistent.

4. Smoking: When the data is controlled for age, there is grade 1 evidence that smoking is not associated with risk of conversion from amnestic MCI to Alzheimer's dementia or any-type MCI to all-cause dementia (unadjusted pooled OR = 0.45; 95% CI, 0.24–0.84) [1].
5. Alcohol: There is grade 2 evidence that heavy alcohol use predicts conversion from any-type MCI to dementia. However, there is inconsistent evidence regarding the moderate alcohol use and the risk for dementia among individuals.
6. Metabolic syndrome: It is defined as ≥3 of the following: abdominal obesity, elevated plasma triglycerides, low HDL cholesterol, hypertension or antihypertensive treatment, and high fasting plasma glucose. There is grade 2 evidence that the metabolic syndrome predicts a greater risk of all-cause dementia among individuals with amnestic MCI [1].

B. Neuropsychiatric Symptoms

1. Depression: Data from epidemiological studies indicates that there is grade 1 evidence that more depressive symptoms predict the conversion from any-type MCI to all-cause dementia. However, data from clinical studies is inconsistent about whether depressive symptoms predict the conversion from amnestic MCI to Alzheimer's dementia or to any-cause dementia [1].
2. Anxiety: Evidence regarding anxiety symptoms being associated with the conversion from amnestic MCI to Alzheimer's dementia and whether apathy predicts the risk of conversion from amnestic MCI to Alzheimer's dementia or from any-type MCI to dementia is large (pooled OR = 20.11; 95% CI, 20.34–0.11).
3. Any neuropsychiatric symptom: Data from clinical studies indicate that there is grade 2 evidence to suggest that the presence of neuropsychiatric symptoms among individuals with any-type MCI predicts the conversion to all-cause dementia.

C. Dietary Factors

1. Mediterranean diet: There is grade 2 evidence that the use of a Mediterranean diet decreases risk of conversion from amnestic MCI to Alzheimer's dementia [1].
2. Folate: There is grade 2 evidence that a lower folate serum level predicts conversion from any-type MCI to all-cause dementia.
3. Homocysteine: There is inconsistent evidence whether higher serum homocysteine level predicts the conversion of individuals with MCI to dementia.
4. Copper: There is grade 2 evidence that higher serum level of copper predicted the conversion from amnestic MCI to Alzheimer's dementia.

D. Education

There is grade 1 evidence from both clinical and epidemiological studies that amount of education does not predict the conversion from any-type MCI to all-cause dementia or from amnestic MCI to Alzheimer's dementia.

E. Others

1. Physical activity: Greater physical activity predicts the conversion from any-type MCI to all-cause dementia in clinical studies.
2. Body mass index (BMI): Low body mass index predicts the conversion from any-type MCI to all-cause dementia in clinical studies.
3. Atrial fibrillation: The presence of atrial fibrillation predicts the conversion from any-type MCI to all-cause dementia in clinical studies.
4. Antidementia drugs: Antidementia drugs reduce the risk of conversion from any-type MCI to all-cause dementia in a clinical study, but not in a higher-quality epidemiological study.
5. Estrogen: Estrogen replacement therapy predicted a shorter time to conversion from any-type MCI to all-cause dementia, but did not increase the overall risk for dementia.
6. Anticholinergic drug: In one epidemiological study, after controlling for age, the use of anticholinergic drugs predicted conversion from any-type MCI to all-cause dementia among women but not in men [1].

Conclusions Available evidence indicates that diabetes increases the risk of conversion to dementia. Other modifiable prognostic factors include prediabetes, metabolic syndrome, neuropsychiatric symptoms, and low dietary folate levels. Additionally, interventions to reduce neuropsychiatric symptoms may reduce the incidence of dementia.

Strengths of the Study

1. The review's strengths include the combination of epidemiological studies and clinical studies, with 62 studies analyzed across 76 articles.
2. The authors stratified evidence by quality (sample representativeness, adequate follow-up, and clear diagnostic criteria). Fourteen studies were considered to be of "high quality."
3. Additionally, the authors stratified study findings' strengths by grade or relationship to other studies' findings in the high-quality category.
4. A variety of clinical variables portray a broad range of possible factors, including cerebrovascular disease, concurrent neuropsychiatric symptoms, and lifestyle.
5. Based on the Newcastle-Ottawa Quality Assessment Scale bias for cohort studies [2], this review is adequate in its comparability and outcome assessment. However, the representation of the study samples (epidemiological studies and clinical studies) is not discussed. Descriptions of high-quality epidemiological studies' demographics would be beneficial to the discussion because the team's designation of "grade 1 evidence" involves the relation of these cohorts to one

another. However, the designation of "high-quality studies" mandated a representative study, so it may be reasonable to assume that the 14 high-quality studies were comparable (Table 59.1).

Limitations

1. The exclusion criteria for studies are minimal (abstracts).
2. Authors address a former review that concluded that preventative treatments in persons with MCI were ineffective in reducing the incidence of dementia. While the clinical utility of addressing modifiable risk factors is appealing, the translation to clinical utility and preventative medicine is lacking [3].
3. The diagnostic criteria for MCI do not specify memory loss in all of the studies. This lack of specificity may confound early signs of dementia as opposed to a diagnosis of MCI.
4. For studies examining alcohol's relationship to the incidence of dementia, heavy alcohol consumers were not represented well in the samples.
5. Studies examining education found no relationship between years of schooling and risk of AD; a possible confound in studies exploring education level would be the degree of socialization in career paths, which may correlate with higher educational levels in some professions.
6. Studies were evaluated against the criteria adopted by the authors.
7. Most study evidence was "grade 2" or supported by a single high-quality study; the only evidence marked by "grade 1" quality is the lack of association of smoking, education, or depression with dementia incidence. The latter findings were insignificant in clinical studies.

Table 59.1 Quality Assessment Scale

Domain	Description	Score (1 or 0)
Selection		
Representativeness of the exposed cohort	No description of the derivations of the cohort	0
Selection of the nonexposed cohort	No description of the derivation of the nonexposed cohort	0
Ascertainment of exposure	Structured interview	1
Demonstration that the outcome of interest was not present at the start of the study	Yes	1
Comparability		
Studies control for	Age, education	2
Outcome		
Assessment of outcome	Record linkage	1
Was follow-up long enough for outcomes to occur?	Yes	1
Subjects lost to follow-up unlikely to introduce bias; small number lost; > % (select an adequate %) follow-up	60%	1

Adapted from Wells et al. [2]

8. Participant follow-up was only 1 year long for the "high-quality" category; strengths of risk relationships may have increased with longer follow-up more representative of clinical practice treating older adults.

Take-Home Points

1. While little is known about preventative approaches to mitigate the risk of dementia in MCI patients, epidemiological studies suggest potentially modifiable risk factors: diabetes, metabolic syndrome, neuropsychiatric symptoms (including depression), and low folate diets.
2. The Mediterranean diet decreased the risk of AD in amnestic MCI patients in one study.

Practical Application of the Take-Home Points

For patients with MCI, dietary approaches and lifestyle modifications in metabolic syndrome and diabetes may ameliorate the risk of dementia. Similarly, treating comorbid depression presents the greatest potential to lessen the risk of AD.

References

1. Cooper C, Sommerlad A, Lyketsos CG, Livingston G. Modifiable predictors of dementia in mild cognitive impairment: a systematic review and meta-analysis. Am J Psychiatry. 2015;172(4):323–34.
2. Wells GA, Shea B, O'Connell D, Peterson J, Welch V, Losos M, Tugwell P. The Newcastle-Ottawa Scale (NOS) for assessing the quality of nonrandomised studies in meta-analyses 2000. https://web.archive.org/web/20210716121605id_/http://www3.med.unipmn.it/dispense_ebm/2009-2010/Corso%20Perfezionamento%20EBM_Faggiano/NOS_oxford.pdf. Accessed on 17 Feb 2022.
3. Cooper C, Li R, Lyketsos C, Livingston G. Treatment for mild cognitive impairment: systematic review. Br J Psychiatry. 2013;203(3):255–64.

Chapter 60
Pharmacological Management of Lewy Body Dementia: A Systematic Review and Meta-analysis

Chadrick E. Lane and Michelle L. Conroy

Authors of the Original Article Chris Stinton, Ian McKeith, John-Paul Taylor, Louise Lafortune, Eneida Mioshi, Elijah Mak, Victoria Cambridge, James Mason, Alan Thomas, John T O'Brien.

Journal Published *American Journal of Psychiatry.*

Year of Publication 2015.

Type of Study Combined systematic review and meta-analysis.

Funding Sources National Institute for Health Research (NIHR).

Objectives To describe several impacts of pharmacologic management in LBD delineated in a combined systematic review and meta-analysis [1].

Methods The authors searched a variety of resources, including online databases, clinical trial registers, and the gray literature (e.g., those materials that may have not been published through traditional academic routes). Furthermore, they explored references listed in related works and consulted with experts; there were no pre-specified criteria for length or language. The selected studies included subjects with

C. E. Lane (✉)
Peter O'Donnell Jr. Brain Institute, Department of Psychiatry, UT Southwestern Medical Center, Dallas, TX, USA
e-mail: Chadrick.lane@utsouthwestern.edu

M. L. Conroy
Yale University School of Medicine, New Haven, CT, USA

VA Connecticut Healthcare System, West Haven, CT, USA
e-mail: Michelle.l.conroy@yale.edu

R. R. Tampi et al. (eds.), *Essential Reviews in Geriatric Psychiatry*,
https://doi.org/10.1007/978-3-030-94960-0_60

diagnoses of DLB, PDD, or LBD and pharmacologic intervention and contained defined outcome metrics.

The studies were categorized by treatment strategy and level of evidence. Methodological quality was graded using the Quality Assessment Tool of Quantitative Studies, with several domains of each study being rated as either weak, moderate, or strong in quality. For the meta-analysis, a random-effects or fixed-effects model was used depending on the degree of study heterogeneity. The authors summarized findings to the best of their ability when data could not be synthesized.

Results Of the 28,568 works that were screened, 633 advanced to further review, 197 met inclusion criteria, and 44 were ultimately analyzed. There was a wide range of pharmacologic agents captured in the analysis, spanning from cholinesterase inhibitors (ChEIs), memantine, armodafinil/modafinil, piracetam, antiparkinsonian medications, antipsychotics, antidepressants, sedatives, anticonvulsants, and herbal treatments. Forest plots demonstrated the effects of ChEIs on global clinical response, cognitive function, and neuropsychiatric symptoms and the effect of memantine on global clinical response. Descriptive summaries detailed relevant findings for the remaining pharmacologic interventions and their outcomes.

ChEIs Subjects who received donepezil and rivastigmine were more likely to have measurable improvement on clinical rating scales [risk ratio (RR) = 1.37, 95% confidence interval (CI), 1.15–1.62]. When assessed for an absence of deterioration, those receiving ChEIs again fared better than those receiving placebo (RR = 1.26, 95% CI, 1.01–1.57). Utilizing changes in clinical impression as a continuous variable, those treated with ChEIs evidenced a mean decrease of 0.55 points, consistent with observed improvements (95% CI, −0.82 to −0.28). Studies of cognitive effects used the Mini-Mental State Examination (MMSE) and showed subjects receiving ChEIs experienced an improvement of 1.26 points (95% CI, 0.66–1.86).

In studies using the ten-item Neuropsychiatric Inventory (NPI-10), ChEIs did not have a statistically significant effect (−1.36, 95% CI, −3.20 to 0.47), although the authors point out there was significant heterogeneity among the studies. Subanalyses of six studies did find effects for donepezil and rivastigmine in the treatment of neuropsychiatric symptoms (NPS) in PDD, but not in DLB. In two studies using the shorter four-item NPI (apathy, depression, delusions, and hallucinations), ChEIs were efficacious in DLB [weighted mean difference (WMD) = −3.36, 95% CI, −5.85 to −0.87], although further subgroup analysis demonstrated benefit from donepezil but not rivastigmine. Treatment with ChEIs potentially offers functional benefits in PDD, though it appeared this effect was driven by rivastigmine and not donepezil.

While studies utilizing galantamine were limited to one each for DLB and PDD, galantamine was favored on measures of cognition and neuropsychiatric symptomatology, although the data on cognitive improvements in DLB were mixed.

A single uncontrolled trial assessing the impact of abrupt withdrawal of ChEIs pointed to worsening cognition in DLB and PDD and increases in neuropsychiatric disturbances in PDD.

Other Agents

Memantine: Studies of memantine included in this paper did not demonstrate significant improvements in cognition, neuropsychiatric symptoms, or function.

Wake promoting agents: Armodafinil may improve wakefulness in DLB, and a retrospective review revealed half of patients treated with armodafinil or modafinil were rated as minimally improved, with another third rated as much improved.

Piracetam: No between-group differences on a number of clinically relevant measures.

Antiparkinsonian agents: While levodopa afforded motor benefits in a percentage of patients with PDD and DLB, it is worth noting a sizable number also developed psychotic symptoms. Levodopa withdrawal did not appear to worsen motor, non-motor, and cognitive measures in a trial of patients with PDD. There were no studies of amantadine in DLB, and one uncontrolled trial in PDD suggests modest improvements in only 2 out of 15 cognitive assessments. Rotigotine, a dopamine agonist, may lessen severity of disability and anxiety in PDD. Selegiline, a monoamine oxidase inhibitor (MAOI), had no benefit in PDD and no studies for DLB were found.

Antipsychotics: Studies of the antipsychotics – clozapine, olanzapine, quetiapine, and risperidone – were analyzed. Clozapine was effective in lowering agitation scores in PDD, weighed against the classic side effects of clozapine including sedation, sialorrhea, and constipation. Efficacy of olanzapine was mixed, suggesting lower doses may have benefit for neuropsychiatric symptoms but this effect is lost beyond 5 mg/day. Studies suggest olanzapine is poorly tolerated in DLB and PDD. Findings for quetiapine were also mixed, with a randomized controlled trial revealing no differences in a number of outcomes, including neuropsychiatric symptoms, cognitive performance, daily functioning, motoric ability, and clinical change. Risperidone appears to be poorly tolerated and ineffective in DLB, although it may have had benefit for neuropsychiatric symptoms and functioning in PDD with psychosis without significant side effects. A caveat of the risperidone in PDD with psychosis study is that it was an uncontrolled trial.

Antidepressants: In a small trial of citalopram in DLB, over 70% of participants withdrew due to an inability to tolerate the drug. Duloxetine, escitalopram, and trazodone may reduce depressive symptoms, although no numeric data were available for these latter two agents.

Sleep promoting agents: Clonazepam and ramelteon may lessen sleep disturbances, with ramelteon also showing improvements in caregiver burden and neuropsychiatric symptoms more broadly.

Anticonvulsants: Single case reports found gabapentin reduced restless leg symptoms and agitation in DLB and PDD, respectively. Case series suggest zonisamide may offer demonstrable benefits for function, caregiver burden, neuropsychiatric symptoms, and motor ability.

Herbals: Yokukansan, an herbal agent, may reduce neuropsychiatric symptoms in DLB and PDD, recognizing that the DLB data was from a randomized crossover trial and the PDD data from an uncontrolled trial.

The authors were unable to find research on patient and caregiver perspectives as they relate to pharmacologic interventions. Cost-effectiveness studies were limited and mixed in their results.

Conclusions In LBD, ChEIs appear to have benefits on outcomes of cognition and neuropsychiatric symptoms, with the evidence being more robust for donepezil and rivastigmine than for galantamine. Memantine does not convincingly provide much clinical benefit. A number of other agents may be useful in the management of LBD, but double-blind randomized controlled trials are lacking in the literature.

Strengths of the Study

1. The authors utilized a systematic review and, when feasible, a meta-analysis of those studies included.
2. Unpublished data, i.e., the gray literature, were included in the search in an attempt to limit publication bias.
3. Studies were assessed on the basis of their methodological rigor and level of evidence.

Limitations of the Study

1. Several studies were of smaller sample sizes, open label, uncontrolled, or limited to case series and single case reports.
2. Some of the analyses were impacted by considerable heterogeneity.
3. Only 9 of 16 studies contained data for the global response proportions, and 5 of 16 studies were useful for calculating the cognitive response proportions.
4. Diagnostic purity in studies may have been variable.
5. For the analysis, there was a need to estimate data when missing and not readily available from the original authors.
6. There is growing uncertainty as to how accurate and useful it is to consider PDD and DLB as separate diagnostic entities. Much of the research included in this paper makes this distinction, which may in fact be arbitrary and could cloud the overall picture.

Take-Home Points

Reasonably high-level evidence supports the use of ChEIs in treating cognitive impairment and neuropsychiatric symptoms due to LBD. Although well tolerated, memantine appears to be of minimal, if any, benefit. A variety of other drugs spanning antidepressants, antiparkinsonian agents, wakefulness-promoting agents, antipsychotics, sleep aids, anticonvulsants, and herbals possess varying degrees of efficacy with a wide range in the quality of their evidence.

Practical Applications of the Take-Home Point

ChEIs may benefit patients experiencing cognitive impairment and neuropsychiatric symptoms due to LBD, while the evidence is more variable for a range of other pharmacologic agents. The use of ChEIs or any other central nervous system (CNS) active pharmacotherapy should weigh the risks and benefits in addition to utilizing shared decision-making between the provider, patient, and/or surrogate decision-maker (s).

Reference

1. Stinton C, McKeith I, Taylor JP, Lafortune L, Mioshi E, Mak E, Cambridge V, Mason J, Thomas A, O'Brien JT. Pharmacological management of Lewy body dementia: a systematic review and meta-analysis. Am J Psychiatry. 2015;172(8):731–42.

Chapter 61
Meta-analysis of Modifiable Risk Factors of Alzheimer's Disease

Emily B. Phelps and Sandra Swantek

Authors of the Original Article Wei Xu, Lan Tan, Hui-Fu Wang, Teng Jiang, Meng-Shan Tan, Lin Tan, Qing-Fei Zhao, Jie-Qiong Li, Jun Wang, Jin-Tai Yu.

Journal Published *Journal of Neurology, Neurosurgery, and Psychiatry.*

Year of Publication 2015.

Type of Study Meta-analysis.

Funding Sources None listed.

Objectives The investigators wanted to evaluate the association between AD and its modifiable risk factors [1].

Methods The investigators followed the Meta-analysis Of Observational Studies in Epidemiology (MOOSE) Group and the PRISMA 2009 guidelines for systematic review and meta-analysis in addition to the Cochrane Collaboration definition of systematic reviews and meta-analysis. They searched PubMed and the Cochrane Database of Systematic Reviews for studies that reported risk factors of AD from August 1968 to July 2014 using the search terms "Alzheimer's disease," "dementia," and "risk factor." The investigators only searched for papers published in English language. The bibliographies of retrieved studies and all relevant articles on

E. B. Phelps
Mount Sinai Hospital, New York, NY, USA
e-mail: Emily.Phelps@mountsinai.edu

S. Swantek (✉)
Rush Medical College, Chicago, IL, USA
e-mail: Sandra_Swantek@Rush.edu

R. R. Tampi et al. (eds.), *Essential Reviews in Geriatric Psychiatry*,
https://doi.org/10.1007/978-3-030-94960-0_61

the topic were searched for additional studies. They included studies if these studies reported on the odds ratio (OR) or relative risk (RR) of AD using a longitudinal cohort study or retrospective case-control study design, the study population was representative of the general population, and the exposures were considered to be positively or negatively associated with a later diagnosis of AD and were potentially modifiable. Any disagreement between authors on which studies to include was resolved by further discussion until an agreement was reached.

Only exposures with significant associations were included. If studies utilized multiple control groups, the authors prioritized randomly selected and healthy controls with no cognitive disease evidence at baseline. The authors prioritized individuals with AD without cerebrovascular disease. The authors stratified the results of continuous or dose-dependent exposures and converted these into categorical classifications. The combined results formulated a pooled effect size for exposures reported across studies. The calculation of a population attributable risk (PAR) used the largest study population as a proxy for the global population.

The investigators assigned three grades of evidence in support of the conclusion based on two elements – the pooled sample size and heterogeneity. Grade I evidence was defined as both pooled population >5000 and lower heterogeneity ($I^2 < 50\%$). Grade II-A evidence was defined as pooled population >5000 but with higher heterogeneity ($I^2 \geq 50\%$). Grade II-B evidence was defined as lower heterogeneity ($I^2 \geq 50\%$) but with pooled population <5000. Grade III evidence was defined as both pooled population <5000 and higher heterogeneity.

Results A total of 351 articles were eligible for inclusion in the systematic review, and 323 of these articles were included in the meta-analysis. Thirteen risk factors demonstrated significant associations: 11 with Grade I evidence and 2 with Grade II-A evidence. There were 23 protective factors: 18 with Grade I evidence and 5 with Grade II-A evidence. No significant association was found for 23 factors: 19 with Grade I evidence and 4 with Grade II-A evidence.

1. Risk Factors

Grade I evidence exists for the following 13 risk factors being associated with an increased risk for AD, noted in descending order of effect size: heavy smoking (55.5–156 pack years), low diastolic blood pressure (DBP) (≤70 mm Hg), high body mass index (BMI) in midlife, carotid atherosclerosis, diabetes mellitus 2 in Asian population, low BMI (≤30), low educational attainment, high total homocysteine levels, depression, systolic blood pressure (SBP) ≥160 mm Hg, and frailty.

Grade II-A evidence exists for the following two risk factors being associated with an increased risk for AD, noted in descending order of effect size: current smoking among the Asian population and neuroticism.

2. Protective Factors

Grade I evidence exists for the following 18 protective factors against the development of AD, noted in descending order of effect size: arthritis, high folate intake, current statin use, coffee/caffeine drinking, cognitive activity, ever use of estrogen, light to moderate drinking, ever alcohol use, cancer, heart disease, metabolic syndrome, antihypertensive medications, high vitamin E intake, high vitamin C intake, nonsteroidal anti-inflammatory drug (NSAID) use, high BMI in late life, current smoking in Western population, and ever-smoking.

Grade II-A evidence exists for the following five protective factors against the development of AD, noted in descending order of effect size: a healthy diet pattern, high AB42/AB40 ratio, fish consumption, high education, and physical activity.

3. No Significant Association

Grade I evidence exists for the following 19 factors having no significant association with the development of AD: docosahexaenoic acid, alcoholism, combination of vitamin E and C, past smoking, suburban area versus rural area, eicosapentaenoic acid, elevated cholesterol level, stroke, diabetes mellitus 2 in Western population, SBP ≥130–140, high density lipoprotein, general anesthesia, low frequency electromagnetic field (EMF), kidney disease, head trauma with or without loss of consciousness, high fasting insulin level, occupational pesticide exposure, high intake of saturated fat, and peripheral arterial disease.

Grade II-A evidence exists for the following four factors having no significant association with the development of AD: no partner versus having a partner, aluminum in drinking water supply, atrial fibrillation, and heart failure.

Publication bias (as assessed via Eggers test and the trim and fill method) was present in ten factors. The bias had barely any effect on the summary estimate for personality (neuroticism) and depression but did influence the summary estimate for high educational attainment, stress, high serum total homocysteine (tHcy) levels, high serum total cholesterol level, docosahexaenoic acid (DHA) consumption, low educational attainment, heavy smoking, and high participation in cognitive activity. However, their adjusted statistical meanings were not altered.

The investigators calculated the population attributable risks (PAR) for the 9 of the 13 risk factors that showed a significant positive association (Grade I and II-A) with the development of AD, for which the global prevalence was available. The significant risk factors where the global prevalence was available included obesity (3.4%), current smoking in the Asian population (34.7–61.1% for men and 0.5–2.6% for women), carotid atherosclerosis (25.4% for men and 26.4% for women), DM-2 in the Asian population (8.2%), low education (≤primary school; 40%), hyperhomocysteine (27.5%), depression (13.2%), hypertension (8.9%), and frailty (4.9–27.3%). These nine potentially modifiable risk factors contribute to roughly 66% of AD cases globally based on their combined PAR.

Conclusions Modifiable risk factors exist for AD across diet, lifestyle, medications, biochemical exposures, mental health, and chronic conditions. Interventions to modify these factors may decrease the incidence of AD.

Strengths of the Study

1. At the time of publication, this study is the most comprehensive review of literature investigating the modifiable risk factors of AD.
2. The authors adhered to rigorous meta-analysis and systematic review standards outlined by the Meta-analysis Of Observational Studies in Epidemiology (MOOSE) Group [2], the PRISMA 2009 guidelines [3], and the Cochrane Collaboration [4]. Studies considered for inclusion met the criteria of the Newcastle-Ottawa scale [5]. Publication bias was assessed via the Egger test and the trim and fill method [6].
3. The studies selected were analyzed using standards for high quality. Please see the Methods section for details of the grading system.
4. Considerations of modifiable risk factors include 67 associations, and priority was assigned to the 36 associations demonstrating significant findings. The authors also excluded 61 additional factors due to inconsistencies in methodology or reporting.
5. Subgroup analyses determined the impact of any single study on the pooled effect sizes. The statistical significance of these factors did not change. This analysis supported the validity of the findings of each included study.
6. The inclusion of a PAR calculation demonstrates that as many as 66% of AD cases may result from modifiable risk factors. This data supports the argument that modifiable risk factors are worth addressing to reduce the incidence of AD.

Limitations

1. The authors included only English language studies. This search parameter may limit the body of data such that other cultural, geographical, and lifestyle factors are unexamined.
2. Since factors were stratified categorically, the exploration of dose-dependent relationships was minimal. However, subgroup analyses demonstrated an increased risk of AD in persons with midlife BMI ≥30 and education ≤6–8 years, implying a dose-dependent relationship.
3. Grades of evidence did not necessarily correspond to statistical significance. As such, some claims of high-grade evidence (increased AD risk associated with factors such as heavy smoking, high systolic blood pressure, and low BMI) are somewhat misleading without statistical significance.
4. The clinical significance is difficult to ascertain or explain for some factors; metabolic syndrome and heart disease are significant protective factors, while high BMI in midlife, diabetes in the Asian population, and carotid atherosclerosis are significant risk factors.

Take-Home Points

Promoting positive health behaviors such as a nutritious diet (folate, vitamins C/E, fish), remaining physically active, addressing depression, engaging in cognitive activity, and limiting alcohol consumption as well as treating underlying metabolic conditions such as hypertension, obesity, and diabetes may contribute to modifying the population's AD risk profile.

Practical Application of the Take-Home Points

Geriatric psychiatrists can play a significant role in advocating for interventions addressing modifiable risk factors. Clinicians may also consider partnering with primary care physicians to amplify health interventions across diet, exercise, meditation choices, and chronic conditions.

References

1. Xu W, Tan L, Wang HF, Jiang T, Tan MS, Tan L, Zhao QF, Li JQ, Wang J, Yu JT. Meta-analysis of modifiable risk factors for Alzheimer's disease. J Neurol Neurosurg Psychiatry. 2015;86(12):1299–306.
2. Stroup DF, Berlin JA, Morton SC, Olkin I, Williamson GD, Rennie D, Moher D, Becker BJ, Sipe TA, Thacker SB. Meta-analysis of observational studies in epidemiology: a proposal for reporting. Meta-analysis Of Observational Studies in Epidemiology (MOOSE) group. JAMA. 2000;283(15):2008–12.
3. Moher D, Shamseer L, Clarke M, Ghersi D, Liberati A, Petticrew M, Shekelle P, Stewart LA, PRISMA-P Group. Preferred reporting items for systematic review and meta-analysis protocols (PRISMA-P) 2015 statement. Syst Rev. 2015;4(1):1.
4. Green S, McDonald S. Cochrane collaboration: more than systematic reviews? Intern Med J. 2005;35(1):3–4.
5. Wells G, Shea B, O'Connell D, Peterson J, Welch V, Losos M, Tugwell P, Ga SW, Zello G, Petersen J. The Newcastle-Ottawa Scale (NOS) for assessing the quality of nonrandomised studies in meta-analyses 2014. https://web.archive.org/web/20210716121605id_/http://www3.med.unipmn.it/dispense_ebm/2009-2010/Corso%20Perfezionamento%20EBM_Faggiano/NOS_oxford.pdf. Accessed on 17 Feb 2022.
6. Duval S, Tweedie R. Trim and fill: a simple funnel-plot-based method of testing and adjusting for publication bias in meta-analysis. Biometrics. 2000;56(2):455–63.

Chapter 62
Memantine for Alzheimer's Disease: An Updated Systematic Review and Meta-analysis

Emily B. Phelps and Sandra Swantek

Authors of the Original Article Taro Kishi, Shinji Matsunaga, Kazuto Oya, Ikuo Nomura, Toshikazu Ikuta, Nakao Iwata.

Journal Published *Journal of Alzheimer's Disease.*

Year of Publication 2017.

Type of Study Systematic review, meta-analysis.

Funding Sources None listed. All authors reported nothing to disclose.

Objectives To conduct a systematic review and meta-analysis of the literature on the efficacy and safety of memantine in AD [1].

Methods This meta-analysis was conducted according to the Preferred Reporting Items for Systematic Reviews and Meta-Analyses (PRISMA) guidelines and was registered with PROSPERO. Two of the authors independently searched the following databases – MEDLINE, Cochrane Library, Scopus, and PsycINFO – without any language restrictions and using specific search terms. They also searched clinical trial registries including clinicaltrials.gov, ISRCTN registry, and International Clinical Trials Registry Platform. The authors only included randomized placebo-controlled or usual case-controlled trials among individuals with AD that lasted for

E. B. Phelps
Mount Sinai Hospital, New York, NY, USA
e-mail: Emily.Phelps@mountsinai.edu

S. Swantek (✉)
Rush Medical College, Chicago, IL, USA
e-mail: Sandra_Swantek@Rush.edu

R. R. Tampi et al. (eds.), *Essential Reviews in Geriatric Psychiatry*,
https://doi.org/10.1007/978-3-030-94960-0_62

more than 2 weeks. The investigators included studies with memantine monotherapy or combination therapy with an acetylcholinesterase inhibitor. The three authors independently selected the studies based on the inclusion/exclusion criteria. Additionally, the references of included articles and review articles were searched for additional published and unpublished studies, including conference abstracts. Two authors independently extracted data from the included studies. Intention-to-treat (ITT) analysis or a full analysis set (FAS) population was completed whenever possible. In situations where such data was unavailable, the results for observed case (OC) analysis were extracted from each of the studies. The investigators contacted the investigators or companies and requested additional data when the information required for a meta-analysis were missing from the relevant studies. The meta-analysis was conducted using Review Manager software. The authors selected a random-effects model for this meta-analysis because of the potential heterogeneity across the different studies. For the dichotomous outcomes, risk ratios (RRs) with 95% confidence intervals (CIs) were calculated. The investigators calculated the number needed to harm (NNH) when the random-effects model showed significant differences between groups. Mean difference (MD) or standard MD (SMD) was used to analyze continuous outcomes. The methodological quality of the trials was assessed using the Cochrane risk-of-bias criteria. The heterogeneity among the studies was assessed using the I^2 statistic with $I^2 \geq 50\%$ reflecting significant heterogeneity. Sensitivity analyses were conducted to detect confounding factors of primary outcomes for efficacy. The authors detected potential publication bias using funnel plots, with Egger's regression test used to detect publication bias in meta-analyses.

The study's primary outcomes were improved cognitive function, a reduction in behavioral disturbances, and all-cause discontinuation. Secondary outcomes were improved cognition and function based on the various standardized scales, treatment discontinuation due to inefficacy, treatment discontinuation due to adverse events, and the incidence of individual adverse events. For studies with three arms (memantine 10 mg a day, memantine 20 mg a day, and placebo), data for the memantine 10 mg a day arm was combined with that of the memantine 20 mg a day arm.

Results The authors identified a total of 30 studies in the literature search: memantine monotherapy versus placebo ($N = 11$) and combination therapy with memantine and cholinesterase inhibitors (ChEIs) versus ChEIs monotherapy ($N = 17$). Seven of the 30 studies were not published in the English language. Three studies did not report whether they provided memantine monotherapy or combination therapy, and these studies were excluded from the meta-analysis. All 11 of the monotherapy studies were RCTs. All but 1 of the 11 studies was sponsored by a pharmaceutical company. Of the 17 combination studies, 12 were RCTs and 5 were open-label studies. All but 4 of the 17 combination studies were sponsored by a pharmaceutical company.

For the monotherapy trials, memantine when compared to placebo showed significant improvements in cognitive function scores ($P < 0.00001$) and behavioral disturbances scores ($P = 0.01$). The investigators did not find any evidence for publication bias for cognitive function scores or behavioral disturbances score in each treatment group. Additionally, they did not detect any heterogeneity with respect to cognitive function scores ($I^2 = 35\%$) or any confounding factors during the sensitivity analyses. For the behavioral disturbances score, the investigators identified heterogeneity ($I^2 = 52\%$). However, among individuals with moderate-severe AD, heterogeneity was not detected ($I^2 = 36\%$). The use of memantine resulted in a significant reduction in the behavioral disturbances score compared to the placebo ($P = 0.003$). Meta-regression analysis indicated that the effect size for the memantine group for cognitive function scores was associated with Mini-Mental State Examination (MMSE) scores at baseline ($P = 0.0136$) and the percentage of male participants ($P = 0.0199$). The investigators identified no significant differences in all-cause discontinuation rates between memantine and placebo treatment groups (RR = 0.94, $P = 0.47$). There was no evidence for publication bias for all-cause discontinuation in each treatment group. The use of memantine was associated with greater incidence of dizziness (RR = 1.53, $P = 0.04$, NNH = 50) and somnolence (RR = 2.36, $P = 0.05$, NNH = not significant) when compared to placebo. The use of memantine was associated with a lower incidence of agitation (RR = 0.70, $P = 0.03$, NNH = not significant), increased blood potassium (RR = 0.20, $P = 0.05$, NNH = not significant), and psychotic symptoms (RR = 0.50, $P = 0.03$, NNH = not significant) when compared to placebo. The investigator did not find any significant differences in other adverse events between the two treatment groups.

In the combination therapy trials, the investigators found a trend toward superiority for combination treatment in improving cognitive function scores compared to ChEI monotherapy ($P = 0.06$). Also, the combination therapy was superior to ChEI monotherapy in reducing behavioral disturbances scores ($P = 0.02$). No publication bias was noted for cognitive function scores, whereas publication bias was identified for the behavior disturbances score ($P = 0.0264$). Combination therapy was superior to ChEI monotherapy for the severe impairment battery (SIB) score, clinical global impression score, verbal fluency scores, and discontinuation due to inefficacy. The investigators noted heterogeneity for cognitive function scores ($I^2 = 56\%$). Subgroup analysis showed superiority for combination therapy over ChEI monotherapy on cognitive function in the memantine extended-release subgroup ($P = 0.007$), donepezil subgroup ($P = 0.006$), and ChEIs other than galantamine subgroup ($P = 0.01$). The combination of memantine and galantamine was inferior to ChEI monotherapy ($P = 0.05$). Heterogeneity was also noted for behavioral disturbances score ($I^2 = 77\%$). The combination therapy was superior to ChEI monotherapy in reducing behavioral disturbances in the double-blind, placebo-controlled subgroup ($P = 0.04$) and the memantine extended-release subgroup ($P = 0.01$). The effect size of combination therapy for the behavioral disturbances score was associated with the study duration ($P = 0.0264$). The investigators found no significant difference in all-cause discontinuation rates between all treatment groups (RR = 1.00, $P = 0.98$). There was no publication bias noted for all-cause discontinuation in each treatment group. The combination treatment was associated with a greater incidence of at least one adverse event (RR = 1.05, $P = 0.05$,

NNH = 33), somnolence (RR = 2.29, $P = 0.008$, NNH = not significant), and weight increase (RR = 2.31, $P = 0.006$, NNH = 33) when compared to ChEI monotherapy. There were no significant differences noted in other adverse events between the treatment groups.

Conclusions This systematic review and meta-analysis indicates that memantine is fairly well tolerated, improves cognition, and reduces behavioral disturbances among individuals with AD both as monotherapy and in combination with ChEIs.

Strengths of the Study

1. According to the Preferred Reporting Items for Systematic Reviews and Meta-Analyses guidelines, this meta-analysis was conducted and was registered with PROSPERO.
2. A total of 30 studies: Memantine monotherapy versus placebo ($N = 11$) and combination therapy with memantine and cholinesterase inhibitors (ChEIs) versus ChEI monotherapy ($N = 17$) were included in the review.
3. The methodological quality of the trials was assessed using the Cochrane risk-of-bias criteria.
4. The heterogeneity among the studies was assessed using the I^2 statistic with $I^2 \geq 50\%$ reflecting significant heterogeneity.
5. Sensitivity analyses were conducted to detect confounding factors of primary outcomes for efficacy.
6. Potential publication bias was detected using funnel plots, with Egger's regression test used to detect publication bias in meta-analyses.

Limitations

1. As 10 of the 11 monotherapy studies were sponsored by a pharmaceutical company and 13 of the 17 combination studies were sponsored by a pharmaceutical company, there could be significant sponsorship bias in this systematic review and meta-analysis.
2. There was significant heterogeneity among the included studies based on differences in patient characteristics, symptom severity, inclusion criteria, race, ethnicity, and study duration.
3. Both the monotherapy and combination studies had a short duration (28.4 weeks and 29.4, respectively) and less male participants (33.9% and 47.0%, respectively).
4. There was publication bias noted for the behavior disturbances score in the combined studies.

Take-Home Points

1. Memantine monotherapy improves cognition and behavioral disturbances when compared to placebo among individuals with AD.
2. In combination with ChEIs, other than galantamine, memorization improves cognition among individuals with AD compared to ChEI monotherapy. Also, the combination therapy was superior to ChEI monotherapy in reducing behavioral disturbances.
3. Memantine monotherapy appears to be as well tolerated as placebo among individuals with AD. Combination therapy of memantine with a ChEI was as well-tolerated as ChEI monotherapy.

Practical Application of the Take-Home Points

Among individuals with AD, memantine monotherapy and combination treatment with a ChEIs other than galantamine improve cognition and behavioral disturbances and are relatively well-tolerated. When combining memantine with a ChEIs among individuals with AD, donepezil would be the preferred ChEI of choice.

Reference

1. Kishi T, Matsunaga S, Oya K, Nomura I, Ikuta T, Iwata N. Memantine for Alzheimer's disease: an updated systematic review and meta-analysis. J Alzheimers Dis. 2017;60(2):401–25.

Chapter 63
Update on the Risk of Motor Vehicle Collision or Driving Impairment with Dementia: A Collaborative International Systematic Review and Meta-analysis

Emily B. Phelps and Sandra Swantek

Authors of the Original Article Justin N Chee, Mark J Rapoport, Frank Molnar, Nathan Herrmann, Desmond O'Neill, Richard Marottoli, Sara Mitchell, Mark Tant, Jamie Dow, Debbie Ayotte, Krista L Lanctôt, Regina McFadden, John-Paul Taylor, Paul C Donaghy, Kirsty Olsen, Sherrilene Classen, Yoassry Elzohairy, David B Carr.

Journal Published *American Journal of Geriatric Psychiatry.*

Year of Publication 2017.

Type of Study Systematic review and meta-analysis.

Funding Sources Canadian Institutes of Health Research (KRS grant 339665).

Objectives To conduct a systematic review and meta-analysis on the risk of motor vehicle collision (MVC) or driving impairment among individuals with dementia as measured by on-road testing in order to update the international guidelines on driving with dementia [1].

Methods The investigators included primary papers that were published between 2005 and 2015. In addition, they searched the bibliographies of systematic reviews for additional studies. The investigators excluded reviews, editorials, conference

E. B. Phelps
Mount Sinai Hospital, New York, NY, USA
e-mail: Emily.Phelps@mountsinai.edu

S. Swantek (✉)
Rush Medical College, Chicago, IL, USA
e-mail: Sandra_Swantek@Rush.edu

R. R. Tampi et al. (eds.), *Essential Reviews in Geriatric Psychiatry*,
https://doi.org/10.1007/978-3-030-94960-0_63

proceedings, dissertations, reports that were not available in English, studies conducted among individuals with mild cognitive impairment (MCI) or among older adults without dementia, and studies that used driving simulators. The also excluded studies that used the same group of participants to report on MVC risk or driving impairment. Authors with relevant publications were not allowed to screen or extract data from their own publications.

The investigators searched Ovid MEDLINE In-Process and Other Non-Indexed Citations (October 13, 2015), Ovid MEDLINE without Revisions (1990–October Week 1, 2015), and Ovid MEDLINE (1990–1995) and subsequently adapted for CINAHL (1990–2015), Scopus (1990–2015), Cochrane Central Register of Controlled Trials (CENTRAL) (1990–2015), EMBASE (1990–2015), PsycINFO (1990–2015), and the Transportation Research Information Database (1990–2015) with the last search being run on October 30, 2015.

The investigators included studies that involved individuals with dementia that was diagnosed using any well-established criteria or as a result of a referral from a healthcare practitioner. In addition, there was no restriction based on the age of the participants or with regard to the severity of dementia. The primary outcome measures for the review were road MVCs (self- or informant-reported data and state/government accident registries and skill performance and road-test failure rates that were determined using on-road driving assessments on formal testing or in naturalistic environments). Eligible studies were independently identified by pairs of reviewers. Any disagreements between reviewers were resolved by consensus or by utilizing a third-party arbiter among the coauthors.

The quality of evidence in each of the included studies was assessed using an article grading guideline (Class I, II, III, or IV) that was developed following an in-person meeting of ten of the coauthors. The specific rating that was assigned to each of the included studies was arrived at by consensus.

The investigators conducted a meta-analysis that compared individuals with and without dementia and computed the risk ratio (RR) and 95% confidence interval (CI) associated with failing an on-road assessment. The meta-analysis was conducted using a DerSimonian and Laird random-effects model. The χ^2 test and I^2 statistic were used to determine the heterogeneity and its magnitude in the included studies.

Results The investigators included a total of nine studies in the final analysis. Eight of the studies were qualitatively described with four of the that presented a failure rate for on-road assessments being quantitatively pooled in a meta-analysis.

The two studies that examined MVC risk among individuals with dementia did not find any difference between the healthy comparison group and individuals with dementia on the percentage of individuals with MVCs or the number of MVCs per year per 10,000 miles driven in the past year (Class I). Another study found that there were no differences between the dementia group and the healthy comparison group in the percentage of individuals with MVCs, MVC rate per driver per year, or total number of MVCs in the 3 years before a baseline assessment (Class I).

However, the total number of MVCs per 1000 miles driven per week was 4.72 times higher among individuals in the dementia group (8.78 MVCs) when compared to the healthy comparison group (1.86 MVCs; $P < 0.01$). The investigators also found that 3 years after the baseline assessment, the percentage of MVCs in the healthy comparison group was 11.0 times higher than that of the dementia group (11% versus 1%; $P < 0.05$). However, this difference was nullified after the distance driven per week was corrected.

Measures of on-road performance were reported in all nine of the included studies. Seven of the nine studies presented driving impairment outcomes, four studies reported on on-road assessment failure rates, and two studies reported on both the outcomes. Among seven of the studies that examined driving impairment, one study was rated as Class I for quality, whereas the other six trials were rated as Class IIb for quality. A total of six of the seven studies showed a reduced performance on at least one measure of driving behavior among individuals with dementia when compared to healthy comparators. The effect sizes in these studies ranged between 0.26 and 3.61. The effect sizes were noted to be large for 19 of the outcomes (landmark/sign identification, number of lost trips, etc.) and medium for 10 of the outcomes (total safety errors, lane observance errors, etc.)

The meta-analysis included four studies that included data for on-road failure rate. Two of the studies were rated as Class I for quality, and two studies were rated as Class IIb for quality. The results indicated that individuals with dementia were much more likely to fail a road assessment than healthy comparison group (RR: 10.77, 95% CI: 3.00–38.62, $z = 3.65$, $P < 0.001$). The investigators did not find any significant heterogeneity among the study findings ($\chi^2 = 1.50$, $P = 0.68$, $I^2 = 0\%$). Additionally, there was no publication bias noted as there were no asymmetries in the funnel plot. One study did not conceptualize marginal or probably safe/unsafe cases separately than passing or failing cases, which differed from the three other studies. When the sensitivity analysis was completed without including data from this study, the results were similar (RR: 6.77, 95% CI: 1.24–36.96, $z = 2.21$, $P < 0.03$). There was no significant heterogeneity noted ($\chi^2 = 0.80$, $P = 0.67$, $I^2 = 0\%$). The two studies that presented failure rates separately for the clinical dementia rating scale (CDR) 0.5, CDR 1, and control participants found that the absolute increase in risk for CDR 0.5 ranged from 11% to 12% which corresponded with a relative risk of 5–11%. The absolute increase in risk for CDR 1 ranged from 18% to 22% which corresponded with a relative risk of 8–20%.

Conclusions Data from two studies indicated that individuals with dementia have a fourfold increase in MVCs per 1000 miles driven per week in the 3 years prior to baseline assessment. Additionally, medium to large effects were noted for the presence of dementia on driving abilities in six of the seven seven recent studies that evaluated driving impairment. Furthermore, individuals with dementia were more likely to fail a road test than healthy controls. Individuals with even mild stages of dementia are at higher risk for failing a performance-based road test and of demonstrating impaired driving abilities on the road.

Strengths of the Study

1. This was a well-designed and well-conducted systematic review and meta-analysis.
2. The results are easy to interpret and the discussion is robust with strengths and weaknesses of the paper being clearly discussed.
3. This study identified an important gap in the literature where there is very little available data on drivers with moderate dementia.

Limitations of the Study

1. Only nine studies included in the final review.
2. The investigators did not search gray literature, i.e., conference presentations and proceedings, dissertations and unpublished manuscripts, and technical reports, and did not include papers that were published in languages other than in English.
3. Individuals with mild cognitive impairment were not included in the review [2].
4. Only one of the included studies was longitudinal.
5. In all the included studies, the control groups were younger than the dementia groups. In addition, there were less men in the control groups when compared to the dementia group, in all but one study.
6. There may be some reporting bias in the studies as many individuals may stop driving independently or are taken off the road prior to an MVC. In addition, there may be underreporting of MVCs among individuals with dementia.
7. There is a significant risk for type II error (error of omission/false negative) as the sample sizes in these studies were small.

Take-Home Points

Individuals with dementia exhibit on-road driving impairment, driving errors, and failure on on-road tests when compared to controls. These risks are most likely due to memory impairment, visuospatial perception difficulties, reduced hand-eye coordination, and delayed reaction time.

Practical Application of the Take-Home Points

Clinicians evaluating individuals with dementia should discuss driving abilities with the individual with dementia and their caregivers. The discussion should involve a review of available evidence regarding this topic, the importance of executive dysfunction, the caregiver concern about driving, and the pros and cons of continued driving as dementia is a progressive illness. Specialized on-road testing should be recommended when driving safety is uncertain in individuals with dementia.

References

1. Chee JN, Rapoport MJ, Molnar F, Herrmann N, O'Neill D, Marottoli R, Mitchell S, Tant M, Dow J, Ayotte D, Lanctôt KL, McFadden R, Taylor JP, Donaghy PC, Olsen K, Classen S, Elzohairy Y, Carr DB. Update on the risk of motor vehicle collision or driving impairment with dementia: a collaborative international systematic review and meta-analysis. Am J Geriatr Psychiatry. 2017;25(12):1376–90.
2. Rapoport MJ, Naglie G, Herrmann N, Zucchero Sarracini C, Mulsant BH, Frank C, Kiss A, Seitz D, Vrkljan B, Masellis M, Tang-Wai D, Pimlott N, Molnar F. Developing physician consensus on the reporting of patients with mild cognitive impairment and mild dementia to transportation authorities in a region with mandatory reporting legislation. Am J Geriatr Psychiatry. 2014;22(12):1530–43.

Chapter 64
Pharmacological Interventions for Apathy in Alzheimer's Disease

Jasmine Singh and Marianne Klugheit

Authors of the original article Myuri T Ruthirakuhan, Nathan Herrmann, Eleenor H Abraham, Sarah Chan and Krista L Lanctôt

Journal published *Cochrane Database of Systematic Reviews*

Year of publication 2018

Type of study systematic review and meta-analysis

Funding sources no external funding sources. National Institute of Health Research (NIHR) via Cochrane infrastructure funding to Cochrane dementia and cognitive impairment group

Objectives

1. The investigators proposed to assess the efficacy and safety of pharmacotherapies for the treatment of apathy among individuals with Alzheimer's disease (AD) [1].
2. The investigators also wanted to assess the effect of pharmacotherapies on apathy for other primary outcomes in the treatment of AD.

J. Singh
Banner Health Tucson, Tucson, AZ, USA
e-mail: jasminesingh@psychiatry.arizona.edu

M. Klugheit (✉)
Banner University of Arizona College of Medicine Department of Psychiatry, Tucson, AZ, USA

Southern AZ VA Health Care System, Tucson, AZ, USA

R. R. Tampi et al. (eds.), *Essential Reviews in Geriatric Psychiatry*,
https://doi.org/10.1007/978-3-030-94960-0_64

Methods The investigators electronically searched the Specialized Register of the Cochrane Dementia and Cognitive Improvement Group (ALOIS), MEDLINE, Embase, CINAHL, PsycINFO, LILACS, ClinicalTrials.gov, and the World Health Organization (WHO) portal, ICTRP, on May 17, 2017, for double-blind, randomized, placebo-controlled trials (RCTs) that investigated apathy as a primary or secondary outcome among individuals with AD. The investigators also included parallel and crossover RCTs that compared two or more medications for treating apathy among individuals with AD or mixed AD.

Three reviewers independently screened citations identified from the literature search. They also independently assessed these articles based on the predetermined criteria. The authors resolved any disagreements by discussion, involving the third reviewer when necessary to resolve disagreements. They contacted the original study authors for further information when necessary.

The three reviewers independently extracted the data from the identified articles using a data extraction form. Missing data was obtained from the study authors whenever possible. One reviewer entered the data into Review Manager 5 (RevMan), and the other reviewer checked data entry for accuracy. Any discrepancies were resolved by consensus.

The risks of bias were assessed by two reviewers independently in accordance with the Cochrane "risk of bias" assessment tool for assessing quality and risk of bias. They then compared the "risk of bias" ratings and resolved discrepancies through discussion with coauthors. The risk of bias based on the assessment tool is divided into three categories: low risk, high risk, and unclear risk. Any studies identified as having a high risk of bias were excluded.

The reviewers used the mean difference with 95% confidence interval (CI) for the measurement of treatment effect from continuous data. For dichotomous data, the measure of treatment effect was the relative risk with a 95% CI. The GRADE rating which takes into account the risk of bias, imprecision, inconsistency, publication bias, and indirectness and then expresses the degree of confidence that the effect estimate is close to the true effect was used to assess the overall quality of evidence for all outcomes.

Results The reviewers included a total of 21 studies involving a total of 6384 participants in the quantitative analyses. All of the trials included were randomized, double-blind, and placebo-controlled. Eighteen of the 21 studies were multicenter trials. All studies included individuals with possible or probable AD according to standardized and accepted diagnostic criteria.

Four studies investigated the effect of a pharmacological treatment on apathy as a primary outcome measure. Three of the studies compared methylphenidate to placebo, whereas the fourth study compared modafinil to placebo.

Methylphenidate appears to improve apathy when assessed using the apathy evaluation scale (AES) [three studies, $n = 145$, mean difference (MD) = −4.99, 95% CI -9.55 to −0.43, low quality evidence], but not when assessed using the neuropsychiatric inventory (NPI)-apathy subscale, which was used by two of the three studies [two studies, $n = 85$, MD = −0.08, 95% CI −3.85 to 3.69, low quality evidence].

Methylphenidate may also improve cognition [three studies, $n = 145$, MD = 1.98, 95% CI 1.06 to 2.91, moderate quality evidence] and probably improves instrumental activities of daily living [one study, $n = 60$, MD = 2.30, 95% CI 0.74 to 3.86, $P = 0.004$, moderate quality evidence] when compared to placebo. The investigators did not find difference between methylphenidate and placebo in the risk of developing an adverse event [three studies, $n = 145$, RR = 1.28, 95% CI 0.67 to 2.42, low quality evidence]. The duration of the study did not change the results in terms of efficacy or the development of adverse effects. The only study of modafinil was small ($n = 22$) and of low quality to definitely determine the effect of modafinil on apathy assessed using the FrSBe-apathy subscale [MD = 0.27, 95% CI −3.51 to 4.05] when compared to placebo. There was only one adverse effect noted in the modafinil group when compared to none in the placebo group.

Seventeen studies investigated apathy as a secondary outcome. There were six studies of cholinesterase inhibitors (ChEIs), one study of ChEI discontinuation, two studies of antipsychotics, one study of antipsychotic discontinuation, two studies of antidepressants, one study of mibampator, 1 study of semagacestat and 3 studies of Cholinesterase inhibitors (ChEIs) may slightly improve apathy when compared to placebo (six studies, $n = 3598$, MD = −0.40, 95% CI −0.80 to −0.00, low quality evidence). When currently approved ChEIs are taken into account, they may have little or no effect on apathy when compared to placebo (three studies, $n = 2531$, MD = −0.21, 95% CI −0.85 to 0.43, $P = 0.29$, low quality evidence). Metrifonate may improve apathy compared to placebo (three studies, $n = 1067$, MD = −0.63, 95% CI −0.98 to −0.29, $P > 0.001$, low quality evidence). Among individuals with moderate AD, ChEIs may slightly improve apathy compared to placebo (four studies, $n = 3100$, MD = −0.43, 95% CI −0.79 to −0.07, $P = 0.02$, low quality evidence). Among individuals with severe AD, ChEIs may improve apathy when compared to placebo (two studies, $n = 498$, MD = −0.36, 95% CI −1.82 to 1.10, $P = 0.63$, low quality evidence).

Only one study that investigated the discontinuation of ChEIs compared to continuation of ChEIs met the inclusion criteria. All participants in this trial were long-term ChEI users, i.e., more than 2 years' duration. Discontinuing ChEIs appeared to improve apathy slightly when compared to continuing the ChEI, based on the NPI-apathy subscale (one study, $n = 40$, MD = 1.11, 95% −0.88 to 3.10, $P = 0.28$, low quality evidence).

Only two studies that compared antipsychotics to placebo with apathy as a secondary outcome met the inclusion criteria and hence a meta-analysis was not done. Antipsychotic use appeared to slightly worsen apathy when compared to placebo [two studies, $n = 1070$, standardized mean difference (SMD) = 0.14, 95% CI −0.00 to 0.28, $P = 0.05$, low quality evidence].

Only one study that compared the continuation of antipsychotics to discontinuation of antipsychotics with apathy as a secondary outcome met the inclusion criteria. The continuation of antipsychotic use may slightly improve apathy when compared to antipsychotic discontinuation (placebo) [one study, $n = 55$, MD = −0.24, 95% CI −0.51 to 0.03, $P = 0.08$, low quality evidence].

Only two studies that compared antidepressants to placebo with apathy as a secondary outcome met the inclusion criteria. It was unclear if antidepressants improve apathy when compared to placebo over the duration of treatment (two studies, $n = 126$, MD = −1.24, 95% −1.44 to −1.04, $P < 0.00001$, low quality evidence).

Only one study that compared mibampator to placebo with apathy as a secondary outcome met the inclusion criteria. It was unclear if mibampator improved apathy when compared to placebo (one study, $n = 132$, MD = −1.20, 95% −1.94 to −0.46, $P = 0.001$, low quality evidence).

Only one study that compared semagacestat to placebo with apathy as a secondary outcome met the inclusion criteria. Semagacestat appeared to worsen apathy when compared to placebo (one study, $n = 939$, MD = 0.20, 95% CI 0.15 to 0.25, $P < 0.001$, low quality evidence).

Only three studies that compared valproate to placebo with apathy as a secondary outcome met the inclusion criteria. There appeared to be little or no difference between treatment groups in the change in apathy over the duration of treatment [three studies, $n = 257$, standardized mean difference (SMD) = 0.02, 95% CI −0.23 to 0.26, $P = 0.88$, low quality evidence].

Conclusions Available data from this systematic review and meta-analysis although of low quality indicates that methylphenidate may improve apathy when compared to placebo among individuals with AD and is well tolerated. Moderate quality of evidence indicates that methylphenidate may also improve both cognition and function among individuals with AD. In studies where apathy was a secondary outcome, this systematic review and meta-analysis found that following evidence: Low quality evidence indicates that the use of ChEI may slightly improve apathy (small effect size) when compared to placebo among individuals with AD. Low quality evidence indicates that similar benefits for ChEI were noted among individuals with both moderate and severe AD. Data from one antipsychotic discontinuation trial indicates that continued antipsychotic use may slightly improve apathy (small effect size) when compared to antipsychotic discontinuation. Low quality of evidence indicates that valproate demonstrated little or no difference in apathy among individuals with AD.

Strengths of Study

1. There was extensive search of the literature using a standardized search strategy.
2. Any conflict in selecting studies for inclusion in this systematic review and meta-analysis was resolved by consensus.
3. The risk of bias among the included studies was limited as the studies were well conducted and well reported.

Limitations of Study

1. Among the included studies where apathy was the primary outcome, the overall quality of the evidence was low. In studies where the apathy was a secondary measure, the nature and quality of the evidence was limited.
2. Ten out of the 21 studies included in the meta-analysis were pharmaceutical industry-sponsored studies. This data may be a source of publication bias as pharmaceutical industry funding is often associated with outcomes that are favorable for the funder of the study.

3. Different scales were used to assess apathy in the included studies, and hence heterogeneity of results is a concern.

Take-home points Apathy is one of the most common neuropsychiatric symptom (NPS) of AD. Available evidence from this systematic review and meta-analysis although of low quality indicates that methylphenidate may improve apathy when compared to placebo among individuals with AD and is well tolerated. Methylphenidate may also improve both cognition and function among these individuals. ChEIs may slightly improve apathy when compared to placebo among individuals with AD and can equally benefit individuals with both moderate and severe AD. One antipsychotic discontinuation trial indicated that continued antipsychotic use may slightly improve apathy when compared to antipsychotic discontinuation among individuals with AD.

When compared to the current systematic review and meta-analysis, how does the evidence in the literature for the pharmacotherapy for apathy in AD stack up? We have included three additional studies that have addressed this question. In a systematic review by Berman et al. [2], the authors reviewed studies that used apathy outcome scales to document results of pharmacologic treatments for apathy. The investigators found that there is limited evidence for the efficiency of pharmacotherapy for treatment of apathy in dementia. The best results were found for acetylcholinesterase inhibitors with some evidence for efficacy for memantine but less evidence for the efficacy for stimulants, calcium antagonists, and antipsychotics. There was no evidence to support the use of antidepressants or anticonvulsants. The quality of research studies included was modest. A systematic review by Harrison et al. [3] evaluated the evidence for the efficacy of pharmacotherapies for apathy in dementia from studies since 2013. The authors did not find benefits for acetylcholinesterase inhibitors and memantine in recent studies. Antidepressants had mixed results with positive effects for apathy shown only for agomelatine whereas stimulants, analgesics, and oxytocin study results were found to be inconclusive. In the antipsychotic review, they found positive effects only in combination with nonpharmacological approaches. The limitations of this review included relatively few studies assessing specifically assessing apathy as an outcome, and none of the studies evaluated outcomes for emotional, motivational, and behavioral components of apathy. A systematic review and meta-analysis conducted by Sepehry et al. [4] that investigated pharmacological therapy for apathy in AD included 15 RCTs of which 11 were analyzed quantitatively. The drugs that were included were cholinesterase inhibitors, memantine, and psychostimulants. The investigators found no significant treatment effect in favor of any of the drugs.

Practical applications of the take-home points When individuals with AD present with apathy as symptoms, the use of methylphenidate may be appropriate in patients who do not have contraindications for the use of this medication which are open angle glaucoma, the concomitant use of monoamine oxidase inhibitors, hypertension, and other cardiovascular disorders. The use of this medication may also benefit cognition and function among individuals with AD. If methylphenidate does not help, ChEIs may benefit these individuals with apathy if this class of medication has not already been tried. A possibility for the treatment of apathy in AD is to combine methylphenidate and ChEIs if no contraindications exist.

References

1. Ruthirakuhan MT, Herrmann N, Abraham EH, Chan S, Lanctôt KL. Pharmacological interventions for apathy in Alzheimer's disease. Cochrane Database Syst Rev. 2018;5(5):CD012197.
2. Berman K, Brodaty H, Withall A, Seeher K. Pharmacologic treatment of apathy in dementia. Am J Geriatr Psychiatry. 2012;20(2):104–22.
3. Harrison F, Aerts L, Brodaty H. Apathy in dementia: systematic review of recent evidence on pharmacological treatments. Curr Psychiatry Rep. 2016;18(11):103.
4. Sepehry AA, Sarai M, Hsiung GR. Pharmacological therapy for apathy in Alzheimer's disease: a systematic review and meta-analysis. Can J Neurol Sci. 2017;44(3):267–75. https://doi.org/10.1017/cjn.2016.4.

Part XI
Sleep Disorders

Chapter 65
Behavioral and Pharmacological Therapies for Late-Life Insomnia: A Randomized Controlled Trial

Maureen Waweru and Seetha Chandrasekhara

Authors of the original article Charles M. Morin, Cheryl Colecchi, Jackie Stone, Rakesh Sood, Douglas Brink

Journal published *Journal of the American Medical Association*

Year of publication 1999

Type of study Randomized controlled study

Funding sources National Institute of Mental Health

Objectives The objective of the study was to evaluate whether behavioral or pharmacological treatment either alone or when combined together would lead to the best outcomes on various sleep measures among older adults with insomnia [1].

Methods Recruitment of participants was accomplished through advertisements and physician inquiries. Participants who were aged 55 or older and reported insomnia (onset latency and/or maintenance disruption) for a minimum of three nights per week for 6 months with at least one negative complaint (fatigue, mood disturbance, impaired functioning) were included. Diagnosis was based off the criteria for primary and chronic insomnia from the *Diagnostic and Statistical Manual for Mental Disorders* (*DSMIII-R*) and also the *International Classification of Sleep Disorders*. Those whose insomnia was related to a medical condition or medication and were

M. Waweru
Hospital at University of Pennsylvania, Philadelphia, PA, USA

S. Chandrasekhara (✉)
Lewis Katz School of Medicine at Temple University, Philadelphia, PA, USA
e-mail: Seetha.Chandrasekhara@tuhs.temple.edu

R. R. Tampi et al. (eds.), *Essential Reviews in Geriatric Psychiatry*,
https://doi.org/10.1007/978-3-030-94960-0_65

diagnosed with sleep apnea (apnea-hypopnea index >15) or periodic limb movement (myoclonic index with arousal >15) or had regular psychotropic (including hypnotic) use were not included. Individuals currently in psychotherapy, with cognitive impairment (Mini-Mental State Examination <23), or with severe psychopathology (including major depression) based on Brief Symptom Inventory self-report and Structured Clinical Interview from the DSMIII-R were excluded from the study.

A multistep screening process was conducted with the first step using a telephonic screen, sleep history interview, medical history (with physical examination), and psychological assessment. Evaluations were conducted by a board-certified sleep specialist, physician, and clinical psychologist who met regularly to ensure that participants met criteria for inclusion. Of the 163 individuals included for further evaluation after recruitment, 48 were excluded due to psychopathology ($n = 9$), medical problems ($n = 6$), another suspected sleep disorder ($n = 9$), lack of meeting insomnia criteria ($n = 3$), or lack of interest/consistent use of sleeping agents ($n = 21$). After the first step, 115 individuals were evaluated using polysomnography which led to a further 37 adults being excluded due to sleep apnea ($n = 23$), periodic limb movements ($n = 6$), a combination of the prior two disorders ($n = 2$), no insomnia recorded ($n = 3$), or another medical/psychiatric condition or lack of interest ($n = 3$). This led to a final 78 participants who provided consent for inclusion.

Demographically, the 78 participants randomized were community-dwelling and had a mean age of 65 years and an average education level of 14.4 years (SD = 2.5 years). More women ($n = 50$, 64.1%) were included for randomization. Participants were mostly married ($n = 53$, 67.9%) with a significant number being retired ($n = 37$, 47.4%). Majority of participants were identified as white ($n = 70$, 89.7%) with a smaller number of Black ($n = 7$, 9%) and Native American ($n = 1$, 1.3%) participants.

Individuals who were randomized reported an average of 16.8 years (SD = 16.9 years) of insomnia which included mixed sleep-onset and maintenance insomnia ($n = 49$, 62.8%), sleep maintenance insomnia ($n = 22$, 28.2%), and sleep-onset insomnia ($n = 5$, 6.4%). Sixty individuals reported previous sleep medication use. Participants were randomized into a cognitive behavioral therapy (CBT) group ($n = 18$), pharmacotherapy (PCT) group ($n = 20$), combined CBT + PCT group ($n = 20$), or placebo group ($n = 20$). CBT was provided by a licensed clinical psychologist or postdoctoral psychology fellow with prior treatment experience in a group format using manual-based treatment including sleep restriction therapy, stimulus control procedures, and education regarding sleep and aging. Due to this, all 78 participants were placed in clusters of four to six individuals within their respective intervention arm. The CBT group was unable to be blinded due to the organization required for treatment. Sessions were recorded and reviewed in order to ensure adherence.

Medication used for treatment of insomnia was temazepam (7.5 mg–30 mg), and participants were informed to use the medication an hour before bedtime. They were also informed to use the medication at minimum two to three nights per week.

All participants randomized to receive medication (both single and combined with CBT) or placebo were blinded, and evaluators were blinded as well. Participants met weekly with a physician for consultation to assess medication use, response, and side effects. Physicians were also able to provide education regarding late-life sleep changes and general encouragement while being careful to not include any behavioral recommendations. Those participants in the placebo group were offered active treatment after the 3-month follow-up period.

Outcome measures from sleep diaries, polysomnography, and clinical rating scales were obtained in order to determine which treatment produced greater short-term and long-term effects on both subjective and objective data. Outpatient treatment lasted 8 weeks with follow-ups conducted at 3, 12, and 24 months. Sleep diary outcome measures (bedtime, arising time, sleep-onset latency, wake after sleep onset, medication intake) were collected from 2 weeks prior to starting treatment, during the 8 weeks of active treatment, and for 2 weeks at the subsequent follow-ups. Main outcome measures were amount of time awake after sleep onset, total wake time, total sleep time, and sleep efficiency (ratio of total time asleep to actual time in bed multiplied by 100). This was used to assess the quality of sleep within participants' home environment and better understand subjective perception of sleep.

Polysomnography was conducted by a blinded, experienced technician for three consecutive nights in a sleep lab within 2 weeks of initiating treatment and at the end of treatment. Outcome measures were averaged from the second and third night of pretreatment and posttreatment measurements to allow for participants to acclimate to the lab environment. Clinical scales included ratings using a five-point scale to assess severity in various areas (sleep onset, sleep maintenance, early morning awakenings, daytime functional interference, noticeable impairment, distress/concern, satisfaction with current sleep pattern). These items were then translated to a composite score of the previously seven stated areas (range 5–35, increased severity with higher score). Follow-up assessments were obtained to determine degree of improvement. The Sleep Impairment Index (SII) as a collateral outcome measure for treatment was completed by participants, their significant others, and a clinician (pre- and posttreatment).

Results Seventy-one of the 78 participants completed the treatment protocol. Six withdrew before the mid-treatment phase which included three participants from the PCT group (discontinued because of adverse effects), one participant from the CBT + PCT group (discontinued due to lack of improvement), and two participants from the placebo group (discontinued due to lack of improvement). One placebo group participant withdrew after completing more than half of the assigned treatment, and mid-treatment data was included in analysis.

No significant differences were noted demographically or clinically for those participants who completed the study compared to those who withdrew. Similar outcomes were calculated when measures of withdrawn participants were included versus not included into statistical analyses, but analyses which did not include withdrawn participants were ultimately used. Therefore, results included a total of 72 participants (18 = CBT, 17 = PCT, 19 = CBT + PCT, 18 = placebo).

Analysis of variance of sleep diary data demonstrated significant time effects on all four dependent measures of wake after sleep onset, sleep efficiency, total wake, and total sleep time (all individual dependent measures $P < 0.001$). The three active groups were significantly more improved than those in the placebo condition using post hoc comparisons at posttreatment ($P < 0.05$). Posttreatment wake after sleep values were significantly lower in the active groups compared to placebo ($P < 0.01$). There was no significant difference between the active treatment groups. Reduction of wake after sleep onset was highest for the CBT + PCT (63.5%) along with improvement of sleep efficiency (20.9%). CBT (55%, 16.5%), PCT (46.5%, 10.3%), and placebo (16.9%, 4.4%) followed in both categories, respectively.

Additionally, variance analysis of polysomnographic data demonstrated significant time effects for the four abovementioned dependent measures ($P < 0.001$ for all). Post hoc comparisons for total wake time and sleep efficiency showed that the CBT + PCT yielded more improvement compared to placebo (both = $P < 0.05$). No significant difference was detected between the three active groups. When analyzing clinical ratings, participants and the CBT and CBT + PCT groups provided significantly improved ratings compared to PCT ($P = 0.01$) or placebo ($P = 0.002$).

The authors also performed post hoc comparisons on the sleep impairment index scale and found that subjects in the CBT and combined conditions rated themselves as significantly more improved, more satisfied, and less distressed and felt less interference with daytime functioning than subjects in the PCT or placebo conditions. Comparisons of significant others' ratings and clinicians' ratings showed no difference among the active treatments. The subjects in the CBT condition rated their improvements higher than those in placebo, and those in the combined group rated their improvements greater than those in PCT or placebo ($P < 0.05$ for all). There was no significant difference between PCT and placebo. Improvements in all active treatment groups were reported by assessments from significant others ($P < 0.05$, all groups) and clinicians ($P < 0.05$, all groups) when compared to placebo.

Follow-up analyses only included active treatment groups. Results showed that treatment was maintained during posttreatment assessment in the CBT group as there was no significant change on any of the dependent variables at any of the follow-ups. However, the PCT group showed significant worsening at 24-month follow-up in total wake time ($P = 0.04$), sleep efficiency ($P = 0.03$), and wake after sleep ($P = 0.03$). The CBT + PCT group also demonstrated significant changes at all three follow-ups on measures of total wake time, sleep efficiency, and wake after sleep onset ($P < 0.05$ for all). This was shown as a worsened sleep pattern over time. Clinical ratings analyses (paired t-tests) showed a less favorable self-reported ratings (higher scores) in the CBT group at 12-month follow-up which did not align with significant others' lower scores at 3- and 12-month follow-up. CBT + PCT participants' ratings were higher at 12-month follow-up. No significance was calculated for the PCT group.

A sleep efficiency of greater than 85% was used to determine clinical significance in order to differentiate impaired versus normal sleep. 64.8% (13/19) of participants in the CBT + PCT group met this criterion at posttreatment. 55.6% (10/18) in the CBT group, 47.1% (8/17) in the PCT group, and 22.2% (4/8) in the placebo group also met this criterion with CBT ($p = 0.04$) and CBT + PCT ($P = 0.005$) demonstrating more clinical significance compared to placebo. Using polysomnographic data, CBT ($n = 10$), PCT ($n = 10$), CBT + PCT ($n = 13$), and placebo ($n = 6$) also demonstrated clinical significance, but the finding was not statistically significant ($P = 0.22$). Using the SII, CBT (78%) and CBT + PCT (75%) no longer met diagnostic criteria for insomnia. 56% of PCT participants and 14% of placebo participants also did not meet insomnia diagnostic criteria at posttreatment. More participants in active treatment met the previous criterion ($P < 0.05$ for all) when compared to placebo.

No significance was determined between adherence to treatment between the groups. No significant difference was found between PCT (average 20 mg/night), CBT + PCT (average 16 mg/night), and placebo (average 20 mg/night) for medicated nights for treatment period. Urine drug screen at baseline found one participant in the CBT + PCT group took benzodiazepines. Posttreatment, urine drug screen confirmed adherence for those in PCT and CBT + PCT groups. One participant in the placebo group had traces of benzodiazepine in their urine at posttreatment collection.

Conclusion The findings of this randomized controlled study showed that late-life insomnia in older adults can be managed short term by both behavioral and pharmacological interventions. Long-term effects were seen in the behavioral treatment group only.

Strengths of the Study

1. Randomized, double-blind, and placebo-controlled study design.
2. Jadad score of 5 which indicates that this was high-quality study [2].

Questions Yes (1) No (0)	Was the study described as random?	Was the randomization scheme described and appropriate?	Was the study described as double-blind?	Was the method of double blinding appropriate? (Were both the patient and the assessor appropriately blinded?)	Was there a description of dropouts and withdrawals?	Total score Range of score quality 0–2 Low 3–5 High
Score	1	1	1	1	1	5

3. The inclusion of behavioral treatment in the study separately evaluated from pharmacological intervention
4. The study sample included only older adults (>64 years).
5. Included ratings from participants, significant others, and clinicians in order to better assess any difference in objective and subjective complaints of insomnia

Limitations of the Study

1. A small sample size of 78 participants.
2. A short study period of only 8 weeks of treatment in all four groups.
3. The study does not elaborate on the nature of the adverse effects noted in the PCT group and combined groups that led to dropouts. Although temazepam has been shown to be well tolerated in older adults, it comes with risks of respiratory depression, coma, profound sedation, cognitive impairment, fall risk, and death.
4. Recruitment of participants by newspaper advertisements and letters to physicians which can contribute to selection bias.
5. Reporting bias by participants when collecting sleep diary data.
6. The study did not mention evaluation of substance use disorders which are likely to affect stages of sleep and be misused in individuals with insomnia.

Take-home points This study was effective in studying both pharmacological and behavioral treatments for late-life insomnia in older adults. Further studies are needed to determine how to combine the adequate short-term and long-term treatments to ensure effective management of symptoms.

Practical applications of the take-home points The study of adequate insomnia treatment options for older adults is difficult given the high risk of adverse effects with psychotropic use in this population. Although temazepam may be better tolerated, benzodiazepines are not first-line treatment given the increased risk of falls, cognitive impairment, respiratory depression, and coma/death. Older adults are more likely to have multiple medications and medical comorbidities, which can affect the metabolism of benzodiazepines increasing risk of side effects. Additionally, the study also investigated the efficacy of behavioral treatment which has been shown to have long-term efficacy in treating chronic insomnia.

References

1. Morin CM, Colecchi C, Stone J, Sood R, Brink D. Behavioral and pharmacological therapies for late-life insomnia: a randomized controlled trial. JAMA. 1999;281(11):991.
2. Jadad AR, Moore RA, Carroll D, Jenkinson C, Reynolds DJ, Gavaghan DJ, McQuay HJ. Assessing the quality of reports of randomized clinical trials: is blinding necessary? Control Clin Trials. 1996;17:1–12.

Chapter 66
Cognitive Behavioral Therapy Versus Zopiclone for the Treatment of Chronic Primary Insomnia in Older Adults: A Randomized Controlled Trial

Andrew Tuck and Paul A. Riordan

Authors of the original article Børge Sivertsen, Siri Omvik, Ståle Pallesen, Bjørn Bjorvatn, Odd E Havik, Gerd Kvale, Geir Høstmark Nielsen, Inger Hilde Nordhu

Journal published *The Journal of the American Medical Association*

Year of publication 2006

Type of study Randomized placebo-controlled trial

Funding sources The University of Bergen, the Meltzer Fund, and the EXTRA funds from the Norwegian Foundation for Health and Rehabilitation. These organizations reportedly played no role in the study's design, conduct, analysis, or publication.

Objectives To compare the short-term efficacy of cognitive behavioral therapy (CBT), zopiclone, and placebo and the long-term efficacy of CBT and zopiclone in the treatment of chronic primary insomnia in older adults [1]

Methods This study recruited 92 Norwegian adults aged 55 years or older with insomnia. Participants were required to have insomnia as defined by *Diagnostic and*

A. Tuck
Department of Psychiatry, Duke University School of Medicine, Durham, NC, USA
e-mail: Andrew.tuck@duke.edu

P. A. Riordan (✉)
Durham Veterans Affairs Medical Center, Department of Psychiatry and Behavioral Sciences, Duke University School of Medicine, Durham, NC, USA
e-mail: paul.riordan@duke.edu

R. R. Tampi et al. (eds.), *Essential Reviews in Geriatric Psychiatry*,
https://doi.org/10.1007/978-3-030-94960-0_66

Statistical Manual of Mental Disorders, fourth edition (*DSM-IV*) criteria, including difficulties falling asleep, staying asleep, and/or waking up early for at least 3 months with associated impairment of daytime functioning [2]. Exclusion criteria included use of hypnotic medication in the previous 4 weeks, current use of antidepressants or antipsychotics, presence of dementia or serious cognitive impairment (defined by Mini-Mental Status Exam scores of <23), or presence of a severe mental disorder (including major depressive disorder) as determined by the Structured Clinical Interview for the *DSM-IV*. Additionally, the study excluded participants if they had sleep apnea or periodic limb movements during sleep, anticipated working night shifts during the study, or had significant somatic conditions felt to prevent participation.

Participants were randomized in a double-blind fashion to insomnia-specific CBT (n = 18), zopiclone (n = 18), or pharmacological placebo treatment using pills identical to the zopiclone (n = 12). The authors chose zopiclone, a GABA-potentiating hypnotic, because of its popularity in Norway, accounting for nearly half of all hypnotic sales at the time. Two participants in the zopiclone arm withdrew immediately after randomization and were not included in intent-to-treat analysis. The CBT group underwent 6 weeks of once-weekly CBT) sessions that followed a manualized, insomnia-specific CBT protocol [3]. Sessions pertained to five topics: (1) sleep hygiene education (to teach what affects sleep, such as alcohol and exercise), (2) sleep restriction (to promote strict schedule of bedtimes and awakening times), (3) stimulus control (to break association between sleep environment with activities that are not sleeping), (4) cognitive therapy (to challenge maladaptive beliefs about sleep), and (5) progressive relaxation technique (to learn a skill to recognize and control muscle tension for relaxation). The zopiclone group took 7.5 milligrams of zopiclone nightly for 6 weeks with the option to continue for an additional 6 months at the end of the 6-week period. Participants in the placebo group were randomly assigned to one of the two treatment groups after 6 weeks. They were not included in the final 6-month intent-to-treat analysis which only compared CBT to zopiclone.

Four primary outcomes were assessed: total wake time, total sleep time, sleep efficiency (the ratio of total sleep time to time spent in bed which was expressed as a percentage in this review), and slow-wave sleep (time spent in stage 3 or stage 4 sleep). Slow-wave sleep is thought to be beneficial for daytime functioning, and no previous studies have assessed whether CBT for insomnia could improve slow-wave sleep. This study assessed these outcomes at three time points: pretreatment, after a 6-week treatment period, and 6 months posttreatment. Each of the four outcomes was assessed by a combination of daily sleep diaries (logged by participants for 2-week periods at each assessment point) and by polysomnography conducted in the participants' homes. Slow-wave sleep was assessed only by polysomnography.

Results

Baseline Characteristics

45 of the original 46 participants completed the 6-week treatment period. The mean age of the sample was 60.8 (SD 5.4) years. The mean duration of insomnia was 14.1 (range 1–43) years. After randomization, some demographic and health characteristics were notably different between groups. For example, the participants in the CBT group were more likely to have previously received treatment for insomnia than the other two groups and were less likely to be on other medications than the placebo group. The participants in the zopiclone group were more likely to be current smokers than the other two groups. At baseline, the mean sleep *efficiency* of the entire sample was 81.0% (SD 10.5) when measured by polysomnography, but only 66.2% (SD 11.8) by subjective reports in the participants' sleep diaries.

Adherence

Participants' adherence to their intervention was measured using a self-reported five-point scale. Adherence was high for all groups (mean of 4.6, SD 0.6) with no significant differences between groups at the end of the treatment period.

Results: End of Treatment Period

At the end of the 6-week treatment period, there were notable differences in outcomes between the two sources of measurement: the sleep diaries and polysomnography. With the sleep diaries, participants as a whole had improvements in total wake time ($P = 0.001$), total sleep time ($P = 0.003$), and sleep efficiency ($P < 0.001$) with no statistically significant differences between groups.

With polysomnography, the CBT group experienced a significantly greater reduction of total wake time by 52%, compared to only a 4% reduction in the zopiclone group and a 16% reduction in the placebo group. The CBT group had about 50 minutes less time awake than the other groups at 6 weeks. Total sleep time did not significantly increase in the sample as a whole and was not different between individual groups. Unlike the reported diary sleep times, polysomnography showed a decrease in total sleep time at 6 weeks for all three groups (although only the zopiclone's decrease was statistically significant with a 17% decrease in total sleep time). For sleep efficiency, CBT outperformed placebo with a 9% improvement compared to −3% ($P = 0.004$), but this was not significantly different from zopiclone, which had a −1% change.

Notably, there was a 27% improvement in slow-wave sleep for the CBT group, compared to a 20% *decrease* for participants taking zopiclone ($P = 0.002$) and 13% less slow-wave sleep for the placebo group ($P = 0.03$).

Results: Six-Month Follow-Up

As measured by their sleep diaries, participants in both the CBT and zopiclone groups experienced statistically significant improvement in total wake time, total sleep time, and sleep efficiency at the 6-month follow-up compared to their baselines (see Table 66.1). Between groups, the only statistically significant difference was the CBT group's shorter average wake time per night compared to the zopiclone group: 69.9 minutes (51% improvement) versus 115.7 minutes (27% improvement) ($P = 0.03$). The CBT group also had better sleep efficiency (83.2%) than the zopiclone group (73.9%), but this did not reach statistical significance ($P = 0.11$).

Table 66.1 Outcomes: percent change and effect size of CBT and zopiclone at 6-month follow-up compared to pretreatment baseline

	Sleep diaries		Polysomnography	
	Cognitive behavioral therapy % improvement (effect size)	Zopiclone % improvement (effect size)	Cognitive behavioral therapy % improvement (effect size)	Zopiclone % improvement (effect size)
Total wake time	51% (1.3)	27% (0.6)	56% (1.7)	10% (0.2)
Total sleep time	13% (0.7)	13% (0.6)	−1.3% (−0.1)	−15% (−0.9)
Sleep efficiency, %	21% (1.2)	17% (0.8)	11% (1.2)	−1% (−0.0)
Slow-wave sleep	–	–	34% (0.7)	−23% (−0.5)

Polysomnography showed that the CBT group had a 56% decrease in total wake time compared to baseline ($P < 0.001$), dropping from a mean of 107.8 minutes nightly down to 47.1 minutes. Total sleep time did not significantly increase compared to baseline (−1.3% change), but sleep efficiency improved from 80.4% at baseline to 90.1% ($P < 0.001$). The average amount of nightly slow-wave sleep also increased in the CBT group by about 21 minutes (34%) over the course of the study ($P < 0.01$).

By polysomnography, the zopiclone group fared poorly. Total sleep time significantly decreased over the course of the study, dropping from a mean of 6.47 hours at baseline to 5.53 hours at 6-month follow-up (15% worsening; $P < 0.05$). Additionally, slow-wave sleep significantly decreased by 17 minutes (23%) compared to the baseline ($P < 0.05$). There were no statistically significant changes compared to baseline in the other two outcomes – total wake time and sleep efficiency. At 6 months, the CBT group statistically outperformed the zopiclone group in three out of four measures: total wake time, sleep efficiency, and slow-wave sleep.

Adverse Events

Participants in the zopiclone group reported a small number of adverse effects which led to one participant withdrawing from the study during the initial treatment period and two withdrawing in the follow-up period. The most common adverse events reported were bitter taste ($n = 6$) and dry mouth ($n = 4$). Participants in the CBT group did not report any adverse effects.

Conclusions CBT for insomnia outperformed zopiclone in both the short-term and long-term treatment of older adults with insomnia. Additionally, CBT was better tolerated than zopiclone.

Strengths of the Study

1. Randomized, double-blind, placebo-controlled design.
2. As indicated by a Jadad score of 4 out of 5, the quality of this trial was high [4].

Questions Yes (1) No (0)	Was the study described as random?	Was the randomization scheme described and appropriate?	Was the study described as double-blind?	Was the method of double blinding appropriate? (Were both the patient and the assessor appropriately blinded?)	Was there a description of dropouts and withdrawals?	Total score Range of score quality 0–2 Low 3–5 High
Score	1	1	0[a]	1	1	4

[a]CBT-I could not be blinded

3. Outcomes were assessed by both sleep diaries and polysomnography. The improvement in slow-wave sleep demonstrated by polysomnography for the CBT group is clinically important since slow-wave sleep is thought to be especially restorative.
4. The sample had high participation including 100% attendance to sessions in the CBT group and high adherence to the interventions being tested.
5. The findings are directly clinically relevant to the population being studied.
6. This is one of the first studies to demonstrate superiority of CBT for insomnia over GABAergic medications. Recent meta-analyses and guidelines continue to show that medications have little clinical benefit for the treatment of chronic insomnia [5].

Limitations of the Study
1. The sample size was small, with only 46 participants included in the intent-to-treat analysis and 12 to 18 participants per group. Due to the small sample size, there may be some confounding factors not accounted for as seen by some differences noted between groups in the baseline characteristics.
2. By its nature, CBT cannot be blinded. There was no "non-pharmacological" control group (e.g., an educational group on sleep hygiene) to compare against CBT.
3. The exclusion of participants with insomnia due to a psychiatric or medical condition may limit generalizability of the findings.
4. By polysomnography, most participants had good sleep efficiency at baseline (79–81%).

Take-home points CBT for insomnia led to improvements over baseline in several sleep-related outcomes in both the short term and long term. CBT was more effective than zopiclone and placebo on several of these measures including total wake time, sleep efficiency, and slow-wave sleep. The zopiclone group experienced decreases in slow-wave sleep and total sleep time as measured by polysomnography. CBT was also better tolerated than zopiclone.

Practical applications of the take-home point When treating older adults with primary insomnia, clinicians should consider CBT first.

References

1. Sivertsen B, Omvik S, Pallesen S, Bjorvatn B, Havik OE, Kvale G, Nielsen GH, Nordhu IH. Cognitive behavioral therapy vs zopiclone for treatment of chronic primary insomnia in older adults: a randomized controlled trial. JAMA. 2006;295(24):2851–8.
2. American Psychiatric Association. Diagnostic and statistical manual of mental disorders, 4th ed. (DSM-IV). The American Psychiatric Association. 1994.
3. Morin CM. Insomnia: psychological assessment and management. New York: Guilford Press; 1993.
4. Jadad AR, Moore RA, Carroll D, Jenkinson C, Reynolds DJ, Gavaghan DJ, McQuay HJ. (1996). Assessing the quality of reports of randomized clinical trials: is blinding necessary? Control Clin Trials. 1996;17(1):1–12.
5. Sateia MJ, Buysse DJ, Krystal AD, Neubauer DN, Heald JL. Clinical practice guideline for the pharmacologic treatment of chronic insomnia in adults: an American Academy of Sleep Medicine clinical practice guideline. J Clin Sleep Med. 2017;13(2):307–49.

Chapter 67
Suvorexant in Elderly Patients with Insomnia: Pooled Analyses of Data from Phase III Randomized Controlled Clinical Trials

Miles Christensen and Paul A. Riordan

Authors of the original article W Joseph Herring, Kathryn M Connor, Ellen Snyder, Duane B Snavely, Ying Zhang, Jill Hutzelmann, Deborah Matzura-Wolfe, Ruth M Benca, Andrew D Krystal, James K Walsh, Christopher Lines, Thomas Roth, David Michelson

Journal published *American Journal of Geriatric Psychiatry*

Year of publication 2017

Type of study Pooled analysis of randomized, double-blind, placebo-controlled trials with parallel groups

Funding sources Merck & Co (developers of suvorexant)

Objectives To evaluate the efficacy and safety of suvorexant in the elderly by pooling the data of elderly participants from three efficacy and three safety randomized, double-blind, placebo-controlled trials [1]

Methods

Patient Selection

All patients included in the trials met criteria for insomnia based on the *DSM-IV*. Investigators excluded persons with poor general health, with major

M. Christensen
Department of Psychiatry, Duke University School of Medicine, Durham, NC, USA
e-mail: miles.christensen@duke.edu

P. A. Riordan (✉)
Durham Veterans Affairs Medical Center, Department of Psychiatry and Behavioral Sciences, Duke University School of Medicine, Durham, NC, USA
e-mail: paul.riordan@duke.edu

R. R. Tampi et al. (eds.), *Essential Reviews in Geriatric Psychiatry*,
https://doi.org/10.1007/978-3-030-94960-0_67

depressive disorder and sleep-related breathing disorders like obstructive sleep apnea.

Enrolment criteria differed according to whether patients had polysomnography (PSG) or not. For participants with sleep diary data only to be enrolled, participants had to report a total sleep time of under 6.5 hours on at least four of the nights in the week prior to the screening survey and report at least 30 minutes of time to sleep onset for at least four of seven nights in the week prior to the screening survey.

A total of 75% of patients also underwent PSG (polysomnography) for over 8 hours. Patients enrolled by PSG criteria were screened with two nights of PSG and had to have a latency onset of persistent sleep of 20 minutes and average wakefulness after persistent sleep onset ≥60 minutes with each night at least >45 minutes. The patients were analyzed separately based on whether they completed the PSG.

Study Design

This study used existing patient data from two phase III randomized, double-blind, placebo-controlled trials with parallel groups and an additional three safety trials by extracting data for elderly participants only (defined as age 65 or older). Elderly patients in these trials were assigned to treatments of 30 mg, 15 mg, or placebo either in a 3:2:3 ratio or 2:1:2 ratio depending on the original trial. All trials had randomized assignment using a computerized allocation system. Study investigators, site staff, patients, PSG scorers, and monitoring staff remained blinded to treatment allocation for all trials included in this pooled analysis.

All hypnotic medications were discontinued before entering trials, with patients provided a 2-week placebo, and then continued to either high-dose suvorexant, intermediate-dose suvorexant, or placebo. Dosing in the original trials was different for elderly and non-elderly patients, with elderly patients receiving either 30 mg or 15 mg of suvorexant compared to 40 mg or 20 mg for non-elderly patients. All trials included monitoring to at least 3 months. The difference in dosing was determined by previous studies that observed differences in plasma exposure based on age. For the run-out phase at the end of treatment (used to monitor withdrawal effects and rebound insomnia), half of those individuals who were initially randomized to suvorexant were again randomized to receive either the same dose of suvorexant or were switched to placebo in a 1:1 ratio. Those individuals who were initially randomized to placebo were continued on placebo (placebo to placebo).

Patients were assigned an electronic diary to use each morning which recorded subjective time to sleep onset (sTSO), subjective total time slept (sTST), and subjective time to wakefulness after persistent sleep onset (sWASO). Values used in the analysis were the mean of the daily values for week 1, the last week of the first month, and the last 2 weeks of the third month. PSG measured objective time to wakefulness after persistent sleep onset (WASO) and latency to onset of persistent sleep (LPS). PSG results were included on day 1 of study participation, the end of month 1, and the end of month 3. The efficacy endpoints were the changes from baseline in these measures of sleep maintenance and sleep onset.

Statistical Analysis
The pooled subgroup analysis included all participants who took at least one dose of the treatment, had baseline data, and had at least one posttreatment efficacy measure. Patients with missing data were included. The investigators used least-squares mean estimates and comparisons of the treatment differences versus placebo in elderly patients with a Satterthwaite's approximation for degrees of freedom. Rebound insomnia and multiple safety endpoints were analyzed separately from those patients that entered the 1-week run-out at the end of their treatment.

Results
The pooled efficacy dataset included 839 patients, and the pooled safety dataset included 1298 patients. At baseline, the patients reported a mean total sleep time of 5 hours and a time to sleep onset of 1 hour. Tables 67.1 and 67.2 summarize the effect of suvorexant on subjective and objective measures of sleep in terms of mean minutes difference.

The safety adverse events were reported separately. There were no important differences in serious adverse events among treatment groups. The most common side effect reported was next day somnolence. There were reports of all of the following clinically important adverse events in at least one patient that were not reported with placebo: hypnopompic or hypnogogic hallucinations ($n = 3$), sleep paralysis ($n = 1$), complex sleep-related behavior ($n = 1$), and suicidal ideation ($n = 1$). Notably it is unclear whether there were differences in motor vehicle accidents/violations with four (2.8%) reported in the 15 mg group, two (0.9%) in the 30 mg group, and two (1.0%) in the placebo group.

Analysis of changes in the Tyrer Withdrawal Symptom Questionnaire score during the first three nights following drug discontinuation showed no significant differences in the number of patients meeting withdrawal criteria for placebo and suvorexant.

Conclusions Elderly individuals comprise a large percentage of those with insomnia, and relatively few RCTs have assessed the use of sleep medications in this population, especially in the setting of long-term use. Suvorexant was shown to be

Table 67.1 Summary of the effect of suvorexant on subjective sleep measures measured as the average change in minutes compared to baseline

Measure	Dose	Week 1	Month 3
Subjective total time slept (sTST)	15 mg	16.7	18.9
Subjective time to sleep onset (sTSO)	15 mg	−6.5	−6.5
Subjective time to wakefulness after persistent sleep onset (sWASO)	15 mg	−9.3	−10.8
Subjective total time slept (sTST)	30 mg	24.9	20.4
Subjective time to sleep onset (sTSO)	30 mg	−9.6	−9.2
Subjective time to wakefulness after persistent sleep onset (sWASO)	30 mg	−10.3	−9.4

Table 67.2 Summary of the effect of suvorexant on polysomnogram sleep measures measured as the average change in minutes compared to baseline

Measure	Dose	Night 1	Month 3
Latency of onset to sleep (LPS)	15 mg	−10.0	−6.2
Wakefulness after sleep onset (WASO)	15 mg	−39.3	−23.4
Latency of onset to sleep (LPS)	30 mg	−17.5	−7.7
Wakefulness after sleep onset (WASO)	30 mg	−49.4	−24.7

effective at increasing time to sleep onset as well as total length of sleep both as reported by study participants and as shown on polysomnography. The investigators reported that the effects of suvorexant on sleep parameters observed earlier in the study were maintained throughout the 3-month period. However, these effects are notably smaller at the 3-month mark, likely indicating some degree of tolerance that develops over time. Compared to GABAergic medications for insomnia, suvorexant appears relatively safer and better tolerated, without a significantly increased risk of dependence or increased risk of falls [2]. There is some evidence that abrupt discontinuation may cause rebound insomnia. Despite blocking orexin receptors, there was no identified cataplexy.

Strengths of the Study

1. The trials this study draws upon were multisite across multiple countries and continents reflective of a diverse sample with primary insomnia.
2. The studies were randomized, double-blind, and placebo-controlled trial design with good methodology. The quality of this study assessed on the basis of Jadad score indicates that this was high-quality study with a score of 5 out of 5 [3].

Questions Yes (1) No (0)	**Was the study described as random?**	**Was the randomization scheme described and appropriate?**	**Was the study described as double-blind?**	**Was the method of double blinding appropriate? (Were both the patient and the assessor appropriately blinded?)**	**Was there a description of dropouts and withdrawals?**	**Total score Range of score quality 0–2 Low 3–5 High**
Score	1	1	1	1	1	5

3. This study contained several primary end points all directly related to sleep initiation and duration of sleep. The end points contained both subjective and objective measures with direct report from patients and polysomnography which showed efficacy across all domains.
4. The study sample included only older adults (≥65 years).
5. Adverse events were carefully assessed.

6. Studies based on subgroup analyses are always complicated to do well, but the authors appear to have adequately accounted for this issue [4].

Limitations of the Study

1. The trial excluded patients with other DSM diagnosis such as major depression which is often comorbid or a cause of poor sleep in the elderly. Due to this fact, it remains unclear if these results are generalizable to these populations. More importantly it is unclear what the safety profile would be in these populations.
2. The doses used in this study (15 mg and 30 mg) for the elderly are not the currently recommended doses in the elderly which is now 10 mg with a maximum dosing of 20 mg. As a result, the study data that is of the most relevance to clinical application is the 15 mg data.
3. This study did show statistical significance with clinical benefit of subjective total sleep time increased by 18.9–20.4 minutes nightly at 3 months which is only a mild improvement, albeit comparable to most other hypnotics [5].

Take-Home Points

1. The data in this pooled group analysis shows that both 30 mg and 15 mg of suvorexant are mildly effective at reducing time to sleep onset and at increasing total amount of time slept in healthy individuals ≥65 years who suffer from primary insomnia.
2. Suvorexant is a generally well-tolerated medication with the most common side effect being daytime somnolence.
3. The pooled data of 15 mg shows a few participants suffered from difficulty with motor vehicle operation, abnormal sleep behavior, or sleep-related hallucinations although it is unclear if this was due to random variation given the relatively low number of study participants who experienced these adverse events.

Practical Applications of the Take-Home Points

1. Suvorexant is a generally well-tolerated and mildly effective medication that can be prescribed safely to elderly patients with primary insomnia.
2. The efficacy and safety of this drug for insomnia due to other conditions in the elderly has not yet been evaluated.

References

1. Herring WJ, Connor KM, Snyder E, Snavely DB, Zhang Y, Hutzelmann J, Matzura-Wolfe D, Benca RM, Krystal AD, Walsh JK, Lines C, Roth T, Michelson D. Suvorexant in elderly patients with insomnia: pooled analyses of data from phase III randomized controlled clinical trials. Am J Geriatr Psychiatry. 2017;25(7):791–802.
2. Park H, Satoh H, Miki A, Urushihara H, Sawada Y. Medications associated with falls in older people: systematic review of publications from a recent 5-year period. Eur J Clin Pharmacol. 2015;71(12):1429–40.

3. Jadad AR, Moore RA, Carroll D, Jenkinson C, Reynolds DJ, Gavaghan DJ, McQuay HJ. Assessing the quality of reports of randomized clinical trials: is blinding necessary? Control Clin Trials. 1996;17:1–12.
4. Hemkens LG, Contopoulos-Ioannidis DG, Ioannidis JPA. Routinely collected data and comparative effectiveness evidence: promises and limitations. CMAJ. 2016;188(8):E158–64.
5. Sateia MJ, Buysse DJ, Krystal AD, Neubauer DN, Heald JL. Clinical practice guideline for the pharmacologic treatment of chronic insomnia in adults: an American Academy of Sleep Medicine Clinical Practice Guideline. J Clin Sleep Med. 2017;13(2):307–49.

Chapter 68
Cognitive Behavioral Therapy for Older Adults with Insomnia and Depression: A Randomized Controlled Trial in Community Mental Health Services

Daniela Vela, Izabella Dutra de Abreu, Megan Tusken, Audrey Eichenberger, and Mary "Molly" Camp

Authors of the original article Paul Sadler, Suzanne McLaren, Britt Klein, Jack Harvey, Megan Jenkins

Journal published *Sleep*

Year of publication 2018

Type of study randomized controlled clinical trial

Funding sources None

Objective The study's objectives were twofold, first to research the effectiveness of cognitive behavioral therapy for insomnia (CBT-I) in older adults with comorbid insomnia and depression and, second, to investigate if an enhanced form of CBT-I produced better results when compared to a standard form of CBT-I [1].

Methods Seventy-two older adults from the community with a mean age of 75 years were initially enrolled in this 8-week randomized controlled clinical trial. The eligibility criteria included age 65 and older, referred to and/or case managed by a community mental health service, DSM-V diagnostic criteria of comorbid insomnia, and major depressive disorder. Exclusion criteria included not meeting DSM-V criteria for insomnia and depression, cognitive impairment as evidenced by a score of less than 24 on the Mini-Mental State Exam (MMSE), changes to

D. Vela · I. D. de Abreu · M. Tusken · A. Eichenberger · M. M. Camp (✉)
UT Southwestern Medical Center at Dallas, Dallas, TX, USA
e-mail: Daniela.Vela@UTSouthwestern.edu; Izabella.DeAbreu@UTSouthwestern.edu; Megan.Tusken@PHHS.org; Audrey.Eichenberger@PHHS.org; Molly.Camp@UTSouthwestern.edu

R. R. Tampi et al. (eds.), *Essential Reviews in Geriatric Psychiatry*,
https://doi.org/10.1007/978-3-030-94960-0_68

psychotropic medication within 4 weeks of the trial and/or change made throughout treatment, current high risk (suicide plan/intent, manic, psychotic), current course of maintenance electroconvulsive therapy (ECT), and current psychotherapy treatment.

The assessment process to establish a diagnosis included two steps. First, provisional and generalist psychologists together conducted a face-to-face semi-structured insomnia interview based on Buysse et al. [2] and Morin and Benca's [3] assessment guidelines for insomnia and the major depression model of the Mini-International Neuropsychiatric Interview [4]. Then multidisciplinary clinical review consensus meetings were held to finalize the diagnosis.

Outcome measures were completed at pretreatment (week 0), posttreatment (week 8), and 3-month follow-up (week 20). The primary measures included the Insomnia Severity Index (ISI) and the Geriatric Depression Scale (GDS). Secondary measures included the sleep-onset latency (SOL), wake time after sleep onset (WASO), total sleep time (TST), sleep efficiency (SE), and sleep quality (SQ) from the consensus sleep diary (CDS). In addition, other secondary measures administered included the Dysfunctional Beliefs and Attitudes About Sleep 10-item Scale (DBAS-10), SLEEP-50 scale, Geriatric Anxiety Inventory-Short Form (GAI-SF), Beck Hopelessness Scale (BHS), and the EuroQol 5-D 3-L Scale (EQ-5D-3L).

Participants were allocated to one of three conditions: CBT-I, enhanced form of CBT-I (CBT-I+), and psychoeducation control group (PCG) using a block/cluster randomization design. Participants were blinded to the condition they were randomly allocated to complete. The standard CBT-I group met with two co-therapists for 8-weekly, 60- to 75-minute sessions. These sessions included therapy worksheets, homework activities, behavioral modification interventions, cognitive restructuring of unhelpful sleep beliefs, and relapse prevention. The CBT-I+ program included three additional CBT strategies that targeted comorbid depression. These strategies included behavioral activation, cognitive reframing for depression, and positive affirmations. These sessions lasted for 75–90 minutes. The PCG included 8-weekly sessions of psychoeducation about sleep, insomnia, and depression. Treatment completion was defined as participating in six out of eight sessions.

Ten provisional and generalist psychologists who were undertaking a geropsychology postgraduate clinical placement conducted the assessments and interventions. Therapists and assessors had opportunities to perform both roles. They each received training and daily supervision. Protocol adherence was monitored through group supervision, audio recordings, and written materials.

Primary and secondary outcome measures were analyzed using linear mixed modeling to test for cluster effects due to program delivery; no cluster effects were found. Dichotomous variables were analyzed using longitudinal logistic regression. Effect sizes using Cohen's d were calculated as well.

Results Sixty-nine out of 72 initially enrolled participants completed the post-assessment measures, and 65 completed the 3-month follow-up. Sixty-six completed the sleep diary at post-assessment, and 60 completed it at follow-up. No significant differences for demographic variables, sleep and mental health characteristics, or treatment expectancy were found between the three conditions (CBT-I, CBT-I+, PCG).

CBT-I and CBT-I+ had significant effects in insomnia and depression as evidenced by reduction in scores measured by the ISI and GDS from pre to post and follow-up, respectively. In contrast, the PCG condition did not have an effect on insomnia or depressive symptoms reduction. When comparing CBT-I and CBT-I+ to PCG, both reduced insomnia severity and depressive symptoms significantly from pre to post.

Large effect sizes were found for both cognitive behavioral interventions in their ability to reduce insomnia and depression symptoms at post and follow-up. When comparing both forms of CBT-I, there were no significant differences in insomnia or depression severity reduction at post or follow-up.

In the CBT-I condition, 71% of participants no longer met DSM-V criteria for comorbid insomnia at post and 68% at follow-up. Eighty-eight percent of these participants no longer met criteria for major depressive disorder at post and 73% at follow-up.

In the CBT-I+ condition, 78% of participants no longer had comorbid insomnia at post and 45% at follow-up. Seventy-eight percent of them no longer met DSM-V criteria for major depressive disorder at post and 64% at follow-up.

In the PCG condition, 27% of participants no longer met criteria for comorbid insomnia at post and 14% at follow-up. Thirty-six percent no longer met criteria for major depressive disorder at post and 19% at follow-up.

Additionally, significant improvements were observed in the various sleep diary measures for CBT-I and CBT-I+ from pre to post. No significant changes were observed during the 3-month follow-up. Both CBT-I and CBT-I+ demonstrated significant improvement from pre to post in measures of anxiety, hopelessness, dysfunctional beliefs about sleep, and physical health. These changes were maintained during the 3-month follow-up.

Conclusions Evidence from this RCT demonstrated that CBT-I and CBT-I+ to be superior to PCG. The second hypothesis, which compared CBT-I and CBT-I+, was not supported. Possible reasons for this include lack of sufficient power in the study to test for equivalence and increased complexity involved in delivering CBT-I+. Overall, we can conclude that older adults with comorbid insomnia and depression attending community mental health settings can benefit from standard CBT-I for the reduction of both insomnia and depression.

Strengths of the Study

1. Block/cluster randomized controlled trial design
2. Posttreatment and 3-month follow-up assessors blinded
3. High retention/completion rate
4. First RCT to include diverse sample of older adults with comorbid insomnia and depression

Limitations of the Study

1. Lack of objective physiological sleep measures, such as actigraphy and polysomnography.
2. Larger sample needed to detect possible differences between CBT-I and CBT-I+ was not achieved.
3. Not including CBT for depression as another treatment group.
4. Potential confound from the quality of the therapist dyad.

Take-Home Points

1. CBT-I is more effective for insomnia than psychoeducation alone.
2. Second, when treating patients with comorbid insomnia and depression, using the standard form of CBT-I may be beneficial for both disorders, and the benefits may continue to be observed 3 months later.

Practical Applications of the Take-Home Points

1. When treating older adults with comorbid insomnia and depression in a community setting, there is no need to expend hours applying both CBT-I and CBT for depression.
2. Based on these results, older adults with comorbid insomnia and depression get benefit for both diagnoses from CBT-I.

References

1. Sadler P, McLaren S, Klein B, Harvey J, Jenkins M. Cognitive behavior therapy for older adults with insomnia and depression: a randomized controlled trial in community mental health services. Sleep. 2018;1:41(8).
2. Buysse DJ, Ancoli-Israel S, Edinger JD, Lichstein KL, Morin CM. Recommendations for a standard research assessment of insomnia. Sleep. 2006;29(9):1155–73.
3. Morin CM, Benca R. Chronic insomnia. Lancet. 2012;379(9821):1129–41. https://doi.org/10.1016/S0140-6736(11)60750-2.
4. Sheehan DV, Lecrubier Y, Sheehan KH, Amorim P, Janavs J, Weiller E, Hergueta T, Baker R, Dunbar GC. The Mini-International Neuropsychiatric Interview (M.I.N.I.): the development and validation of a structured diagnostic psychiatric interview for DSM-IV and ICD-10. J Clin Psychiatry. 1998;59 Suppl 20:22–33; quiz 34–57.

Part XII
Suicides

Chapter 69
Medical Illness and the Risk of Suicide in the Elderly

Andrew Wong, Vahid Pasovic, Adan Aslam Khan, and Esther Akinyemi

Authors of the original article David N Juurlink, Nathan Herrmann, John P Szalai, Alexander Kopp, Donald A Redelmeier

Journal publisher *Archives of Internal Medicine*

Year of publication 2004

Type of study Population-based case-control study

Funding sources Ontario Mental Health Foundation

Objectives To assess the relationship between specific common illnesses and suicide in the elderly using a population-based case-control study [1]

Methods The study was based out of Ontario, Canada, where all patients have universal access to health insurance and are thus registered in databases for prescription drug coverage, physician services, and hospital care. The investigators identified consecutive cases of suicide in Ontario residents who were 66 years of age or older, occurring over a 9-year period (January 1, 1992, to December 31, 2000), from the records of the Office of the Chief Coroner of Ontario. In the province, all suspected cases of suicide are reported, and those with clear evidence of intent in the opinion of the coroner (such as a suicide note, previous threats or episodes of self-harm, or other evidence) are deemed suicides. Demographic information about each completed suicide was collected from the Registered Persons Database of Ontario.

A. Wong · V. Pasovic · A. A. Khan · E. Akinyemi (✉)
Henry Ford Health System, Detroit, MI, USA
e-mail: vpasovi1@hfhs.org; EAkinye2@hfhs.org

R. R. Tampi et al. (eds.), *Essential Reviews in Geriatric Psychiatry*,
https://doi.org/10.1007/978-3-030-94960-0_69

For each individual who completed suicide, four control patients were selected from the Registered Persons Database, matched by age, sex, and residential income quintile. Controls had to have visited an optometrist or dentist at least once within the year of the suicide date to ensure they were residing in the province and alive at the time. Case suicide patients were able to serve as controls in the period preceding their death as well.

Investigators analyzed the prescription medication records of case and control patients in the 6-month period prior to the suicide date using the Ontario Drug Benefit program which contains prescription records for all elderly residents of Ontario. Specific drugs or drug combinations served as markers of the presence of each illness, of which they focused on 17. These were ischemic heart disease, congestive heart failure, chronic lung disease, hyperacidity syndromes, seizure disorder, Parkinson's disease, diabetes mellitus, rheumatoid arthritis, urinary incontinence, psychoses, depression, anxiety and sleep disorders, bipolar disorder, breast cancer, prostate cancer, moderate pain, and severe pain. They used marker medications for each illness selected by the consensus of three clinicians. Investigators did not use physician diagnoses or hospital discharge diagnoses as they felt it to be unreliable. The investigators also used three control illnesses for which they did not expect an association with suicide. These were glaucoma, gout, and hypothyroidism. Dyslipidemia was included based on previous reports that treatment of this was associated with reduced risk of suicide. Investigators excluded illnesses that could not be discerned from others based on the medication records.

The primary analysis used conditional logistic regression to estimate the odds ratio and 95% confidence interval for suicide associated with specific illnesses. Illnesses bearing a relationship with suicide in the univariate analysis were included in the multivariate model to adjust for the influence of other illnesses on the relationship. Additionally, the relationship between the number of illnesses and suicide risk was explored. Analyses were repeated using modifications to test the robustness of the findings. In one, control selection process was repeated without requirement of recent visit to doctor or optometrist. In another, cases could not serve as controls for themselves prior to suicide. In a third, the cohort was stratified by sex, age, and income quintile. Finally, a post hoc analysis was performed for the relationship between specific illnesses and the chosen method of suicide.

Results In the 9-year study interval, a total of 1354 suicides in adults 66 years or older were identified in Ontario. However, 25 cases were not able to be analyzed due to invalid health records, erroneous identifying data, or residence outside of Ontario. Therefore, 1329 suicide cases were used in the study.

Death by firearms was the most frequent mechanism of suicide among all cases and the most common method used by men. Women most often committed suicide by poisoning. Hanging was the second most frequent cause of death among both genders. Mechanisms of suicide did not differ year by year throughout the 9-year study period.

Table 69.1 Medical illnesses associated with increased risk of suicide

Diagnoses	Odds ratio (95%)	Confidence interval
Congestive heart failure	1.73	1.33–2.24
Chronic obstructive lung disease	1.62	1.37–1.92
Hyperacidity syndromes	1.26	1.09–1.47
Seizure disorder	2.95	1.89–4.61
Urinary incontinence	2.02	1.29–3.17
Anxiety disorders	4.65	4.07–5.32
Depression	6.44	5.45–7.61
Psychotic disorders	5.09	3.94–6.59
Bipolar disorder	9.20	4.38–19.33
Moderate pain	1.91	1.66–2.20
Severe pain	7.52	4.93–11.46

Eleven of the 15 prespecified illnesses were associated with a significant increased risk of suicide in the univariate analyses as seen in the table below (Table 69.1).

Investigators found no association between increase in suicide risk among patients with the control illnesses of hypothyroidism, glaucoma, and gout. As previously expected, treatment of dyslipidemia was associated with a reduced risk of suicide. In the multivariate analyses, nine conditions were found to be independent predictors of an increased risk of suicide. These included all the above except for diabetes and hyperacidity syndromes. Bipolar disorder, depression, and severe pain were associated with the largest risk of suicide.

The investigators observed a strong association between the cumulative number of illnesses and the estimated relative risk of suicide. Patients with three illnesses had approximately threefold increase in relative risk of suicide; patients with five illnesses had approximately fivefold increase in risk compared to patients with no illness. Patients with the greatest number of illnesses ($\geq$7) have about a ninefold higher risk of suicide than those without illness.

Investigators also looked at healthcare visits by patients prior to suicide. Elderly patients who committed suicide were almost twice as likely to have visited a physician in the week before death (45% vs. 24%; $P < 0.001$), and most patients had visited a physician in the month before death (73% vs. 49%, $P < 0.001$). The five most common diagnoses listed in the week before suicide included anxiety, unspecified gastrointestinal symptoms, depression, unspecified cardiac symptoms, and hypertension.

Investigators noted clustering among illnesses and mechanisms of suicide. Patients with severe pain and congestive heart failure were more likely to kill themselves with a firearm. Patients with Parkinson's disease were more likely to commit suicide via suffocation. Patients with psychotic disorders were less likely to use a firearm.

Conclusions This study shows a significant association between suicide in the elderly and several common medical and psychiatric illnesses, which is cumulative with the number of illnesses. Additionally, most elderly patients who commit suicide have recent contact with the healthcare system, giving potential room for intervention.

Strengths of the Study

- This study utilized a large population sample with each case matched with four controls based on age, sex, and household income due to access to provincial databases
- The study used control illnesses
- There was the ability to explore many associations at the individual patient level
- The statistical analysis was robust including univariate and multivariate model of analyses
- There was repetition of analyses using several modifications to test robustness of findings

Limitations of the Study

- The deaths from suicide may be misclassified in the database from the Office of the Chief Coroner of Ontario especially in elderly if it was concealed or misattributed to medical illness, thus underestimating risk factors contributing to suicide.
- The use of prescriptions as markers for certain illness – some medications may be used for multiple illnesses, and some illnesses are not associated with specific drugs (e.g., malignancies may vary in pharmacological treatment).
- The study did not account for psychosocial factors contributing to suicide in elderly including bereavement, isolation, and burden of disability.
- The study did not account for substance use issues contributing to suicide in elderly.
- The study did not account for medications which contribute to an increase risk of suicide.
- The study did not account for unrecognized illness which can be common in elderly, e.g., depression.
- In the sample demographics, the study did not comment on race/ethnicity.

Take-home points The study underscores the importance of screening for suicide in medically and mentally ill older adults and engaging in risk reduction interventions such as restriction to firearms and medications for these patients.

Practical applications of the take-home points Elderly patients who suffer from chronic common illnesses are at increased risk for suicide. The more chronic illnesses a patient suffers from, the higher risk of suicide. It is important for physicians to assess suicide risk at each appointment including acute risk factors such as firearm access.

Reference

1. Juurlink DN, Herrmann N, Szalai JP, Kopp A, Redelmeier DA. Medical illness and the risk of suicide in the elderly. Arch Intern Med. 2004;164:1179–84.

Chapter 70
The Risk of Suicide with Selective Serotonin Reuptake Inhibitors in the Elderly

Adan Aslam Khan, Andrew Wong, Vahid Pasovic, and Esther Akinyemi

Authors of the original article David N. Jurrlink, MD, PhD, Muhammed M. Mamdani, Pharm.D, MA, MPH, Alexander Kopp, BA, Donald A. Redelmeier MD, MSc

Journal publisher *American Journal of Psychiatry*

Year of publication 2006

Type of study Comparative study

Funding sources Supported by a grant from the Ontario Mental Health Foundation. Dr. Jurrlink was supported by the New Investigator Award from the Canadian Institutes of Health Research and by the University of Toronto Drug Safety Research Group. Dr. Mamdani was supported by the New Investigator Award from the Canadian Institutes of Health Research. Dr. Redelmeier was supported by a Career Scientist Award from the Ontario Ministry of Health and a Canada Research Chair in Medical Decision Sciences.

Objectives To assess the relationship between initiating treatment with SSRI antidepressants and completed suicide in older adults [1]

Methods This was a population-based study conducted in Ontario, Canada, where all residents ≥65 years have universal access to health insurance for services including prescription drug coverage, physicians' services, and hospital care. Over a 9-year study period (Jan 1, 1992–Dec 31, 2000), cases of suicide were identified

A. A. Khan · A. Wong · V. Pasovic · E. Akinyemi (✉)
Henry Ford Health System, Detroit, MI, USA
e-mail: vpasovi1@hfhs.org; EAkinye2@hfhs.org

R. R. Tampi et al. (eds.), *Essential Reviews in Geriatric Psychiatry*,
https://doi.org/10.1007/978-3-030-94960-0_70

among Ontario residents aged ≥66 years using records from the Office of the Chief Coroner for Ontario. Individuals aged ≥65 years were excluded, and the first year of eligibility (at age 65) for prescription medication benefits was not examined to avoid incomplete medication records. The date of suicide was the index date for all analyses. The final matched analyses included 1138 suicide cases and 4552 comparison subjects.

A comparison patient group was identified from the general population using the propensity score method. A propensity score was calculated for each individual predicting the suicide outcome by balancing multiple characteristics between the suicide cases and comparison subjects. In this score, multiple elements (such as demographic characteristics, medical and psychiatric disorders, admission to a psychiatric facility during the previous year, care by a psychiatrist in the previous year, days in hospital during previous year, and suicide attempt in the previous year) were identified to minimize the difference between the two groups. Propensity scores were also calculated for all possible comparison patients (for each case at every index site) to account for changes in patterns of antidepressant use over the study period. Once these scores were calculated, all eligible comparison patients (if they were within 0.2 standard deviations of the propensity score) were identified. From this group, four comparison subjects (per suicide case) were randomly selected. Subjects ($n = 191$) with propensity scores that were too high to match four comparison subjects were excluded from the matched analyses but retained for descriptive purposes.

The Ontario Drug Benefit program collects comprehensive prescription records (<1% missing data) dispensed to elderly residents in Ontario. Prescription records of suicide cases and comparison groups were examined through this program. Selective serotonin reuptake inhibitor (SSRI) antidepressants included fluoxetine, fluvoxamine, paroxetine, sertraline, and citalopram. Other antidepressants included secondary amine cyclic antidepressants (desipramine, nortriptyline, protriptyline, maprotiline, and amoxapine), tertiary amine cyclic antidepressants (amitriptyline, imipramine, doxepin, trimipramine, and clomipramine), and miscellaneous antidepressants (venlafaxine, trazodone, bupropion, and nefazodone). Monoamine oxidase inhibitors (MAO-I) were not examined due to their infrequent use, and mirtazapine was not studied as it was not insured during most of the study period.

In the primary analyses, "new antidepressant use" was defined as no use of an antidepressant in the same class for the previous 6 months. For the primary analysis, a conditional logistic regression was used to estimate the odds ratio (OR) and 95% confidence interval (CI) for suicide associated with the new use of an antidepressant at monthly intervals from the start of the treatment. Multivariate analysis was used to adjust for rural place of residence (using home postal code), estimated residential income quintile, previous suicide attempt, the number of prescription medications dispensed in the previous year, evidence of alcohol abuse (using prescription records, physician diagnosis codes, or hospital discharged records from the previous year), malignancy, anxiety or sleep disorder, bipolar disorder, depression or other mood disorder, agitation or psychosis, poisoning or other injury, provision of care by a psychiatrist, or admission to a psychiatric facility. For statistical significance, all test used a two-tailed P-value of 0.05.

Results A total of 1354 cases of suicide (≥66 years) were identified among Ontario residents during the study period. Of the total group, 25 (2%) were excluded because of having an invalid health card number, erroneous identifying data, or principal residence outside of Ontario. A total of 191 (14%) were excluded as their scores were too high to be matched to the comparison subjects. A total of 1138 suicide cases were analyzed using 4552 comparison subjects with comparable demographic characteristics and patterns of illness. Many individuals who died by suicide were men living in an urban setting (80%), and a small percentage of the total group of suicide cases had seen a psychiatrist in the preceding year (13%). The most common methods of suicide were death from a firearm ($n = 370$), hanging ($n = 318$), and self-poisoning ($n = 285$). Of the total 1329 suicide cases (including the 191 individuals whose scores were too high to be matched to a comparison group), 68% ($n = 907$) did not receive antidepressant therapy 6 months before death.

The investigators found that the risk of suicide in the first month of treatment with an SSRI is fivefold higher than that with other antidepressants ($P = 0.0009$), but no difference is seen with continued therapy. This comparison was noted after adjustments were made through a multivariate analysis.

Tertiary amines may be used for illnesses other than depression (such as neuropathic pain, pruritis, migraine). Findings did not change significantly when tertiary amines were excluded from the group of non-SSRI antidepressants. Venlafaxine is an antidepressant that blocks serotonin and norepinephrine reuptake (SNRI) at higher doses. Consistent results were obtained when venlafaxine was categorized as an SSRI antidepressant. These findings were also consistent when amoxapine and maprotiline (which are structurally different from other secondary amine cyclic antidepressants) were excluded from the analysis and when clomipramine (which selectively interferes with serotonin transport) was excluded from the group of tertiary amine cyclic antidepressants.

During the secondary analysis, the "new antidepressant use" was defined as no use of any other antidepressant in the previous 6 months. The findings of this analysis were consistent with the original results and persisted in the replicated analysis. In most aspects, in the first month of treatment with an SSRI antidepressant (in comparison with non-SSRI antidepressants), there was noted to be a disproportionate increase in suicide among the elderly population. These results were consistent within a series of subgroup analyses stratified by demographic characteristics, mental health history, and patterns of medical illness. The only exception was that this finding was not found among women.

The investigators also reported that relative to non-SSRI antidepressant treatment, suicides of a violent nature were more strongly associated with SSRI antidepressant treatment during early therapy ($P = 0.0016$). Suicides of a violent nature were described as hanging, gunshot, jumping, stabbing, vehicle collision, blunt trauma, explosion, electrocution, and self-immolation. Nonviolent suicides were equally common among patients treated with SSRI and non-SSRI antidepressants.

The absolute risk of suicide during the first month of treatment was calculated to be low in both the group receiving treatment with an SSRI antidepressant (1 in 3353) and non-SSRI antidepressant (1 in 16,037). Additionally, the authors note that the risk of suicide due to an antidepressant is probably lower, as many of the suicides in the first month of treatment likely resulted from depression rather than as an adverse effect of treatment.

Conclusions This study shows a substantial increase in the relative risk of suicide only within the first month of SSRI treatment compared to other antidepressants which did not persist. Proposed mechanisms include improving aspects of depression such as psychomotor retardation "energizing the patient to suicide," the development of akathisia-like symptoms, agitation or dysphoria, and use of SSRI antidepressants in patients at high risk for suicide as they are safer in overdose. However, this was considered less likely as physicians may be unable to identify high-risk patients in the elderly population, comparison patients were matched on important characteristics, and consistent results were found in this study regardless of previous psychiatric treatment. Additionally, the higher risk was not noted beyond the first month of treatment with an SSRI antidepressant. The investigators explain that if depression explained their findings, then the persistent risk should have been identified with SSRI therapy as they rarely abate after the first month of treatment.

This study also showed that the absolute risk of suicide during initial treatment with an SSRI antidepressant was very low. The majority of patients treated with SSRI antidepressants do not attempt suicide, although in rare instances an idiosyncratic response may occur and individuals may experience suicidal ideation during the first weeks of therapy. The etiology of this is unknown and may have a pharmacogenetic contribution. It was also noted that there was an undertreatment of depression in the elderly as a significant proportion of individuals (two-thirds) that died by suicide were not receiving an antidepressant.

Lastly, this study shows increased risk of violent suicides with SSRI antidepressant treatment compared to other antidepressants.

Strengths of the Study

1. This study had a large sample size.
2. The study duration long.
3. There were many covariables were assessed during multivariable analysis to minimize confounding effects.

Limitations of the Study

1. A large proportion of the population were males from urban settings.
2. The availability of mental health resources and access to psychiatrist/psychotropic medications were not addressed.
3. There was no direct measure of antidepressant doses, duration of treatment, or adherence to treatment.
4. The severity of depression in each group of treatment could not be assessed.

5. Other important variables including pain control, social support, and bereavement that may contribute to mood symptoms and increase risk of suicidality were not measured.
6. A portion of the group was excluded as the scores were "too high" to be matched to comparison subjects. This may have resulted in selection bias.
7. It is unclear what constitutes early therapy for violent suicide with SSRI treatment.

Take-home points In elderly patients, there has been a significant undertreatment of depression and increased suicide risk. The risks of undertreatment are often greater than the risks of treatment with an SSRI antidepressant. At the onset of treatment with an SSRI antidepressant, it is important to educate patients and family of the increased risk of suicide in the first month, and keeping the environment safe, as well as monitor individuals closely during this period.

Practical applications of the take-home points Among elderly patients with depression and increased suicide risk, SSRI antidepressant is an option for treatment. Close monitoring of tolerability, mood symptoms, and suicide risk, especially at the onset of treatment, is fundamental in the care of these individuals. Additionally, limiting access to violent means of suicide should also be an integral part of treatment planning.

Reference

1. Juurlink DN, Mamdani MM, Kopp A, Redelmeier DA. The risk of suicide with selective serotonin reuptake inhibitors in the elderly. Am J Psychiatry. 2006;163(5):813–21.

Part XIII
Substance Use Disorders

Chapter 71
Naltrexone as an Adjunctive Treatment for Older Patients with Alcohol Dependence

Paroma Mitra

Authors of the original article David Oslin, MD, Joseph G. Liberto, MD, John O'Brien, MSW, Stacy Krois, Jennifer Norbeck, MSW

Journal published *The American Journal of Geriatric Psychiatry*

Year of publication 1997

Type of study double-blind, randomized, placebo-controlled efficacy study

Funding sources DuPont Merck Pharmaceuticals

Objectives to examine the efficacy of naltrexone as an adjunct for alcohol dependence in older adults [1]

Methods Forty-four individuals were recruited for participation in the study from the Baltimore Veterans Affairs Medical Centre. Individuals between ages of 50 and 70 years with a diagnosis of alcohol dependence as per DSM III-R were included in the study.

Individuals were excluded from participation if they had used a psychoactive substance other than alcohol, caffeine, or nicotine up to 6 weeks before the study or used opioids within 7 days before initiation of naltrexone. They were also excluded if they presented with a positive drug screen for opioids, amphetamines, cocaine, benzodiazepines, or barbiturates at the start of the study. Other exclusion criteria included severe medical conditions, especially severe hepatic diseases, severe

P. Mitra (✉)
NYU School of Medicine, Bellevue Hospital Center, New York, NY, USA

R. R. Tampi et al. (eds.), *Essential Reviews in Geriatric Psychiatry*,
https://doi.org/10.1007/978-3-030-94960-0_71

dementia, seizure disorder, and psychosis, or if deemed by a physician to be a danger to self and others.

Study participants were randomized to receive either naltrexone or placebo. Naltrexone was given in doses of 100 mg on Mondays and Wednesdays and 150 mg on Fridays. All participants also received group therapy weekly and check-ins with a case manager twice every month. Medical and psychiatric care were monitored by a psychiatrist in an outpatient geriatric substance use disorder clinic.

Participants were assessed at baseline and monthly using the Addiction Severity Index (ASI), blood chemistries, and vital signs. Physical adverse effects, medication adherence, and compliance with group therapy sessions were examined. Investigators also checked for cravings and feelings of depression and anxiety using a visual analog scale. Clinically significant drinking (relapse) was the primary outcome measure. It was defined as a report of consuming five or more drinks on one occasion, or a report of drinking five or more times in a week, or a blood alcohol concentration (BAC) of 100 mg/dl.

Results The mean age of participants in both groups was approximately 58 years. The treatment and placebo groups did not differ at baseline in terms of age, race, years of education, marital status, or medical history. The severity of drinking, as measured by the number of drinks per occasion (10.0 +/− 8.1 in the placebo group and 11.4 +/− 6.4 in the naltrexone group), and average ASI score (0.48 +/− 0.17) were similar. Treatment compliance was measured by group attendance, the duration of study participation, and medication adherence. Subjects in the naltrexone group attended approximately 7.2 +/− 3.6 group therapy sessions, and those in the placebo group attended 7.0 + 4.1 sessions, and this was not statistically significant. Participants in the naltrexone group completed an average of 10.3 ± 2.6 weeks of the study, and the placebo group completed an average of 9.5 ± 4.0 weeks, and this difference was not observed to be significant.

There were adverse effects reported by both groups, but there was no difference in either the symptoms observed or the duration of adverse effects. The most common adverse effects were sleep disturbances and anxiety, followed by headaches, joint pains, nausea, and vomiting. Gamma-glutamyl transferase (GGT), aspartate aminotransferase (AST) levels, and blood chemistries did not differ between the naltrexone- and placebo-treated groups over the course of the study.

The primary effect demonstrated was a reduction in relapse when an individual sampled any amount of alcohol. Three out of the six participants relapsed while being on naloxone, while all eight participants who drank some alcohol and only on placebo relapsed, an outcome that was statistically significant and clinically relevant ($P = 0.024$). Total abstinence was achieved by 68.2% of all the subjects during the time of participation in the study. The naltrexone-treated group drank approximately 1.9% of study days, whereas individuals in placebo group drank approximately 6.5% of the study days. This was however not observed to be statistically significant ($P = 0.275$). There were similarly no differences in abstinence rates between the naltrexone- and placebo-treated groups ($P = 0.659$). Time to first drink was measured using survival analysis, and naltrexone was not deemed to be effective in prolonging abstinence when compared with placebo ($P = 0.532$).

Participants in both groups demonstrated relapse to clinically significant alcohol consumption but without a significant difference ($P = 0.117$). A total of 14.3% of the participants in the naltrexone-treated group relapsed, whereas 34.8% of those in the placebo-treated group relapsed. There was a significant overall reduction in the score on the alcohol sub-score of the ASI ($P < 0.001$), and there were no significant differences between the two groups in the same. All participants reported a significant decrease in depression ($P = 0.036$), but there were no significant changes between the two groups in self-rated craving, depression, or anxiety scores.

Out of 44 participants,17 did not complete the study. They had a higher rate being arrested for driving under influence (DUI) when compared to those who did not complete the study ($P = 0.009$). The subjects who did not complete the study did not attend as many group sessions compared to those who did complete the study ($P < 0.001$).

Those who did not complete the study missed a larger percentage of doses of study medications compared to those who completed the study (22% vs. 7.4%, $P = 0.002$). There were no differences in abstinence rates between those who completed the study and those who dropped out ($P = 0.211$).

Conclusions

1. In a group of older adults with alcohol use disorder, naltrexone is well tolerated and reduced relapse on sampling with alcohol [2].
2. The study anticipated negative impact on liver enzymes due to naltrexone, but this was not observed. On the contrary, improvement in liver enzymes was observed.
3. Use of naltrexone is likely to decrease the need for psychosocial treatment, thereby limiting costs.

Strengths of the Study

1. The study is randomized and double-blind in nature.
2. Baseline measures were included, not just measures of addiction but also blood chemistries.
3. The study demonstrated efficacy in relapse prevention, consistent with previous literature [3, 4].
4. The quality of study assessed on the basis of Jadad score indicates that this was a high-quality study with a score of 5 out of 5 [4].

Questions Yes (1) No (0)	Was the study described as random?	Was the randomization scheme described and appropriate?	Was the study described as double-blind?	Was the method of double blinding appropriate? (Were both the patient and the assessor appropriately blinded?)	Was there a description of dropouts and withdrawals?	Total score Range of score quality 0–2 Low 3–5 High
Score	1	1	1	1	1	5

Limitations of the Study

1. The sample size was small in both groups.
2. A total of 17 participants dropped out of the study, and follow-up could not be conducted for many of them.
3. The follow-up period was only for 12 weeks. Therefore, longer-term outcomes cannot be discerned, and this is significant given the chronic nature of alcohol use disorder. Additionally, adverse effects that occur later in the course of treatment are likely to have been missed in this study.
4. Only male veterans participated in the study, so the findings are not generalizable to older women and to older men who are not veterans.
5. Outcomes are measured by self-reports. Collateral assessment and biochemical markers of alcohol use were not used, and this may have led to an underestimation of alcohol consumption.

Take-Home Points

1. Naltrexone must be considered as an adjunctive treatment for alcohol use disorder in older adults.
2. Naltrexone should be administered carefully with close monitoring in patients with prior hepatic disease.

Practical Applications of the Take-Home Points

1. Offer naltrexone to prevent relapse of alcohol use in older adults.
2. Measure hepatic enzymes before starting the medication and monitor these regularly.
3. Offer psychosocial supports to individual with alcohol use.

References

1. Oslin D, Liberto JG, O'Brien J, Krois S, Norbeck J. Naltrexone as an adjunctive treatment for older patients with alcohol dependence. Am J Geriatr Psychiatry. 1997;5(4):324–32.
2. Volpicelli JR, Alterman AI, Hayashida M, O'Brien CP. Naltrexone in the treatment of alcohol dependence. Arch Gen Psychiatry. 1992;49(11):876–80.
3. O'Malley SS, Jaffe AJ, Chang G, Schottenfeld RS, Meyer RE, Rounsaville B. Naltrexone and coping skills therapy for alcohol dependence. A controlled study. Arch Gen Psychiatry. 1992;49(11):881–7.
4. Jadad AR, Moore RA, Carroll D, Jenkinson C, Reynolds DJ, Gavaghan DJ, McQuay HJ. Assessing the quality of reports of randomized clinical trials: is blinding necessary? Control Clin Trials. 1996;17(1):1–12.

Chapter 72
Older Adult Patients with Both Psychiatric and Substance Abuse Disorders: Prevalence and Health Service Use

Ankit Jain and Paroma Mitra

Authors of the original article Holly G. Prigerson, Ph.D, Rani A. Desai, Ph.D, and Robert A. Rosenheck, MD

Journal published *Psychiatric Quarterly*

Year of publication 2001

Type of study Cross-sectional survey

Funding sources Supported in part by NIMH grant MH56529, a Claude D. Pepper Older Americans Independence Center grant P60-AG-10469, and a grant by the American Foundation on Suicide Prevention

Objectives To determine the prevalence of dual diagnosis across age groups in a national sample of mental health patients and to examine the characteristics and health service utilization associated with being an older patient with both psychiatric and substance abuse disorders [1]

Methods Data was obtained from three sources. First, records from a cross-sectional sample of outpatients were obtained from a national survey of patients treated in VA mental health clinics during a prespecified 2-week period. The second source was the Patient Treatment File (PTF), which is a discharge abstract of all completed episodes of inpatient care in the VA system. The third source was a combined database from two service use files: the PTF, for inpatient care, and the

A. Jain
Hershey Medical Center, Penn State College of Medicine, Hershey, PA, USA

P. Mitra (✉)
NYU School of Medicine, Bellevue Hospital Center, New York, NY, USA

R. R. Tampi et al. (eds.), *Essential Reviews in Geriatric Psychiatry*,
https://doi.org/10.1007/978-3-030-94960-0_72

Outpatient Care File (OPC) for outpatient care that includes all hospital and outpatient services provided by the VA. From each of the abovementioned sources, information about the diagnosis and treatment of psychiatric and substance use disorders were obtained.

The primary independent variable of interest was the dual diagnosis. Health service utilization indicators were the primary outcome variables of interest. Seven key utilization indicators were identified and calculated, namely, inpatient substance use, inpatient psychiatric, medical, and surgical services and outpatient general psychiatric, medical/surgical, and substance use.

The sample was divided into the following age groups: patients under 55 years of age, patients 55–64 years old, patients 65–74 years old, and patients over the age of 75. Patients were then stratified into four groups, namely, older adults dually diagnosed, older. adults not dually diagnosed, not older adults but dually diagnosed, and not older adults not dually diagnosed. Individuals over the age of 55 years were considered older adults or "elderly." The X^2 statistic was utilized to test for differences between the age groups in the frequency of psychiatric disorders, substance use disorders, and concurrent psychiatric and substance use disorders. Analysis of covariance models was used to compare the four patient groups on each of the seven service utilization indicators, controlling for variables such as sex, race, service-connected disability, substance use only and psychiatric disorder only diagnoses, and the main effects of age and dual diagnosis.

Results

Overall, the number of veterans receiving treatment in mental health programs at the Department of Veterans Affairs was inversely associated with age. The proportion of the sample with only a psychiatric diagnosis increased significantly with advancing age. Ninety percent of the individuals over the age of 65 years had a psychiatric diagnosis. However, comorbid psychiatric and substance use diagnoses decreased with age, from 30.4% among those under 55 years to merely 4.4% in the oldest group. Similarly, a purely substance use diagnosis also decreased with age, from being observed in 11.3% of the sample among those under age 55, but this was far lower at 3.7% among those over the age of 74 years.

Here is a summary of findings with respect to diagnosis:

1. Schizophrenia: Dually diagnosed individuals were significantly less likely to have a diagnosis of schizophrenia in both young and old age groups, compared to those who were not dually diagnosed. Among older adults, a diagnosis of schizophrenia was observed in 17.1% of those who were dually diagnosed and 25.15% of those who were not dually diagnosed, and this was statistically significant. Schizophrenia was the most frequent primary diagnosis (17.1%), followed by major depression (14.5%) among the older adults who were dually diagnosed.
2. Bipolar disorder: The rates of bipolar disorder did not significantly differ among older adults, irrespective of whether or not they were dually diagnosed (7.9% in those who were dually diagnosed vs. 7.17% among those who were not). However, in the younger group, the dually diagnosed (5.77%) were significantly less likely to have bipolar disorder compared to those who were not dually diagnosed (7.79%).

3. Major depressive disorder (MDD): MDD was observed to be the second most common primary psychiatric diagnosis among dually diagnosed older adults (14.5%). Although it was expected that there would be higher rates of affective disorders among the elderly who were dually diagnosed, no significant differences in the occurrence of major depressive disorder emerged among the four groups.
4. Post-traumatic stress disorder (PTSD): PTSD was observed less frequently among older adults in both groups (6.8% among those dually diagnosed vs. 8.9% among those who were not, and this difference was significant). Among younger individuals, the prevalence of PTSD was comparatively higher in both groups (15.67% among dually diagnosed individuals and 18.01% among those who were not), and the difference was significant.
5. Organic brain syndrome: Significantly higher rates of organic brain syndrome (11.6%) were found among dually diagnosed older adults when compared to older adults who were not dually diagnosed (7.95%). Predictably, the prevalence was lower in younger individuals, although it was significantly higher in the non-dually diagnosed group (2.44% vs. 1.69%).
6. Substance use disorders: Alcohol use disorder was the most frequent substance use disorder noted among the older adults who were dually diagnosed (81% versus 26% for the use of other substances). In younger dually diagnosed individuals, the rates were relatively similar (approximately 65%) for alcohol and other substance use disorders.

Here is a summary of findings with respect to service utilization:

1. Inpatient substance use services: Dually diagnosed older adults used inpatient substance use treatment services significantly more than the non-dually diagnosed older adults (1.5 versus 0.6 days, respectively). Dually diagnosed younger patients (5.58 days) also utilized more inpatient substance use services as compared to non-dually diagnosed younger patient (1.15 days), a significant pattern akin to older adults.
2. Inpatient psychiatric services: The quantum of inpatient psychiatric services utilized were predictably higher among individuals who were not dually diagnosed (13.67 days among younger and 10.52 days among older adults).
3. Inpatient medical and surgical services: Dually diagnosed individuals had lower utilization of inpatient medical and surgical services in both age groups, but these differences were not observed to be statistically significant.
4. Outpatient general psychiatric services: Dually diagnosed older adults utilized services significantly higher than non-dually diagnosed (41.3 versus 27.98 visits, respectively). The utilization of services by younger individuals was overall somewhat lower than their older counterparts but followed a similar diagnostic pattern.
5. Outpatient medical and surgical services: No statistically significant differences were demonstrated in the service utilization among the two diagnostic groups. However, as expected, older patients had higher rates of accessing outpatient medical and surgical service compared to younger patients.
6. Outpatient substance use service: Younger dually diagnosed individuals utilized this service the highest (21.35 visits), followed by dually diagnosed older adults

(9.69 visits), significantly higher than the negligible utilization among non-dually diagnosed younger (0.57 visits) and older adults (0.84 visits). The difference across groups was observed to be statistically significant.

Conclusions This cross-sectional survey demonstrated that the rates of dual diagnosis decreased as age advanced. However, dually diagnosed older adults were a group with high service utilization. They utilized inpatient and outpatient substance use treatment services more than older adults who were not dually diagnosed. Notably, this group also utilized outpatient general psychiatric treatment services significantly more than all the other comparison groups.

Strengths of the Study

1. The survey had a large sample size of 91,752 individuals.
2. The investigators carefully classified patients by age group and diagnosis, so patterns can be clearly discerned between the four different groups.

Limitations of the Study

1. Accuracy of diagnosis depends on the reliability of clinical assessment, since the survey relied on preexisting records.
2. This is a cross-sectional study spanning a period of 2 weeks. Longitudinal changes in service utilization will not be captured using this study design.
3. Inpatient service use is likely to vary depending on the availability of inpatient beds in a given region, so it might not fully reflect diagnostic severity or treatment need.
4. Given that this is purely a VA-based study, we do not know whether and to what extent individuals in this sample utilized non-VA health system services.
5. The study sample consists of a disproportionately male population, so the generalizability of the findings is called into question.

Take-Home Points

1. It is imperative to maintain a high risk of suspicion and screen for substance use among older adults
2. Timely diagnosis and treatment of substance use earlier in life can positively impact both medical and psychiatric health service utilization later in life.

Practical Applications of the Take-Home Point

All older adults who present with mental health symptoms must be screened for substance use and treated for the same. This can decrease their need for accessing mental health and medical-surgical services later in life.

Reference

1. Prigerson HG, Desai RA, Rosenheck RA. Older adult patients with both psychiatric and substance abuse disorders: prevalence and health service use. Psychiatry Q. 2001;72(1):1–18.

Chapter 73
Five-Year Alcohol and Drug Treatment Outcomes of Older Adults Versus Middle-Aged and Younger Adults in a Managed Care Program

Paroma Mitra

Authors of the original article Derek D Satre, Jennifer R Mertens, Patricia A Areán, Constance Weisner

Journal published Addiction

Year of publication 2004

Type of study Five-year-long prospective randomized study

Funding sources This study was funded by the National Institute on Alcohol Abuse and Alcoholism (R37 AA10359) and the National Institute on Drug Abuse (R01 DA10572).

Objectives To investigate 5-year treatment outcomes of older adults in comparison with middle-aged and younger adults receiving treatment at a private, nonprofit, managed care chemical dependency program [1]

Methods Study participants aged 18 years and older were recruited from the Kaiser Permanente Sacramento Chemical Dependency Recovery Program (CDRP). Exclusion criteria included active psychosis and a diagnosis of dementia or intellectual disability. Of the 1312 patients contacted for the study, 1204 agreed to participate. Approximately 62% of the participants were randomized into one of the two following treatments: an outpatient day program or a hospital program. Both treatments included participation in a 12-step program, group therapy, psychoeducation, supportive therapy, relapse prevention interventions, and family therapy.

P. Mitra (✉)
NYU School of Medicine, Bellevue Hospital Center, New York, NY, USA

R. R. Tampi et al. (eds.), *Essential Reviews in Geriatric Psychiatry*,
https://doi.org/10.1007/978-3-030-94960-0_73

Individual therapy and psychopharmacologic therapy were offered if participants were interested.

In the hospital program, participants were required to attend 6 hours a day during the first 3 weeks. From weeks 4 to 8, participants then attended 1.5 hours a day for 4 days a week. In contrast, participants in the outpatient program attended 1.5 hours a day for 3 days a week for 8 weeks. All participants then participated in aftercare at week 9 and then were followed up weekly for 10 months. A participant was considered a "dropout" after missing seven continuous days for the first 8 weeks and 30 days after the first 8 weeks. Average length of stay in the hospital and outpatient programs were 10.5 weeks and 8.5 weeks, respectively.

Of those randomized into a treatment group, 63% were grouped into the older adult cohort (aged 55 years and older), 60% into the middle-aged adult cohort (aged 40–54 years), and 63% into the younger adult cohort (aged 18–39 years). The authors reported no significant baseline differences between the groups. A percentage of participants recruited at intake were not randomized due to personal preferences or if they required specific treatment conditions per the staff's clinical judgment.

The investigators used an "intention-to-treat" study design so that all participants recruited from the baseline/intake visit would be included in the authors' analysis. Approximately 76% ($N = 916$) out of the 1204 patients who initially agreed to participate at intake started treatment. Data was collected during a 1-hour telephone intake interview and during a 5-year follow-up interview. The authors reported that 925 of the initial 1204 participants (77%) returned to complete the 5-year follow-up interview. The primary outcome was measured at intake and in the 5-year follow-up interview using the Addiction Severity Index (ASI) to assess addiction severity. The authors also collected the following information for analysis: age, ethnicity, gender, education, employment/income, social network, 12-step program participation (measured through the Alcoholics Anonymous Affiliation Scale), abstinence (i.e., total abstinence from drugs and alcohol over the past 30 days and at the 5-year interview), and whether or not they met the Diagnostic and Statistical Manual of Mental Disorders fourth edition (DSM-IV) criteria for substance use and/or dependence. The authors also took note of readmission frequency which was defined as having at least three visits to a chemical dependency program between 1 and 5 years post-intake with less than or equal to 30 days' time in between each visit. Random urine drug tests and breathalysers were instituted weekly for 4 weeks and then monthly for a year to help confirm abstinence measures.

The authors used chi-squared and univariate analysis (ANOVA) tests to determine if there was a statistically significant difference between the groups in regard to categorical and continuous variables, respectively.

Results The ASI score was significantly higher in deceased patients (mean ASI score of 0.625) compared to alive patients (mean ASI score of 0.442) at the 5-year follow-up ($P < 0.001$).

Individual characteristics by age group: Older adults were more likely to be diagnosed with alcohol dependence compared to younger and middle-aged adults and less likely to be diagnosed with drug dependence ($P < 0.01$). Older adults were also less likely to be diagnosed with combined alcohol and drug dependence ($P < 0.01$) and were more likely than younger adults to report abstinence from drugs and alcohol in the previous month ($P = 0.02$). A total of 52% of older adults reported total abstinence from drugs and alcohol in the previous month compared to 40% of younger adults who reported total abstinence from drugs and alcohol in the previous month.

Variables associated independently with abstinence: The variables for all age groups that were significant for abstinence included female gender ($P = 0.003$), longer treatment retention ($P < 0.001$), and having no close family/friends who encouraged alcohol or drug use in the past 5 years ($P < 0.001$).

Analysis of gender differences: Older women were more likely to be abstinent compared to older men ($P = 0.007$) and more abstinent compared to younger women ($P = 0.04$). Notably older adults tended to stay in treatment compared to younger adults ($P = 0.03$).

Extra treatment factors: Regarding characteristics of participants external to treatment, older adults were reported to have fewer close friends than younger adults ($P < 0.001$) or middle-aged adults ($P = 0.001$). Older adults were also less likely than younger adults to report having family or friends who encouraged use (8% vs. 17%; $P = 0.04$). Lastly, older adults were reported to be more likely to be married compared to younger adults (59% vs. 39%; $P = 0.002$).

When measures of 12-step affiliation were reported, older adults were stated to be less likely than middle-aged adults to have considered themselves a member of a 12-step group ($P = 0.015$) with 19% of older adults as compared to 42% of middle-aged adults reporting to have contacted a 12-step member for assistance with recovery.

Conclusions This study indicates that abstinence rates of older adults appear higher than those of younger adult cohorts though there were no significant age differences found among those dependent only on alcohol. Mortality was associated with a higher rate of alcohol use. Age was not found to be a significant factor in abstinence though social networks that encourage substance use were (older adults were found to be less likely than younger adults to have social circles that encouraged substance use). Older adults were also reported to be more likely to need an adequate and supportive social network posttreatment to maintain abstinence. Longer treatment duration was found to reflect a better outcome, and older adults remained in treatment longer than younger cohorts. When observing for gender differences between older women and men, older women stayed in treatment longer and were noted to have a more supportive network. Notably, older adults were found to exhibit less reliance on 12-step programs.

Strengths of the Study

1. Long-term, 5-year study.
2. Interventions integrated medical and behavioral health treatment.
3. Comparison of different age categories.
4. High retention and follow-up rate.

5. Authors also investigated effect of social support networks and alcoholic anonymous groups.
6. Intention-to-treat analysis to account for attrition.

Limitations of the Study

1. Sample size of the older group is small (n = 65) with only a small number of women recruited (n = 17) compared to the larger younger (n = 564) and middle-aged (n = 296) cohorts.
2. No adjustment for significance level for multiple comparisons.
3. Mortality could confound abstinence rates in older adults as alcohol dependence in this age group was highly associated with higher mortality.
4. They included both randomized and nonrandomized participants.
5. Investigation occurred in a private medical facility where participants were recruited from a population of private insurance and would likely have less severe substance use compared to the general population.
6. Their term of readmission is loosely used. "Readmission" was defined as having at least three visits with no more than 30 days' gap between each visit to a chemical dependency program between 1 and 5 years after intake within the Kaiser Permanente Program. Readmissions outside the Kaiser Permanente network could be communicated by self-reports. Readmission however does not indicate relapse and also includes brief supportive therapy visits.

Take-home points Older adults exhibited better outcomes in terms of abstinence during this 5-year study compared to younger cohorts. Additionally, older women appeared to demonstrate better outcomes than older men and younger women. Social networks appear to be important in maintaining abstinence in older adults. Providing resources like information regarding local alcoholics anonymous and narcotics anonymous meetings in the region and exploring barriers to attending these groups could be beneficial.

Practical applications of the take-home points Older adults should be screened for alcohol and drug use in all settings, in both primary care and behavioral health settings. If alcohol or drug use is suspected, use of screening tools is recommended and referral to treatments encouraged if found to be clinically indicated.

Reference

1. Satre DD, Mertens JR, Areán PA, Weisner C. Five-year alcohol and drug treatment outcomes of older adults versus middle-aged and younger adults in a managed care program. Addiction. 2004;99(10):1286–97.

Chapter 74
Treatment of Late-Life Depression Complicated by Alcohol Dependence

Paroma Mitra

Authors of the original article David Oslin

Journal published *American Journal of Geriatric Psychiatry*

Year of publication 2005

Type of study randomized double-blind study

Funding sources National Institute of Mental Health and Department of Veterans Affairs MERP Award

Objectives The investigator wanted to assess whether the combination of naltrexone and sertraline is effective in the treatment of major depression and alcohol dependence among older adults [1].

Methods This study enrolled a total of 74 outpatients for a 12-week randomized placebo-controlled trial. The study participants were recruited from clinic referrals or through local media advertisements. The inclusion criteria for this study were as follows: age ≥55 years, meeting the DSM-IV criteria for alcohol dependence, meeting the DSM-IV criteria for a major depressive disorder (MDD) or substance-induced depressive disorder, and the successful completion of detoxification from alcohol which was defined as a minimum of three consecutive days of abstinence before the start of the study medication. Participants also had to continue to meet the diagnostic criteria for a depressive disorder in order to start on sertraline. Additionally, the participant should have met the diagnostic criteria for MDD prior to meeting the criteria for alcohol dependence, or the depressive symptoms were persisting during a 3-month period of abstinence from alcohol. Exclusion criteria were as follows: current DSM-IV diagnosis of a psychoactive substance dependence other than either alcohol or nicotine and the evidence for opioid use in the past 30 days which was evaluated both by self-report and/or urine drug screen at the

P. Mitra (✉)
NYU School of Medicine, Bellevue Hospital Center, New York, NY, USA

R. R. Tampi et al. (eds.), *Essential Reviews in Geriatric Psychiatry*,
https://doi.org/10.1007/978-3-030-94960-0_74

time of entry into treatment for the study. Additional exclusion criteria were the presence of severe medical or physical illnesses including AIDS, active hepatitis, or significant hepatocellular injury as identified by elevated total bilirubin levels.

After the participants completed detoxification from alcohol, they were randomized to receive either naltrexone 50 mg a day or placebo in addition to a compliance-enhancement therapy called Biopsychosocial evaluation, Report to the patient, Empathetic approach, Needs assessment, Direct advice to the patient, and Assessment of progress (BRENDA) which was conducted by a nurse (RN or master's level). The stratification of participants for randomization was done by gender and recruitment site in a block design. Following a period of 1 week of treatment with naltrexone or placebo, the participants were started on sertraline 50 mg a day for 1 week with an increase to 100 mg a day as tolerated. To improve and to assess adherence, the study medication was provided in blister cards. BRENDA sessions were conducted initially weekly for 8 weeks and biweekly thereafter.

The rating scales that were used in the study were as follows: the Hamilton Rating Scale for Depression (Ham-D), the Mini-Mental State Exam (MMSE), the Time-Line Follow-Back (TLFB) method of assessing alcohol consumption, the Addiction Severity Index (ASI), and the Medical Outcomes Study Short Form (SF-36). During each study visit, the Ham-D and TLFB were administered, whereas the ASI and SF-36 were administered every month.

A nurse assessed therapy attendance and adherence to the study medication via self-report of medication use and by pill counts. The nurse also monitored adverse events weekly, and this information was reviewed with the principal investigator. Systematic Assessment for Treatment Emergent Effects (SAFTEE) was used to collect reports of adverse events at baseline and at each clinical visit. The definition of adverse events was symptoms that were new or indicated a worsening of a baseline complaint.

The quantity of alcohol used was recorded in standard drinks which was equal to a 12-oz beer, a 6-oz glass of wine, or a 1½-oz shot of hard liquor.

Means and standard deviations (SD) were the descriptive analyses for continuous variables, whereas frequencies were used for categorical variables. The continuous variables were compared using the student *t*-test, and categorical variables were compared using the chi-squared test. To assess the relationship between treatment response (remission of depression and lack of drinking relapse) and treatment assignment (naltrexone versus placebo), the logistic-regression analyses were applied. The covariates that were used were pretreatment drinking variables and depression severity (Ham-D score). Logistic-regression models were constructed to assess the effect of drinking during treatment on depression response. To assess the effects of treatment assignment on the time-to-relapse to significant drinking, Cox regression analyses were constructed. Response measures were Ham-D <10 for remission of depression and drinking more than four standard drinks in 1 day for men or more than three drinks for women to signify a relapse to heavy drinking. Participants who withdrew from the study were considered to have a poor treatment response in the primary outcome analysis.

Results All 74 of the participants who were recruited into the study were randomized. A majority of the participants (79.7%) were white men. A total of 66.2% of the participants were white and 44.6% were married. The participants had an average age of 63.4 (SD: 6.3) years. The demographic variables did not show any significant differences between the two treatment groups. On average, participants used alcohol for 39.6 (SD: 10.8). The drinking-to-intoxication among the participants was on average 17.3 (SD: 9.9) years. In the 90 days preceding the detoxification period, majority of the participants (67.5%, SD: 33.3%) had heavy alcohol use.

No previous formal treatment for alcohol dependence was noted among 51.4% subjects who were randomized into the study, whereas 17.6% that had participated had one previous treatment, and more than one previous treatment was seen in 29.7% of the participants. Only 27.0% of the participants had ever received outpatient mental health treatment. At the time of screening, only 25.7% of the participants were receiving an antidepressant, and the lifetime suicide attempt was noted in 8.1% of the participants. Alcohol-induced depression was noted in 63.5% of the participants. Major depressive disorder independent of alcohol use was diagnosed in 31.1% of the participants. The etiology for depression was indeterminate in 5.4% of the cases. Participants randomized to naltrexone were less depressed ($P = 0.011$), had fewer drinks on a given drinking day ($P = 0.006$), and had fewer days of heavy drinking before randomization ($P = 0.032$).

Attendance for at least 80% of the weekly therapy visits for 3 months was achieved by 83.8% of the participants. The proportion of participants who completed treatment was similar between the naltrexone and the placebo groups [81.1% vs. 89.2%, odds ratio (OR) = 1.16; 95% confidence interval (CI): 0.28–4.9, $P = 0.838$]. In the naltrexone/placebo group, participants were compliant with medications on 83.3% of the study days, whereas in the sertraline group, they were compliant in 79.1% of the study days. There was no difference in the proportion of participants who were compliant to medications in the naltrexone/placebo (83.3%, OR = 1.11, 95% CI: 0.32–3.84, $P = 0.864$) versus the sertraline group (79.1%, OR = 1.54, 95% CI: 0.47–5.07, $P = 0.475$).

As for new or worsening of adverse events during treatment, headache was reported in 58.1% of the participants which was followed by anxiety in 51.4%, nausea in 41.9%, decreased sexual functioning in 39.2%, and vomiting in 24.3% of the participants. These adverse events were not more common in the naltrexone group when compared to the placebo group. Additionally, these symptoms were not related to either the completion of the study or to compliance with medications.

In the study, 52.7% of the participants attained remission from depression with 66.2% of the participants not relapsing to alcohol use. A total of 48.6% of the participants were abstinent from alcohol for 12 weeks. The percentage of individuals who relapsed was no different between the naltrexone and placebo groups (35.1% vs. 32.4, OR = 1.25, 95% CI: 0.042–3.70, $P = 0.690$). The percentage of individuals who were abstinent from alcohol use were no different between the naltrexone and placebo groups (43.2% vs. 54.1%, OR = 1.34, 95% CI: 0.49–3.68, $P = 0.575$).

Depression remitted in 51.4% of individuals in the naltrexone group versus 54.1% of the individuals in the placebo group (OR = 1.25, 95% CI: 0.46–3.44, $P = 0.665$). Overall improvement was seen in 40.5% of individuals in the naltrexone group when compared to 43.2% of individuals in the placebo group (OR = 1.40, 95% CI: 0.48–4.03, $P = 0.537$). It was also noted that the time to the first day of heavy drinking (relapse) was not significantly different between the two groups ($P = 0.839$). It was noted that 25% of the women treated in the naltrexone group had a favorable response when compared to 71.4% in the placebo group (OR = 13.95; 95% CI: 1.02–190.30, $P = 0.048$), and lesser improvement in depression was the contributing factor.

When comparing individuals who relapsed on alcohol use to individuals who did not relapse on alcohol use, the proportion of individuals in both groups who completed treatment were no different (84% vs. 83.7%, OR = 1.11, 95% CI: 0.28–4.42, $P = 0.886$). However, the proportion of individuals who had a remission of depression was greater in the group of individuals who did not relapse to drinking when compared to individuals who relapsed to drinking (63.3% vs. 32%, OR = 3.83, 95% CI: 1.36–10.81, $P = 0.011$). Additionally, the Ham-D score at the end of the trial was lower in the group that did not relapse on alcohol use when compared to the individuals who relapsed (8.8 vs. 12.7, $P = 0.013$). There was no difference in the group that was abstinent from alcohol versus those individuals who had any use of alcohol on the proportion of individuals completing treatment (86.1% vs. 81.61%, OR = 0.77, 95% CI: 0.20–2.91, $P = 0.696$), proportion of individuals who had a remission of depression (55.6% vs. 50.0%, OR = 1.22, 95% CI: 0.48–3.11, $P = 0.684$), and the Ham-D scores at the end of the trial (10.3 vs 11.0, $P = 0.663$). It was noted that there were lower rates of improvements in depression (OR = 2.29, 95% CI: 1.34–3.90, $P = 0.02$) and reduction in Ham-D scores ($P < 0.001$) that were associated with more frequent bouts of heavy drinking during the trial. Any drinking on more than 2 days of the study was associated with a poorer response to depression (OR = 4.00, 95% CI: 1.44–10.82, $P = 0.008$).

Conclusions This trial indicates that the addition of naltrexone to a combination of sertraline and psychosocial support did not improve either symptoms of depression or decrease the consumption of alcohol when compared to treatment with sertraline and psychosocial support. It was noted that any relapse to heavy drinking was associated with a decrease in response to treatment for depression in the participants of this trial.

Strengths of the Study

1. This is a randomized double-blind study.
2. This is one of the few pharmacotherapy studies for substance use disorders among older adults available in the literature.
3. The quality of study assessed on the basis of Jadad score indicates that this was a high-quality study with a score of 5 out of 5 [2].

Questions Yes (1) No (0)	Was the study described as random?	Was the randomization scheme described and appropriate?	Was the study described as double-blind?	Was the method of double blinding appropriate? (Were both the patient and the assessor appropriately blinded?)	Was there a description of dropouts and withdrawals?	Total score Range of score quality 0–2 Low 3–5 High
Score	1	1	1	1	1	5

4. This study provides impetus to evaluate the rationale and process for developing future studies including designing combination treatments for common comorbid psychiatric disorders.

Limitations of the Study

1. The outcome measures for this study were fairly conservative including the proportion of individuals who had a remission of symptoms of depression and the lack of relapse to heavy drinking of alcohol.
2. The sample size was small ($n = 74$).
3. There were relatively few women in the study (<20%).
4. There was a significant lack of diversity among the participants (Caucasians = 66.25%).
5. The study had a relatively short duration of follow-up (3 months).
6. The dosing of sertraline (100 mg a day) was fairly conservative.

Take-home points The addition of naltrexone to a combination of sertraline and individualized psychosocial support did not improve treatment responses for either depression or alcohol consumption among older adults. However, reducing the heavy use of alcohol improved outcomes for the treatment of depression among these individuals.

Practical applications of the take-home points Among older adults who have comorbid depression and alcohol use disorder, reducing the frequency and quantity of consumption of alcohol will improve treatment outcomes for depression.

References

1. Oslin DW. Treatment of late-life depression complicated by alcohol dependence. Am J Geriatr Psychiatry. 2005;13(6):491–500.
2. Jadad AR, Moore RA, Carroll D, Jenkinson C, Reynolds DJ, Gavaghan DJ, McQuay HJ. Assessing the quality of reports of randomized clinical trials: is blinding necessary? Control Clin Trials. 1996;17:1–12.

Chapter 75
Screening and Brief Intervention for Substance Misuse Among Older Adults: The Florida BRITE Project

Paroma Mitra

Authors of the original article Lawrence Schonfeld, Bellinda L King-Kallimanis, Darran M Duchene, Roy L Etheridge, Julio R Herrera, Kristen L Barry, Nancy Lynn

Journal published *American Journal of Public Health*

Year of publication 2010

Type of study Prospective study

Funding sources The BRITE pilot program was funded by the state of Florida.

Objectives The objective of the study was to develop and examine the effectiveness of the Florida Brief Intervention and Treatment for Elders (BRITE), a state-funded program comprising of screening for substance use and providing brief intervention [1].

Methods Four agencies from four different counties were selected for the project, on the basis of the older adult population in the counties and existing services for both aging and substance use disorders in these agencies. BRITE counselors were certified addiction specialists, mental health counselors, counselors, social workers, or nurses who were trained in screening and intervention techniques to be employed in the project. The following steps were followed:

A. *Prescreening*: Referrals were received from primary care providers, families, and other service providers. The BRITE counselors used a brief prescreening interview which addressed general health, life stressors, consumption of alco-

P. Mitra (✉)
NYU School of Medicine, Bellevue Hospital Center, New York, NY, USA

R. R. Tampi et al. (eds.), *Essential Reviews in Geriatric Psychiatry*,
https://doi.org/10.1007/978-3-030-94960-0_75

hol, depression, anxiety, and treatment of mental illnesses. Individuals with positive screens were then invited to participate in the study.

B. *Screening*: The interview detailed upon reasons for referral, six domains of problems associated with substance use, general treatment history, as well as screening for depression and suicidal thoughts. Information regarding consumption of alcohol, illicit drugs, and over-the-counter and prescription medications was systematically obtained, as described below.

   1. Alcohol use: The first three questions of the Alcohol Use Disorders Identification Test (AUDIT) were used to derive information regarding frequency and quantity of use [2, 3]. If alcohol use had occurred within the past year, the ten-item Short Michigan Alcoholism Screening Test, Geriatric Version (the (SMAST-G), was used. A score of 2 or higher on SMAST-G was flagged [4].
   2. Prescription medications: A 17-item questionnaire was specifically developed for this purpose. This included information regarding prescription issues (such as consumption of more than one medication; prescriptions for pain, anxiety, or sleep; receiving prescriptions from multiple doctors), adverse effects of medications, healthcare personnel expressing concern about medication use, need for reminders for medication use, improper use of medications, and borrowing medications from others. The responses obtained as well as the subjective impressions of interviewers to the responses obtained were used to determine the need for intervention.
   3. Over-the-counter medications: There were eight self-report items regarding the use of analgesics, sleeping aids, herbal remedies, etc. Similar to prescription medications, individuals were flagged for intervention, depending on the responses obtained.
   4. Illicit drugs: The interviewer asked whether the subject had used any form of illicit drug in the past year. Any positive response triggered a flag in the screening system.
   5. Depression screen: The 15-item Short Geriatric Depression Scale (SGDS) was used [5]. A score over 4 was considered significant and flagged.
   6. Suicide risk: All participants were screened for suicide risk, using a questionnaire specifically developed for the BRITE project. Questions regarding thoughts of death, suicidal intent, and plan were asked. Suicidal ideation within the past year resulted in referral to a mental health professional.

   Intervention was conducted in the form of brief intervention, brief treatment, and follow-up, as detailed below.

C. *Brief intervention*: Treatment protocols were initiated using Treatment Improvement Protocols developed by Substance Abuse and Mental Health Services Administration (SAMSHA), namely, protocols 26 and 34. BRITE counselors were trained to use a brief intervention that involved one to five sessions delivered in the older adult's home. Motivational interviewing techniques were used to understand and elicit behavioral changes related to substance use.

The intervention comprised of discussion regarding one's future goals for living and one's health habits, understanding of the motivation to quit or reduce the consumption of substances, education about the association of substance use and general health, and medication interactions. The adults would be discharged from treatment upon completion of the recommended workbook and based on the amount of material retained, as deemed by the counselor.

D. *Brief treatment*: Treatment protocols were initiated using a 16-session relapse prevention guide developed by SAMSHA. This comprised of functional analysis of substance use and cognitive behavioral methods to understand triggers for use such as loneliness, social pressure, depression, anxiety, and anger and learn alternative ways of managing them. Completion of the protocol was gauged based on performance on quizzes which indicated retention of information by the individual.

E. *Follow-up*: Individuals were rescreened at 30 and 90 days post-discharge using similar questions as the initial screening.

Results Demographics: A total of 3497 individuals were screened. Almost 70% of the individuals were women, the mean age was 75 years, and about 54% of the respondents were reported to be living alone.

1. Alcohol use. Screening and referral information: 339 individuals (9.7% of those who were screened) were referred with concerns about their alcohol use. Approximately 18% of individuals referred for other purposes screened positive for alcohol use, totaling 556 individuals referred for alcohol use. Out of the 68.8% of the individuals screened, 18.2% consumed more than three drinks a day (total = 102 individuals). Out of the individuals screened, 17.8% consumed six or more alcoholic drinks on one occasion (99 individuals).

Outcomes: A total of 244 individuals received services, and 114 people were rescreened 3 months later. For 109 individuals, the mean scores on SMAST-G had significantly decreased at the time of discharge ($P < 0.001$).

2. Illicit drug use. Screening and referral information: About 1.14% of the total sample or 40 individuals were referred for use of illicit substances.

Outcomes: A total of 32 individuals received services. A total of 12 were rescreened at discharge. Nine individuals (75%) had no flags and showed improvement upon discharge. Three remained unchanged at discharge. Illicit substance use in two individuals was only identified at discharge.

3. Prescription medication misuse. Screening and referral information: Out of the 3497 individuals screened, 26.4% (925 individuals) were referred for medication misuse. 29.5% of those referred were prescribed pain medications, 22.9% anxiolytics, 21.7% sleeping medications, and 2.7% medications for "loneliness or sadness." As many as 16.8% of those referred had difficulties remembering medications they were taking. Approximately 32% of those screened were noted to

have required further education about their prescriptions, about 15.6% did not know the purpose of medications, 10.2% used incorrect doses, and 8.2% consumed medications for incorrect indications.

Outcomes: A total of 398 individuals received treatment. Sixty (32.1%) of the 187 individuals for whom follow-up data is available demonstrated improvement at discharge, whereas 67.9% of the individuals remained unchanged. About 87 individuals were identified for prescription medication misuse only at the time of discharge.

4. Over-the-counter medications. Screening and referral information: A total of 7.8% of those screened or 272 individuals were referred for over-the-counter medication use. About 44% of them required further education about the use of the medications. Notably, about 50% reportedly did not discuss the use of over-the-counter medications and supplements with their physicians.

Outcomes: A total of 24 individuals received services. Twenty-three individuals (95.8%) improved at discharge. One individual stayed the same at discharge. Two (4.2%) individuals were identified only at discharge.

5. Depression and suicide risk. Screening and referral information: About 64.3% (2248) of individuals referred to BRITE were referred for depression. 1050 individuals screened positively for depression. About 22.3% screened for moderate depression and 7.7% for severe depression. 49.1% of the individuals who screened positively on the S-MAST G (about 49.1%) scored moderately on the depression scale. Also 36.8% of older adults needing education about prescription medications, 7.8% of older adults requiring intervention for OTC medication use, and 4% of people flagged for illicit drug use also had depression scores on the GDS in the moderate-to-severe range.

Outcomes: A total of 433 individuals received services. When compared to the baseline (5.56 +/− 3.58), there was a significant reduction in the mean GDS scores at the time of discharge from the brief intervention (3.22 +/− 2.87) for the 323 individuals for whom this information was available. Similarly, there was a statistically significant reduction in the mean scores as well as at the time of the 30-day follow-up (2.8 +/−2.57) for 203 individuals who had follow-up data available. At the time of 30-day follow-up, 48.3% scored in the moderate or severe range on the SGDS, 31.9% reduced their score to none or mild, and 42.1% remained at none or mild. About 0.2% of the 3467 people were referred for suicide risk. However, 62 people screened positive when history of suicidal thoughts in the past few months was inquired. Only 18 of these individuals received any follow-up.

Conclusions The Florida BRITE study was the first of its kind to conduct screening and provide interventions for substance use and depression among a large number of older adults. It demonstrated a low-cost approach to the needs of older adults. It also identified screening methods that could be used effectively in the community to identify substance use that might otherwise be missed in routine clinical encounters.

Strengths of the Study

1. The project utilized evidence-based protocols from SAMHSA.
2. The project was able to triple the number of older adults in Florida who received substance use treatment services.
3. BRITE counselors were trained in the use of screening and intervention techniques for substance use. They received 4 hours of training and follow-up training sessions. They were encouraged to use brief intervention training and offer sessions immediately to persons flagged for substance misuse. They were also trained to refer as needed for higher level of care whether it was for detox/rehab services or mental health services.
4. The study highlights the application of the intervention in treating depression and substance use.
5. The prescreening and screening questions are detailed and applicable to any community setting.

Limitations of the Study

1. The authors have explained that there was a flaw in the data analysis system during the first year. Some of the data flagged for discharge and follow-up after the intervention were missing. This accounted for the low numbers that were entered for analysis to demonstrate the effect of the intervention.
2. The length of follow-up is 3 months, a duration that is short, given the chronicity of substance use.
3. Only a very small percentage of individuals who experienced suicidal thoughts in the past few months were followed up.

Take-Home Points

1. Screening and intervention can be conducted in a variety of community settings.
2. There is a strong concordance between depression and the use of substances or the misuse of medications.
3. A significant number of older adults need education about the indications and dosing regimen of their medications, including over-the-counter medications and supplements.

Practical applications of the take-home points Screening for substance use in older adults is vital, and it may be carried out in multiple settings. It is important to regularly educate older adults about their medications, the doses, and their indications and inquire about the use of herbal supplements. Treatment of mood symptoms and substance use positively impact each other.

References

1. Schonfeld L, King-Kallimanis BL, Duchene DM, Etheridge RL, Herrera JR, Barry KL, Lynn N. Screening and brief intervention for substance misuse among older adults: the Florida BRITE project. Am J Public Health. 2010;100(1):108–14.

2. Bush K, Kivlahan DR, McDonell MB, Fihn SD, Bradley KA. The AUDIT alcohol consumption questions (AUDIT-C): an effective brief screening test for problem drinking. Ambulatory Care Quality Improvement Project (ACQUIP). Alcohol Use Disorders Identification Test. Arch Intern Med. 1998;158(16):1789–95.
3. Fihn SD, McDonell MB, Diehr P, Anderson SM, Bradley KA, Au DH, Spertus JA, Burman M, Reiber GE, Kiefe CI, Cody M, Sanders KM, Whooley MA, Rosenfeld K, Baczek LA, Sauvigne A. Effects of sustained audit/feedback on self-reported health status of primary care patients. Am J Med. 2004;116(4):241–8.
4. Naegle MA. Screening for alcohol use and misuse in older adults: using the Short Michigan Alcoholism Screening Test–Geriatric Version. Am J Nurs. 2008;108(11):50–8; quiz 58–9.
5. Montorio I, Izal M. The Geriatric Depression Scale: a review of its development and utility. Int Psychogeriatr. 1996;8(1):103–12.

Index

R. R. Tampi et al. (eds.), *Essential Reviews in Geriatric Psychiatry*,
https://doi.org/10.1007/978-3-030-94960-0

GPSR Compliance

The European Union's (EU) General Product Safety Regulation (GPSR) is a set of rules that requires consumer products to be safe and our obligations to ensure this.

If you have any concerns about our products, you can contact us on ProductSafety@springernature.com

In case Publisher is established outside the EU, the EU authorized representative is:

Springer Nature Customer Service Center GmbH
Europaplatz 3
69115 Heidelberg, Germany

Batch number: 10732076

Printed by Printforce, the Netherlands